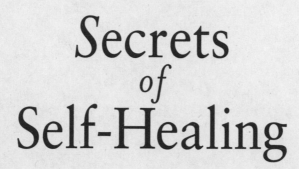

Secrets
of
Self-Healing

Avery

a member of Penguin Group (USA) Inc.

New York

Secrets
of
Self-Healing

HARNESS NATURE'S POWER TO HEAL COMMON AILMENTS,
BOOST YOUR VITALITY, *and* ACHIEVE OPTIMUM WELLNESS

Dr. Maoshing Ni

Published by the Penguin Group

Penguin Group (USA) Inc., 375 Hudson Street, New York, New York 10014, USA • Penguin Group (Canada), 90 Eglinton Avenue East, Suite 700, Toronto, Ontario M4P 2Y3, Canada (a division of Pearson Canada Inc.) • Penguin Books Ltd, 80 Strand, London WC2R 0RL, England • Penguin Ireland, 25 St Stephen's Green, Dublin 2, Ireland (a division of Penguin Books Ltd) • Penguin Group (Australia), 250 Camberwell Road, Camberwell, Victoria 3124, Australia (a division of Pearson Australia Group Pty Ltd) • Penguin Books India Pvt Ltd, 11 Community Centre, Panchsheel Park, New Delhi–110 017, India • Penguin Group (NZ), 67 Apollo Drive, Rosedale, North Shore 0632, New Zealand (a division of Pearson New Zealand Ltd) • Penguin Books (South Africa) (Pty) Ltd, 24 Sturdee Avenue, Rosebank, Johannesburg 2196, South Africa

Penguin Books Ltd, Registered Offices: 80 Strand, London WC2R 0RL, England

First trade paperback edition 2008
Text copyright © 2008 by Maoshing Ni
Compilation copyright © 2008 by Dr. Maoshing Ni and Authorscape Inc.

Most Avery books are available at special quantity discounts for bulk purchase for sales promotions, premiums, fundraising, and educational needs. Special books or book excerpts also can be created to fit specific needs. For details, write Penguin Group (USA) Inc. Special Markets, 375 Hudson Street, New York, NY 10014.

The Library of Congress catalogued the hardcover as follows:

Ni, Maoshing.
Secrets of self-healing : harness nature's power to heal common ailments, boost your vitality, and achieve optimum wellness / Maoshing Ni.
p.   cm.
ISBN 978-1-58333-296-2
1. Medicine, Chinese.   2. Integrative medicine.   3. Self-care, Health.   4. Healing.   I. Title.
R601.N52   2008   2007038534
610—dc22

ISBN 978-1-58333-337-2 (paperback edition)

Printed in the United States of America
10 9 8 7 6 5 4 3 2 1

BOOK DESIGN BY Laurie Dolphin
ACUPRESSURE ILLUSTRATIONS BY Patty Wu

. . . .

FOR YO SAN, WHOSE STRENGTH AND PERSEVERANCE
SAVED THE FAMILY LINEAGE FROM EXTINCTION,
WHOSE LOVE OF HUMANITY MADE PUBLIC A
MEDICAL TRADITION PREVIOUSLY CLOSED TO THE
OUTSIDE WORLD, AND WHOSE LIFE EMBODIED
THE PRINCIPLES OF HEALTH, SELF-HEALING,
AND SPIRITUAL SELF-CULTIVATION

❧ CONTENTS ❧

CONTENTS

PART 2: SELF-HEALING REMEDIES FOR COMMON AILMENTS

HOW TO USE THIS BOOK

IN PART 1, I DISCUSS THE PHILOSOPHY OF health and natural healing. It is important to familiarize yourself with these principles so that you can correctly apply the suggested remedies in Part 2. For each common ailment listed in Part 2, I provide diet, supplement, and herbal therapy suggestions along with exercise, acupressure, and things to avoid.

As you use the advice for each condition, please keep in mind the following:

• The philosophy of self-healing does not exclude working with a medical doctor. In fact, I encourage you to build a healing partnership with both your Western and your Wellness Medicine physicians. Always consult your doctor before beginning any health program.

• Shop and eat organic whenever possible. You can find most of the foods that I recommend at grocery and health food stores and farmers' markets. A few of the ethnic or other special foods, if not available at grocery stores, may be found at Asian markets, online, and from specialty restaurants.

• For supplements, unless noted otherwise, the dosages I recommend are daily amounts for adults of average weight and height. For dosing tailored to individual health needs, you should consult a licensed practitioner. You can find supplements at health food and vitamin stores, health practitioners' offices, and online. For a complete source of professional-grade vitamin supplements, visit www.healingpeople.com.

• Healing herbs should be used in formulations customized for individual needs. The herbs recommended in Part 2 are a good starting point for a discussion with a licensed practitioner. Most herbs can be purchased at health food and vitamin stores, health practitioners' offices, and online. For a good source of high-quality Chinese herbs, visit www.acupuncture.com. For more information on the herbs mentioned in this book, visit www.ask drmao.com.

• The exercises and meditations suggested in Part 2 are of varying degrees of difficulty. Illustrations or video clips of the exercises can be viewed at www.askdrmao.com.

• Acupressure is based on the 5,000-year-old practice of acupuncture. For more information on the acupoints mentioned in this book, and for a directory of licensed practitioners of this ancient art, visit www .acupuncture.com.

• In Part 2, I suggest avoiding various drugs for their potential side effects, which may interfere with your healing program. Do not stop taking any prescription drugs without consulting your doctor. Bring to your doctor's attention the side effects you are experiencing and ask for a medication without the undesirable side effects or a natural alternative.

• Take responsibility for your health. Ask, learn, and accumulate knowledge about health, wellness, and longevity.

Secrets
of
Self-Healing

PART 1

THE PATH TO SELF-HEALING

America's health care system is in crisis precisely because we systematically neglect wellness and prevention.

—TOM HARKIN, U.S. SENATOR, IOWA

DOCTORS DON'T HAVE ALL THE ANSWERS. I learned this more than twenty years ago as a young resident in a hospital affiliated with Shanghai Medical University. I was assigned to the outpatient clinic for gastrointestinal disorders, and one day when I was making my treatment rounds at the clinic I saw a patient who was suffering from a case of stomach acid reflux that was keeping him up all night. He had been medicated with all kinds of acid blockers for two months, without relief. As our conversation carried on, the woman who sat next to him in the waiting room barked out, "Drink potato juice in the morning to get rid of it. It sure got rid of mine." I thought to myself, I am the doctor. What does she know about stomach problems? The next week, when I saw the patient again, he said he had used the potato juice remedy and his acid reflux was 90 percent better. I was humbled.

I knew about many useful natural remedies that had been handed down over the generations, and I learned about others from my patients. I began researching the healing properties of potatoes and other foods. I learned that the potato is not only rich in magnesium and other minerals, but it is also an alkalizing food, meaning it neutralizes acid in the stomach. More recently the potato was discovered to contain compounds called kukoamines that can help lower blood pressure. This knowledge led me to ask, What if everyone learned how to take care of their health problems without fancy drugs and a minimum of invasive treatments? Wouldn't that produce a healthier and happier population? The search for answers led to the publication of my first book, in 1987, called *The Tao of Nutrition*.

Just as planet Earth restores a fire-scarred forest with new saplings, each and every being comes with its own intrinsic healing capability. Humans, since time immemorial, have activated this power of self-healing through natural means. They have chanted, danced, prayed, touched, and used plants to restore themselves and others to health. Virtually every culture in the world has developed natural healing traditions that were in popular use until about a hundred years ago. But in the past century this knowledge has nearly disappeared from our collective memory.

. . . .

AMERICA'S HEALTH CARE CRISIS

AMERICA'S MEDICAL SYSTEM IS DOMINATED by the pharmaceutical, insurance, and biotechnology industries. Both doctors and patients are often left powerless and disillusioned. On the one hand patients are taught to be dependent on their doctors, but on the other, health care providers are overstretched while the insurance industry and HMOs dictate that they should spend still less time with their patients. Trapped in this morass are the nearly quarter of a million Americans who perish each year as a result of medical mistakes, neglect, and drug- or procedure-related side effects. All the while health care costs are spiraling out of control due to untenable economic models. The current health care crisis has exacted a heavy toll on society and individuals alike, sapping productivity and vitality and provoking angst.

Health care consumers have increasingly become frustrated with the broken-down system and are seeking alternative healing methods.

The result is a renaissance of traditional medical systems that promises to empower consumers with knowledge and choices. The growth and emergence of alternative healing practices in the last decade have been driven by consumers whose needs have not changed since the days of their ancestors. The health care industry would be better advised to listen to what the consumers of their products and services want rather than force on them from above a system that serves its own self-interest.

We can take a balanced approach in which the best of the world's medical traditions work side by side for the benefit of the patient. That approach, in fact, has been practiced in China for several decades. Chinese doctors empower their patients by educating them about nutrition and diet therapy. Doctors form lifelong relationships with their patients, allowing them to have input and control over their own health and well-being. The system has worked, and it is a necessity since the government would not be able to support a Western-style health care system for its 1.4 billion patients. I think the two approaches can and should be married to form a comprehensive and successful health care system. (Ironically, as I was finishing this book, the press was reporting that Chinese consumers are increasingly asking for brand-name Western drugs as a result of both marketing efforts by drug companies and China's modernization drive. If China isn't careful, it could find itself in the same crisis the United States is in.)

. . . .

THE NEW PARADIGM OF INTEGRATIVE MEDICINE

RECENTLY, THE TERM "INTEGRATIVE MEDICINE" has been coined to describe the new medical paradigm of offering a multidisciplinary approach to health care. Integrative medicine is a fusion of all medical traditions for the welfare of the patient. It is nondiscriminatory in practice, and it has the potential to best serve patients' needs.

In addition to Western allopathic medicine, Chinese medicine is gaining recognition as an important health tradition. It has been in continuous practice among a large population for thousands of years, and today it serves close to 2 billion people in China and throughout Asia. Its success rests on a naturalistic philosophy of health and medicine that focuses on treating the person—rather than solely the disease—with natural means such as diet and nutrition, herbal medicine, acupuncture, and bodywork. Chinese medicine is less invasive than Western medicine, too. The relative lack of side effects combined with its mind-body approach has made Chinese medicine a popular choice for people looking for alternatives to traditional Western health care. But instead of a flat-out rejection of Western medicine, why not integrate the best of both worlds?

I believe that integrative medicine is the answer to solving the American health care crisis because it involves you, the patient, as the stakeholder in the health care system. By educating you and encouraging you to participate in your own health care through lifestyle and dietary changes, stress management, and self-healing, the need for expensive medical procedures and drugs will decline. Your satisfaction will rise from having more control over your health. In exchange, your health insurance premiums will drop because utilization costs will drop. That is more money in your pocket—which is good for the economy. The science and drug industries would be directed more at prevention and wellness, innovating toward improving the quality and length of people's lives. The reward of integrative medicine is a society of happier and healthier people responsible for their own health and well-being, as well as lower-cost, excellent health care.

THE WELLNESS MEDICINE APPROACH

WHILE THIS BOOK DOES NOT PRETEND to be the ultimate solution to America's health care dilemma, it is my personal effort to help move the process forward. I introduce time-tested and evidence-based health knowledge that will help you gain more control over your health and wellness. This body of knowledge springs from 5,000 years of Chinese medical tradition, which emphasizes prevention and wellness. Therefore, I use the term *Tao of Wellness* to describe its concepts and practices for everyday living. *Tao* means "the Way," and the philosophical tradition of Taoism is the underpinning of Chinese medicine. Part 1 of this book covers the naturalistic philosophy of Wellness Medicine and its principles and applications. Wellness Medicine embraces a variety of safe, effective diagnostic and treatment options.

The seven key concepts of Wellness Medicine are optimal health, whole person, prevention, self-healing, personalized care, healing partnership, and integration.

• Optimal health is the goal of Wellness Medicine. It is the active pursuit of the best level of functioning and balance of an individual's whole being: body, mind, and spirit.

• Treating the whole person is the focus of Wellness Medicine, including a person's inner and outer life and his or her relationship to people and the environment. Disease is a symptom of life out of balance.

• Taking care of yourself before a problem arises is at the heart of Wellness Medicine. Practitioners promote healthy lifestyles, energy balance, and prevention of illness instead of disease treatment.

• The power of self-healing is innate in all of us. The aim of the Wellness Medicine practitioner is to educate patients to use this power to enhance the healing process.

• Personalizing health care to you, the individual, is key to effective healing. Wellness Medicine recognizes that each person is unique and has a different nature. Your individualized needs require a customized approach to health care.

• Wellness Medicine is relationship-centered care. The ideal healing partnership, practitioner-patient relationship, encourages the practitioner to listen to and guide the patient toward personal responsibility and full participation in the healing process.

• Effective integration of Eastern and Western medical traditions offers the best available treatment options. Wellness Medicine promotes the use of natural, noninvasive healing practices as the first line of health care, but it will not hesitate to use chemical and invasive medicine when necessary and critical.

THE UNIVERSAL LAW AND YOU

I WILL DISCUSS THE IRREFUTABLE UNIVERSAL LAW that governs the universe and its inhabitants and how violation of the universal law upsets the delicate balance and leads to disharmony and disease. A simple and obvious example of this is a very macho patient of mine from Michigan. He went outdoors in below-zero weather wearing only a T-shirt. He caught a cold and ended up with pneumonia. Understanding how the universal law works and living in accordance with it will help you prevent illness. In the above example, excess yin, represented by coldness, constricted energy and blood flow, thereby denying the patient's usual immunity from protecting his respiratory system. By increasing yang, or warming energy, in his body right after exposure to cold by drinking ginger and cinnamon tea, he would have been able to better counter the presence of the cold factor. Of course, dressing appropriately would have been my advice beforehand.

. . . .

TAKING STOCK: YOUR HEALTH INVENTORY

THE FIRST STEP TOWARD BECOMING AN ACTIVE PARTICIPANT in your health care is gaining knowledge of your constitutional archetype. This will make you aware of your physical and emotional tendencies. There are five constitutional archetypes, based on the five elements: fire, earth, metal, water, and wood. Being aware of your archetype and learning to take an inventory of your symptoms and signs regularly can greatly enhance your program of health and wellness. For instance, a student of mine recently learned that his constitution was predominantly the wood element. He also learned that wood element archetype people are prone to high blood pressure, heart disease, headaches, eye problems, and impatience. He noticed that he had been easily agitated, flying off the handle and experiencing headaches and palpitations. This level of awareness prompted him to immediately contact me to have his blood pressure checked and to have an electrocardiogram. I found that his blood pressure was elevated and that there was a slight murmur in his heartbeat, so I sent him to a cardiologist colleague of mine. A test revealed an arrhythmia; luckily it was benign. As a result of early detection, his blood pressure returned to normal with stress-release meditation, not medication. The patient took care of the problem while it was small instead of waiting until after a stroke or heart attack. That is the value of taking your health inventory.

. . . .

FIVE PRINCIPLES OF SELF-HEALING AND WELLNESS

Once you've learned about the universal law and how to take your health inventory, the chapters that follow will present the five principles of self-healing and wellness. By learning these concepts and practices, you will acquire powerful tools for maintaining and restoring your optimal health. The five principles are:

- diet and nutrition

- herbs and supplements

- exercise and acupressure

- lifestyle and environment

- mind and spirit

. . . .

DIET AND NUTRITION

DIET AND NUTRITION ARE AT THE TOP OF THE LIST because what you eat affects your health more than anything else. Countless studies have confirmed the healing powers of food—ordinary foods that we eat every day and extraordinary foods that contain powerful compounds useful for the prevention of disease and improving your organ functions. In the Chinese medical tradition, diet and nutrition are considered the most basic of healing modalities.

Over several millennia, the knowledge of nutritional healing has spread far and wide in China. It is common for the Chinese people to swap nutritional remedies with one another. Many of the home remedies presented in Part 2 of this book have survived the test of time and have been confirmed by scientific studies.

. . . .

HERBS AND SUPPLEMENTS

HERBS AND NUTRITIONAL SUPPLEMENTS are both preventive and therapeutic modalities, with the former being prevalent in every culture throughout the world and the latter having become popular with the advent of nutritional science research. Chinese herbal medicine is one of the oldest, most systematized, and most researched natural healing systems in the world. The sweeping number of herbs in its collection— at least 10,000 natural substances—is mind-boggling. However, there are only three to four hundred herbs in common usage. Chinese herbal medicine divides herbs into three categories: tonic, medicinal, and potent. Among a Chinese centenarian group that I researched, the common use of tonic herbs in their diet served not only to maintain health and vigor but also to combat disease if it gained a foothold. The medicinal herbs are used to correct imbalances. The potent herbs are to be dispensed for urgent or severe medical conditions only by expert herbal practitioners.

The success of Chinese herbal medicine's long-recorded remedies has motivated Western pharmaceutical companies to set up research and development centers in China to exploit drug discovery opportunities. One such endeavor focuses on artemisinin, a compound extracted from the Chinese herb artemisia. It has been used for the last two millennia for malaria, and it has been shown to be the only effective treatment for drug-resistant malaria in Africa, according to the World Health Organization. Traditionally, during the rainy mosquito season, households in the regions of China that are prone to malaria would boil artemisia along with other herbs to help prevent contraction of the disease. The herb is also used during the flu season to boost immune function. Studies show that artemisia also possesses antiviral and anticancer properties.

Nutritional supplements have become part of many people's daily regimen for maintaining health and wellness. Much research on vitamins and nutrients in recent years has contributed to the rising popularity of supplements. Supplementing a varied diet rich in essential nutrients with additional natural compounds can enhance and support your health. By learning about nutritional supplements and working with a knowledgeable Wellness Medicine practitioner, you will have another powerful self-healing method within your reach.

EXERCISE AND ACUPRESSURE

IN MANY YEARS OF CLINICAL PRACTICE AND RESEARCH on centenarians, I have never met a healthy person or centenarian who lived a physically inactive life. Exercise is critical to attaining your health and wellness goals. Aerobic exercise stimulates the cardiovascular system. Aerobic activities include brisk walking, hiking, jogging, swimming, bicycling, stair climbing, and many other activities. Don't overlook dancing, rollerblading, and other fun activities that are also good for your heart and circulation. Regular exercise is key to preventing and even reversing non-insulin-dependent diabetes, which afflicts more than 12 million Americans each year and is the fastest-growing disease in industrialized countries throughout the world.

Unique to China are gentler types of movement arts that promote energy, balance of function, and a calm mind. I call them mind-body exercises, and they include tai chi, qi gong, and Dao In Qi Gong. These have traditionally been associated with health and longevity. Many recent studies have confirmed their balancing action on blood pressure, blood sugar, cholesterol, equilibrium, and other conditions. One of my late tai chi teachers in China was in his early nineties when I met him. Though he ate about a pound and a half of fatty beef every day, he also practiced about two hours of tai chi every day, and his cholesterol and vital signs were perfectly normal. I am not suggesting that you eat a lot of red meat, I'm merely illustrating the benefits of mind-body exercise. Mind-body exercise works through a system of energy communication within the body—by deliberately activating the flow of energy and removing blockages, communication is restored and organ functions return to their optimal level.

This energy communication system underlies the Chinese medical system of acupuncture, in which needle stimulation and activation of certain acupoints in the body's energy communication network elicit specific and intended physiological responses. Integrating acupuncture into your health and wellness program can help you maintain healthy energy flow, and it can prevent and treat physical imbalances. If you are unable to work with a licensed practitioner of acupuncture, you can use self-healing acupressure tips found in Part 2. By using a finger instead of a needle to stimulate the acupoints, you will still be able to activate the acupoints for their intended effects. Recently a patient's eight-year-old child came in with a headache. I used acupressure on an acupoint in the web between her thumb and index finger called Valley of Harmony. Within five minutes her headache was gone. Acupressure is that simple and accessible.

. . . .

LIFESTYLE AND ENVIRONMENT

YOUR LIFESTYLE AND ENVIRONMENT INFLUENCE your health and well-being. Engaging in the activities that make your body supple, your mind clear, and your spirit content is the secret of the centenarians. Simplifying your lifestyle and developing healthy habits will not only contribute to an increased quality of life but will also help you avoid illness. For example, taking a power nap in the early afternoon both refreshes you and will lower your risk of heart disease and stroke. How about taking a walk after dinner rather than sitting on your couch? The benefits may include less heartburn and indigestion, better energy, and improved circulation.

A healthy lifestyle reduces the likelihood that your bad genes will get expressed. This is an important element in the nature versus nurture equation. Nature refers to natural law, in this case your genetic makeup, and nurture refers to what people do to facilitate nature. For instance, a mother feeds her baby to help him or her grow.

Nurture has to do with the physical environment, which can either support or derail your health plan. Environmental factors subliminally influence your mood, bodily function, and physical energy.

For example, on the way to work one day, I noticed that the sky was cloudy—an unusual sight for always sunny southern California. Among the patients I saw that day, about ten of them complained of headache and pressure in their sinuses that had come on within the last twenty-four hours. I knew then that the low-pressure weather system had been building and these patients were suffering the effects. By learning the rhythms of nature and the way they affect your health, you can become proactive in adapting to environmental changes and thus prevent illness.

A change in weather is more apparent than other environmental factors, like sick-building syndrome, for instance. The out-gassing of formaldehyde from furniture and carpeting, other indoor pollution, and inadequate oxygen contribute to some $10 billion of lost productivity—not to mention the illnesses related to the exposure. What about *your* environment? Your community can be either health promoting or stress inducing. If you are looking for health and wellness, surround yourself with people who are supportive and uplifting and share positive values.

An even more subtle environmental influence is the energy lines that crisscross the surface of our planet. These lines have long been recognized as an invisible but powerful influence on our health, well-being, and success in life. This is the basis for the Chinese science of feng shui, the practice of arranging your physical space to optimize positive energy flow in all aspects of your life. Similar to the practice of restoring flow to the body's energy communication network or meridians in acupuncture, arranging your living and working environment in harmony with the earth's meridians will enhance the quality of your life.

MIND AND SPIRIT

AN ANCIENT CHINESE SAYING WARNS US, "Fortune and disaster do not come through gates, but man himself invites their arrival." This saying reveals that energy of a specific vibrational frequency responds to and attracts energies of the corresponding frequency. Thus your experience is determined by the energy you embody. The power of the mind should never be underestimated. Subtle energy may be expressed by your conscious mind as ideas, concepts, and behavior, or through your unconscious mind as subtle impressions absorbed through the senses. It has long been observed and now confirmed that there is a personality profile of people who are prone to develop cancer, called personality type C. The type C person tends to be melancholic, depressed, and excessively worried. Years ago I had the pleasure of working with the late Norman Cousins, whose research showed that the mind has a powerful influence on many physiological functions, including a significant influence on the immune system. He demonstrated that an increase in the immune killer cells that attack cancer occurred in people who experienced thirty minutes of deep belly laughter every day for twelve weeks. His work became the foundation for the field of psychoneuroimmunology. Proper training of your mind is fundamental to effective self-healing.

Among all of the precious rewards of life, inner peace is the most worthy and is the most essential element of spiritual growth. No matter what your religious faith, cultivating yourself spiritually and strengthening your connection to the universal divine will bring you inner peace and the ability to cope with life's troubles, including illness and personal loss. Your spiritual clarity will serve to guide you in your life's quest for health, healing, and happiness.

I hope that in reading this book you will become empowered with knowledge and understanding about your health so that you can take care of yourself, and at the same time communicate clearly with your health care practitioner. By having access to and integrating the medical systems of East and West to serve your needs, you will have the best of both worlds. I am convinced that everyone needs appropriate support throughout their lives, so when you have built your effective healing partnerships with professionals you respect and trust, it will surely lessen suffering and bring more peace and enjoyment to your life.

I offer many natural remedies in the chapters ahead. But when it comes to self-healing, nothing comes close to the healing power of love. Love is the power to connect. All lives and things in the universe are part of one interconnected whole. Love opens hearts and engenders compassion. Wellness Medicine recognizes that the healing power of love breaks down blockages and separation, eases pain, comforts loss, and unites humanity with the universal divine. When you cultivate self-love, like a mother's unconditional love for her child, there is nothing that you wouldn't do to get yourself well. Likewise, universal love among all people will help heal the strife and the suffering in our world. I believe that world peace cannot exist until each and every citizen of the world learns to heal themselves.

This book is my humble offering toward that dream.

CHAPTER 1

THE TAO OF WELLNESS
The Naturalistic Philosophy
of Self-Healing

The sages of ancient times emphasized not the treatment of disease, but rather the prevention of its occurrence. To administer medicines to diseases that have already developed, and to suppress revolts that have already begun is comparable to the behavior of one who begins to dig a well after he has become thirsty and of one who begins to forge his weapons after he has already engaged in battle. Would these actions not be too late?

—*THE YELLOW EMPEROR'S CLASSIC OF MEDICINE*

FROM THE POINT OF VIEW OF WESTERN MEDICINE, health is merely the absence of disease. But with Wellness Medicine, it is possible to discover energy imbalances long before they turn into overt disease. Foreseeing and preventing disease before it manifests as painful or distressing physical and mental symptoms is the essence of Wellness Medicine. By taking a preventive route, you can consistently enjoy a feeling of well-being with an abundance of physical and mental energy.

I have helped patients who were not ill by Western medical standard, but who were suffering from fatigue, difficulty concentrating, body aches, and other symptoms that decreased their zest for life. Not sick enough to be bedridden but not well enough to enjoy a good quality of life, these patients are stuck in health limbo. By healing imbalances through diet, supplements, herbs, acupressure, mind-body exercise, and modification of lifestyle and mental habits, or through the use of acupuncture, bodywork, and other healing arts, you can not only eliminate the minor health problems that you have today but also spare yourself the consequences of developing diseases later on.

THE SUBTLE ESSENCE OF ALL CREATION AND THE UNIVERSAL LAW

TO GAIN MASTERY OVER OUR LIVES and achieve optimal health, it is necessary to have a basic understanding of the nature of energy. Vital energy, life force, or *qi*—as the ancient Chinese referred to it—is formless, yet it is the subtle breath of life that permeates and vitalizes the universe. Energy envelops us and fills us. Just as a fish is unaware of the fact that it lives in water, we are unaware of the inexhaustible sea of energy that supports our lives. The Sun is an obvious expression of this energy. It provides fuel for plant life, it activates biological clocks in humans and other organisms, and its energy can even be converted to electricity for use in our homes and offices. But most of the energy around us is imperceptible—that is why we call it *subtle energy.*

Subtle energy gives birth to life. Everything that exists is an expression or projection of that energy in varying states or frequencies. Ancient cultures throughout the world recognized the subtle energy that circulates through the organs and muscles, and that permeates every tissue and cell of the body. It is the life force and the breath of life in all living organisms. The Hindus called it *prana*, the Hebrews called it *ruach,* and the Greeks called it *psyche* or *pneuma.* Human beings are the embodiment of all the different energies of the universe, including those of the Sun, the Moon, the stars, and the Earth. Acupuncture, for example, is a precise science that deals with the processing, storage, distribution, and functioning of vital energy in the human organism as well as the relationship of this energy with the cosmos. By stimulating acupoints on the body, acupuncture subtly affects the circulation of energy on profound psycho-physiological levels.

The Yellow Emperor, the father of Chinese medicine, wrote in *The Yellow Emperor's Classic of Medicine*—which dates back nearly 5,000 years, and is the seminal work upon which all subsequent works on Chinese health and healing were based—"In Heaven there is qi and on Earth form. When the two interplay there is life." Qi is the essence of the universe and the law of all movement. Without a basic understanding of qi, any medical treatment is at best incomplete.

When qi gathers, it is called matter. When qi diffuses, it is called space. When qi animates form it is called life. When qi separates and withdraws from form, it is called death. When qi flows, there is health. When qi is blocked, there is sickness and disease. Qi embraces all things, circulates through them, and sustains them. The planets depend on it for their light and motion, weather is formed by it, and seasons are caused by it. Qi activates and maintains all life.

We can now record and measure subtle energy. For instance, an electroencephalogram (EEG) records "noise" from brain waves that transmit signals from brain cells to tissues. Subtle energy is informational—that is, it carries a specific signal or message similar to how voices or data are carried by electrical current through copper wires or by bursts of light through fiber-optic cables. Our bodies are absorptive, reflective, and generative of informational energy fields. For example, studies show that when a qi gong master is emitting energy toward a subject, there is a consistent shift of EEG brain wave patterns to the alpha state in the subject. Energy animates all the processes of the body: the digestion and assimilation of the food we eat, the inhalation and exhalation of air, the circulation of blood, the dissemination of fluids throughout the body, and, finally, the excretion of waste products of our metabolism. The energy of the various organs also enables the five senses to perform their functions.

The energy in the human body does not have a fixed form. Sometimes it appears in clear, invisible forms. It can show up as thermal energy in fevers, or in a vaporized form in the moistening of the palms, or in an ionized state during the practice of mind-body exercises that affect energy circulation—especially tai chi. Under other conditions the energy is murky but visible, and it can appear in liquid states such as sweat, diarrhea, a runny nose, seminal and vaginal discharge, tears, or saliva, when your mouth is watering. The forms the energy takes depend on internal and external factors in your life and environment, such as your emotional state or the climate. Wellness Medicine treats and takes into consideration all the vital functions of a human being at the same time: physical energy, emotional energy, mental energy, willpower, and spiritual energy.

From the inner workings of the smallest cell or molecule to weather patterns and the movements of the planets in our solar system, all existence is regulated by the same cosmic principles, which are expressed through subtle energy. By understanding the evolution and cycles of energy movement that occur internally, we can gain insight into the nature of the universe. Similarly, through studying the nature of the universe, we can gain insight into our own inner nature. By bringing into the light the workings of subtle energy, we can reconnect with our nature and learn the art of rectifying imbalances in our relationship to the world.

For example, as diurnal creatures humans follow the cycle of the sun. We're awake and productive during daylight hours and we rest at night. If we violate this natural order, we will surely become ill. Studies show that night-shift workers, whose most productive time is in opposition to the natural circadian rhythm, suffer higher rates of cancer and heart disease than those who work during the day. A patient of mine whose job keeps him awake most nights suffers from an irregular heartbeat with no apparent cause. His is a case in which his heart and body are out of sync with the natural law.

. . . .

YIN AND YANG

THE YELLOW EMPEROR SAYS, "Yin/yang is the Way of Heaven and Earth, the fundamental principle of the myriad things, the father and mother of change and transformation, the root of inception and destruction."

Ancient Chinese sages observed the cyclic phases of energy evolution and movement as the combination of two distinctly opposite yet complementary energetic states called *yin* and *yang*. The yin-yang system provides a basis for the analysis of all phenomena by sorting energy into two complementary groups. Creation may be viewed as the organization of the undifferentiated primal energy, polarizing the primal energy into the distinct yin and yang categories. The act of creation may be thought of as an expansion of the primal energy outward from a center. However, for organization to take place, there must also be a counterbalancing contractive force. If the centrifugal or contraction force (yin) and centripetal or expansion force (yang) were not equally balanced, nothing could exist. The structure of an atom illustrates the significance of this balance. If the tendency of the electrons to propel themselves away from the nucleus were not counterbalanced by the attractive force of the protons, the atom would disintegrate. On a much larger scale, this principle functions to hold together our solar system and the billions of galaxies in the universe.

There is no facet of life to which the forces of yin and yang do not apply. Yin and yang express the polar aspects and interrelationships of everything, and the balances of yin and yang are dynamic, not static. For instance, I use the principle of restoring yin-yang balance to help my patients with thyroid conditions—in the case of hypothyroid conditions there is excess yin, and in hyperthyroid conditions there is an excess yang. Likewise, yin or yang can be either deficient or excessive, as in my patients who are overnourished and obese or malnourished and anorexic—both are extreme states of yin and yang. So yin and yang represent two broad categories of opposites that complement each other, such as negative and positive, destructive and creative, inert and active, gross and subtle, actual and potential.

CORRESPONDENCES OF YIN AND YANG

YIN	YANG
Moon	Sun
Earth	Heaven

YIN	YANG
Form	Function
Dark	Light
Deficient	Excess
Depression	Mania
Night	Day
Feminine	Masculine
Contraction	Expansion
Cold	Hot
Interior	Exterior
Slow	Fast
Negative	Positive
Water	Fire
Quiescence	Movement
Autumn, Winter	Spring, Summer
Responsive	Aggressive

These correspondences can continue ad infinitum.

In health and in disease prevention, the application of the universal law of yin and yang to everyday life will help you maintain balance and harmony. Yin and yang are akin to a scale. Take the simple example of body temperature. When you are cold, there is an imbalance tipping the scale toward yin. Your instinctive reaction is to warm up by, say, putting on more clothing to increase yang, tipping the scale back to balance. Or you could warm up by increasing circulation via exercise—movement is an expression of yang. Likewise, when your body is hot or feverish, cooling it off by drinking water, using an ice pack, or inducing perspiration will recalibrate the yin-yang scale from a yang-heavy imbalance to a balance between the two poles.

THE FIVE-ELEMENT NETWORK

THE EVOLUTION OF THE UNIVERSE is not a linear process. Beyond recognizing yin and yang, which describe the process of energy evolution and polarization, the ancient Chinese sages also discerned five basic types of energy transformation. They called the five phases water, wood, fire, earth, and metal. This system, which I will also refer to as the five-element network, provides a complete and systematic symbolism for the interrelationships and cyclical transformations of all existence.

Life is not static. Rather, all life processes are constantly fluctuating between complementary polarities, and there exists in nature a system of checks and balances. Homeostasis is the self-regulating system of controls that maintains the internal environment of living things, and that regulates the balance between the internal and the external. This self-regulation is where the five-element network comes in.

In nature we see homeostasis at work in the delicate cycle of ecology. The life-giving quality of water energy gives rise to forests of wood energy. Lightning strikes forests and engenders fire energy. Through this process the soil is enriched and layered, producing earth energy. Over time, glaciers that contain metal energy cover the earth. Finally, the glaciers melt and water is created all over again—the five-phase cycle of energy transformation begins anew. This is natural law at work.

However, when the natural order is disrupted—often as a result of human intervention—ecological homeostasis becomes threatened. Take the unnatural, rampant burning of rain forests to make room for farming and industry. The carbon dioxide produced by both the fire and the burning of fossil fuel by industry gives rise to global warming, causing the ice caps in Antarctica to melt prematurely. Sea levels rise around the world, threatening not just humans who live near the oceans but arctic flora and fauna, including polar bears, whose habitats are lost.

All living things are homeostatic, otherwise they could not survive. The more complex an organism is, the more vital the process of homeostasis is. When homeostasis fails, an organism suffers and ultimately dies. In humans, if the normal cycle of energy transformation is disturbed, sickness and disease appear. The fundamental goal of Wellness Medicine is the maintenance of homeostasis through yin-yang balance and the five phases of energy.

Each phase has both dynamic and static characteristics. The metal element, for example, when viewed as dynamic yields such actions as contracting, organizing, and changing. Viewed as static, the metal element is exemplified by tools, autumn, and the lung–large intestine network. (More on the different organ networks below.) Some actions associated with the dynamic aspect of the wood element are upward, expansive, and controlling, whereas in its static aspect, the wood element is represented by varieties of vegetation, spring, and the liver-gallbladder network. The water element in its dynamic state represents downward, enduring, and cooling actions. Its static form is represented by fluids, winter, and the kidney-bladder network. The fire element is exemplified in its active state as explosive, warming, and excitable, and in its static state as fire, summer, and the heart–small intestine and pericardium–triple warmer network. The earth element demonstrates its dynamic states through stability, maturity, and centering and its static state through mass, humidity, and the spleen-stomach network.

The energies embodied by an individual and the energies of the cosmos follow the same natural laws. Thus the principles of yin and yang and the five phases of energy evolution operate within the human

FIVE-ELEMENT OR FIVE-PHASE CORRESPONDENCES

WOOD	FIRE	EARTH	METAL	WATER
Spring	Summer	Late Summer	Autumn	Winter
Wind	Heat	Damp	Dryness	Cold
Green	Red	Yellow	White	Black
Sour	Bitter	Sweet	Pungent	Salty
Liver–	Heart–Small	Spleen–	Lung–	Kidney–
Gallbladder	Intestine and	Pancreas–	Large	Bladder
	Pericardium–	Stomach	Intestines	
	Triple Warmer			
Anger	Joy	Worry	Sadness	Fear
Eyes	Tongue	Mouth	Nose	Ears
Wheat	Corn	Rye	Rice	Beans
Vegetation	Fire	Soil	Tools	Fluid
Tendons	Blood	Muscles	Skin	Bones
Ligament	Vessels	Flesh	Hair	Marrow
Soul	Spirit	Logic	Courage	Will

body just as they do in the vast body of the cosmos. The ultimate function of the five-element network is to establish equilibrium of the yang and yin energies and to bring harmony to the entire universe. The five-element network forms a complete system, which is self-contained, self-regulating, and self-renewing.

The five-element network has a corresponding internal organ network: Wood corresponds with the liver and gallbladder; fire corresponds with the heart, small intestine, pericardium, and triple warmer (the thermal energy and fluid circulations within the body's three cavities); earth corresponds with the spleen, pancreas, and stomach; metal corresponds with the lungs and large intestine; and water corresponds with the kidneys and bladder.

In applied Wellness Medicine practices such as acupuncture and herbal medicine, the five-element network is an important tool for the diagnosis and treatment of disease. It is also the basis for an understanding of how the organs interact with one another. Through important indications such as the condition of the eyes, skin, palms, tongue, facial tone, the intricate reading of the pulse waves at the wrist, and general inquiries about lifestyle and habits, a comprehensive view of your health can be obtained. In this way, disturbances in your energy system can be recognized before they manifest as acute symptoms, and the real causes of disease can be treated directly. I'll show you how to take a complete inventory of your health in Chapter 2.

We can also apply yin and yang and the five-element network to mind and spirit. Mind and spirit are very subtle states of energy. Emotion is a heavier form of mental energy that can be expressed in various modes. Anger, for example, is a manifestation of the wood energy, fear of the water energy, sadness of the metal energy, worry of the earth energy, and joy and anxiety of the fire energy. When the emotions shift from one to another in response to various stimuli throughout the day, the energy flows smoothly and health is maintained. When a single emotion dominates, however, the creative cycle of the five-element network is disrupted, internal energies stagnate, and disease manifests.

· ·

CONSTITUTIONAL ARCHETYPES

BY USING THE FIVE-ELEMENT NETWORK AS A GUIDE, you can identify your personality and health tendencies and determine your constitutional archetype. Understanding your constitution will help you make necessary changes, both physically and in mind and spirit, enabling you to continuously improve your state of well-being.

WOOD ARCHETYPE

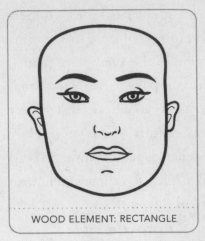

WOOD ELEMENT: RECTANGLE

Facial Structure: Rectangular, muscular, and slightly green in complexion.

Personality Profile: Wood-archetype people tend to be highly motivated and have very strong personalities. Sometimes identified as the type A personality, they can appear to be high energy, confident, intense, smart, decisive, responsible, and authoritative. Therefore, wood-type people tend to command respect and make good managers, but they are also prone to stubbornness and inflexibility, and can be overbearing and controlling.

Health Tendencies: Wood-archetype people are prone to conditions of the liver and the nervous system, affecting the brain, throat, bronchial passage, esophagus, and stomach. They tend to suffer from frequent headaches, eye disorders, nerve pain, neck and shoulder pain, throat constriction, acid reflux disorder, and high blood pressure. Spring is the season that corresponds to the wood element, so wood-archetype people tend to experience their illness during the windy season of spring.

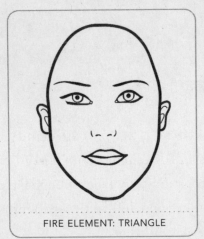

FIRE ELEMENT: TRIANGLE

FIRE ARCHETYPE

Facial Structure: Triangular face that narrows at the chin with prominent features and slight reddish complexion.

Personality Profile: Fire-archetype people tend to be very passionate, excitable, sensitive, and impatient. They are very quick studies, have an eye for detail, and are driven, ambitious, and persistent but frustrate quickly and do not easily adapt to change. They tend to be sociable and articulate, but because of a strong ego they may have a hard time getting along with others. This may lead to loneliness.

Health Tendencies: Fire-archetype people tend to suffer from circulatory and cardiovascular problems such as hypertension and heart conditions, varicose and spider veins, anxiety, insomnia, excess worry, palpitations, stress, neck and shoulder tightness and soreness, toothache, constipation, and menstrual problems in women. The season that affects their health the most is summer, with its hot weather adding fuel to the fire.

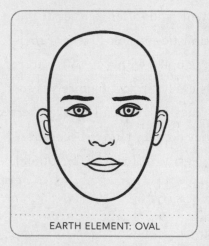

EARTH ELEMENT: OVAL

EARTH ARCHETYPE

Facial Structure: Oval, full, fleshy, and slightly yellow in complexion.

Personality Profile: This type is sincere, easygoing, giving, and nurturing. Thus earth-archetype people make friends easily. They act in a conservative, deliberate, methodical way and tend not to be initiators. They are also imaginative but prone to overintellectualization. Because of their easygoing personality, they may at times become pushovers.

Health Tendencies: The earth-type person tends to have digestive and intestinal problems, including disorders of the pancreas, stomach, spleen, and large and small intestines. Conditions may include stomach and duodenal ulcer, inflammation of the intestines, diarrhea, constipation, bloating, water retention, weak muscles, and low energy. Late summer or monsoon summer is associated with the earth element, so earth types tend to experience imbalances during the wet season.

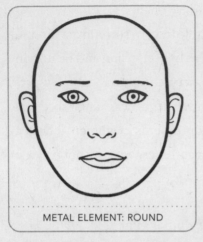

METAL ELEMENT: ROUND

METAL ARCHETYPE

Facial Structure: Round, wide shape with a prominent nose, and fair in complexion.

Personality Profile: Metal-archetype people tend to be intellectual, articulate, rational, meticulous, and very organized. When they focus their energy on a single task, they are persistent and often successful to the end. But because they are often optimistic and able to see the myriad possibilities, excessive deliberating coupled with a curious nature can cause them to change their minds easily, spread themselves too thin, and become scattered and unfocused. They tend to overexert and because they are so good at what they do, they tend to become obsessive and overextended. They are easily influenced by others. However, metal people are often motivated by the prospect of self-improvement.

Health Tendencies: Metal-type people are prone to respiratory conditions such as sinusitis, allergies, asthma, and laryngitis, as well as colitis and upper back pain. They are also prone to colds and flu as well as skin trauma, and they are sensitive to diseases of the mouth, teeth, skin, and bone marrow. Metal people will most likely experience imbalances or flare-ups during autumn, with its falling leaves and drying weather.

WATER ARCHETYPE

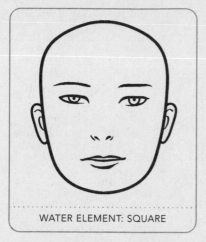

WATER ELEMENT: SQUARE

Facial Structure: Square, filled-out face, large ears, and dark complexion. Personality Profile: Water-type people tend to possess leadership qualities and are able to rally others to their cause. They like to please others and they get along with most people. Water-type people have amazing willpower and endurance, and are hard-working to boot. However, they can appear to be timid at times, hesitant and unsure of themselves. Therefore, water-type people can become too dependent on others or become extreme in their decision making, alienating those around them.

Health Tendencies: Water-archetype people tend to be prone to urinary-genital and reproductive problems with the kidneys, bladder, urinary tract, ovaries, testes, hormonal system, impotence, and infertility, as well as lower back and aging issues. Winter is the season connected with the water element, and water people tend to get sick during the cold weather of winter.

THE FIVE ELEMENTS AND THE HUMAN ORGAN NETWORKS

THERE ARE VAST DIFFERENCES BETWEEN HOW Western medicine and Eastern medicine understand the functioning of the body. Western medicine looks at the human body as a structure that may be taken apart like a piece of machinery to determine how it works. This approach implies that the form brings about the function. The Eastern approach, on the other hand, deals with an individual life as an interrelationship of body, mind, and spirit.

From this perspective we recognize that in the natural development of human life, all structure and form follow from function. Wellness Medicine deals not just with fixed, tangible entities but with functional systems, much as the immune system, which involves actions of the spleen, bone marrow, and the lymphatic and other glands, does. It is these energy systems in the body that enable a person to breathe, digest food, move, and think. The dynamic interplay of these energies is responsible for all the functions and expressions of the body, mind, and spirit.

When I use the term "organ," I'm not simply referring to an anatomical entity but rather to a functional energy network, which may or may not, as in the case of the triple warmer, include a physical counterpart. Therefore, statements about a certain organ network can under no circumstances be made to agree completely with statements about the corresponding organ in Western medicine.

Each organ represents a specific phase in the cycle of energy evolution, so the definition of an organ is not limited to just the physical organ within the body. It also includes the physical, emotional, and spiritual qualities of the person, as well as the organ's correspondences in the external universe according to the five-element network. The ancient understanding of these correspondences laid the foundation for healing with diet, color, and sound.

Since each element corresponds to a particular energy frequency that is affected by light and sound energies, colors and sounds have been used to help balance the energy within each element or organ network. For example, wood (liver) network disorders can show up as vision problems. By having patients visualize the color green or look at dense greenery, the eye muscles will often relax and vision may improve. Analyzing the content of a patient's dreams can also be a valuable diagnostic tool because dreams frequently reveal the nature of disturbances in body, mind, and spirit.

THE HEART–SMALL INTESTINE NETWORK

The heart sphere is the control center of the body. It includes the invisible mind and the visible organ, the heart. It is considered the sovereign ruler of the body because it is the residence of the directing energy called *shen*, the spirit or divine energy of the individual. Shen participates in and regulates the activities of all the other spheres of the entire being. The heart sphere directs the working of the blood vessels and the pulses. When the energy of this sphere ascends upward to the brain, it functions as the mind. When it descends downward to the other organs, it functions as the balancing center of the organism.

Bitter is the corresponding flavor of the heart sphere, scarlet is its color, and the scorched smell is its corresponding odor. The sound of "hah" activates the heart. The heart and mind correspond with the faculty of speech. The emotions that correspond with the heart sphere are joy or pleasure and love. Laughter is its corresponding vocal expression. If the energy of the heart sphere is disturbed, it may express itself in the following dream themes (taken from *The Yellow Emperor's Classic of Medicine*): "If the energy in the heart is exhausted, in dreams one will look for fire and yang things. At the right moment one even dreams of fire and blazes," or "If the heart energy is abundant, one easily laughs in dreams or is afraid; or one may see blazing flames. If there is an acute deficiency of energy in the heart, in one's dream there may appear hills of ashes and gray mountains."

The small intestine corresponds with the fire phase in the cycle of energy evolution. It has the same general correspondences as the heart sphere, which is its paired sphere. Its main function is to separate the pure nutritive energy from the impure, and to transport the waste downward. If the energy of the small intestine is disturbed, it may be evidenced by the following dream theme from *The Yellow Emperor*: "If an extreme deficiency of energy exists within the small intestine, one will dream of populous town districts and of main thoroughfares."

Diseases of the heart–small intestine network, which includes the mind and the anatomical organ of the heart, tend to produce the following symptoms: fearfulness, trembling in the heart, insomnia, general restlessness, mumbling to oneself, dizziness and fainting spells, constipation, abdominal pain, diarrhea, blood in the urine, painful urination, excessive sadness, or sometimes raucous, incessant laughter. Because the heart sphere is the master of the other spheres, any disease affecting it will quickly disturb all other functions.

THE PERICARDIUM–TRIPLE WARMER NETWORK

The pericardium sphere has two functions: to protect the heart sphere and to maintain the order of its energy. The anatomical correspondence of the pericardium sphere is the fatty membrane that encases the heart. Like the heart sphere, the pericardium corresponds with the fire phase in the cycle of energy evolution. Yet whereas the heart and its paired sphere, the small intestine, are known as the "emperor fire," the pericardium and its paired energy network, the triple warmer, are known as the "ministerial fire." All of the fire spheres share the same general correspondences according to the five phases of energy evolution.

The triple warmer corresponds with the fire phase in the cycle of energy evolution. Its paired organ is the pericardium and it shares the same general correspondences as the other three fire spheres. The triple warmer is not a single organ, but rather a group of physiological functions involving three groups of organs. The upper warmer involves the lungs and the heart; the middle warmer involves the stomach, spleen, and liver; and the lower warmer involves the kidneys, large and small intestines, and bladder. Although the triple warmer does not have a separate organ, its energy network extends through the membranes of the body cavities. The membranes combined with the fat deposits provide a protection for the organs and regulate body temperature. The triple warmer holds and adjusts the heat necessary for the various processes of energy transformation that take place in the body. It also influences the supply of subtle energy, blood, and other fluids for the muscles, skin, and the other eleven organ spheres. It is involved with the regulation of the body's energy network in the form of thermal energy circulation, which flows parallel to the circulation of the lymphatic fluid, blood, and other liquid energies. The triple warmer is the source of the body's protective energy. The corresponding sound for the triple warmer is "hee." A disturbance of the pericardium–triple warmer network may express itself in the following dream themes from *The Yellow Emperor's Classic of Medicine:* "If an extreme deficiency exists, one dreams of falling, and if excess is present, then one dreams of flying."

Disease of the pericardium–triple warmer network is evidenced by symptoms of dizziness, loss of voice, delirium, fever, chills, and hot, burning urination.

THE LIVER–GALLBLADDER NETWORK

The main functions of the liver are to cleanse and regulate the supply of blood to the rest of the body and to maintain the body's defense mechanisms. The liver also regulates the functions of the nervous system and is the storehouse of secondary energy. When a person is easily fatigued, it indicates that his or her liver energy is depleted and must be restored by food and rest. The liver sphere corresponds with the wood phase in the cycle of energy evolution. The sour flavor corresponds with the liver, as does the color green and the smell of urine. Its corresponding sound is "shih." The liver outwardly manifests itself in the nails. The specific body openings and the corresponding senses are the eyes. By observing the appearance of the nails and the sharpness of sight, we may gather information about the functional condition of this sphere. Tears are the secreted fluid that is a manifestation of the energy of the liver.

The emotion that corresponds with the liver is anger. Shouting is its corresponding vocal expression. If the energy of the liver is exhausted, one will be overcome by fear; if it is excessive, by anger. If the energy of the liver is disturbed, it may be expressed in the following dream topics from *The Yellow Emperor:* "If the energy is exhausted in dreaming, one will see mushrooms. At the right moment one has the sensation of lying under a tree and not daring to get up," or "If the energy is deficient and the direction of its flow is hence reversed, one dreams of trees in a mountain forest."

The gallbladder participates in digestion and the transformation of nutrients. It corresponds with the wood phase of energy evolution. Its paired sphere is the liver; thus, it shares the liver's same general correspondences. A disturbance of gallbladder energy may express itself in dreams: "If an extreme deficiency exists in the gallbladder, one dreams of being engaged in fights and battles or that one cuts open one's own body."

Diseases of the liver-gallbladder network tend to produce the following symptoms: outbursts of anger, impatience, migraine or tension headaches, dizziness, redness of the face and eyes, blurred vision, glaucoma, abdominal pain and bloating, nausea, belching, and soft, ridged nails.

THE SPLEEN-PANCREAS-STOMACH NETWORK

In the Chinese medical system, the spleen includes functions that according to Western physiology are attributed to the pancreas. The primary function of the spleen is to control the transformation, distribution, and storage of nourishment and energy for the entire body. In other words, it is intimately associated with the digestive system of conventional physiology. The spleen works in conjunction with the stomach, its paired yang sphere, to perform the role of digestion and absorption. The spleen also transforms the liquid from food and distributes it to the other organs for absorption. The physiological function of the spleen is the regulation of blood volume. It stores the nourishing energy of the body and it has an essential role in both imagination and creativity.

The spleen corresponds with the earth phase of energy evolution. The flavor corresponding to the spleen is sweet; the color is yellow; the smell is fragrant. "Hoo" is its corresponding sound. The extension of the energy of the spleen is the muscle fat and its outward manifestation is the lips. Its corresponding body opening is the mouth and its sense organ is the tongue. Saliva is a manifestation of the energy of the spleen.

The emotions that correspond with the spleen are worry and obsession. Singing is its vocal manifestation. If the energy of the spleen is disturbed, it may be expressed in the following dream topics from *The Yellow Emperor:* "If the energy of the spleen is exhausted, one dreams of lacking food and drink. At the right moment one dreams of erecting walls and buildings," or "If the energy is abundant in the spleen, one dreams that one chants and plays music, yet one's body is heavy and one cannot rise. If acute deficiency of energy exists, in one's dream there appear hills and marshes, ruined buildings and storms."

The stomach is referred to as the sea of nourishment. It governs digestion. The spleen, which is its paired sphere, is in charge of distributing and circulating the essences from the food. Because of the stomach's central position and the importance of its role as the depository of nourishment for the body, any disease of the stomach will quickly be reflected in the other organs in the network. The stomach corresponds with the earth phase in the cycle of energy evolution. It shares the same general correspondences as its paired organ, the spleen. A disturbance of the stomach energy may be expressed in the following dream theme: "If an extreme deficiency exists in the stomach energy, one dreams of eating and drinking."

Imbalance in the spleen-pancreas-stomach network tends to produce the following symptoms: indigestion, acid reflux, abdominal pain, bloating and distention, lack of appetite, diarrhea, constipation, and tiredness.

THE LUNG–LARGE INTESTINE NETWORK

The lung represents the respiratory system, and influences not only the rhythm of the pulse but all energetic processes in the body as well. The breathing function and the energy exchange it has with the external world are both fundamental factors in human life. More important, the lung represents the first line of defense against invading pathogens. Its corresponding organ, the large intestine, also functions in synchrony within the crucial function of immunity. The lung corresponds with the metal phase of energy evolution. Hot, spicy flavors correspond with it, as does the color white and the smell of raw fish. "Si" is its corresponding sound. The paired yang sphere of the lungs is the large intestine. The extension of the energy of the lungs is the skin and its external manifestation is body hair. The corresponding body opening as well as its sense organ is the nose. Consequently, the bodily fluid that corresponds with the lungs is the mucus secreted by the nose.

The emotion that corresponds with the lungs is sorrow or grief. Weeping is its corresponding vocal expression. If the energy of the lungs is disturbed, it may be expressed in the following dream: "If the energy of the lungs is exhausted, this causes white objects to appear in dreams, or cruel people," or "If there is an excess of energy in the lungs one will be frightened in dreams, cry or soar through the air. If there is an extreme deficiency of lung energy, one dreams of soaring through the air or sees strange objects made out of metal."

The large intestine functions as a means by which food is assimilated and food residue passed. It is in charge of transporting and transforming these residues. The large intestine is responsible for the elimination and absorption of fluids. It also corresponds with the metal phase in the cycle of energy evolution. It is paired with the lung and shares its general correspondences. If the energy of the large intestine is disturbed, it may be expressed in the following dream themes: "If an extreme deficiency in the large intestine exists, one dreams of fields and rural landscapes."

Imbalance of the lung–large intestine network tends to show up as: cough, asthma, sinus problems, shortness of breath, constipation, skin breakouts, allergies, and food intolerances.

THE KIDNEY-BLADDER NETWORK

The kidney has two functions: to control the fluid in the body and to store essence. There are two kinds of essence that the kidneys store. The first is the essence derived from food and air and is the basic nourishment of life. This can be released on demand to any organ within the network. The second kind of essence that the kidneys store is reproductive essence, the basic substances of human reproduction. These essences are formed from the action of the prenatal, inherited energy upon the energy refined from food.

The kidneys correspond with the water phase of energy evolution. Salty flavor corresponds with it, as does the color black and the odor of decay. The sound "foo" is its corresponding sound. The kidneys correspond with the sense of hearing, and the paired organ of the kidneys is the bladder. The extension of the energy of the kidneys within the body is to the bone and marrow. The kidneys outwardly manifest their energy in the hair of the head. The corresponding body openings are the urethra and the anus, and the sense organ is the ears. The bodily fluid that is a manifestation of the kidney energy is urine.

The emotion that corresponds with the kidneys is fear. Groaning is its corresponding vocal expression. If the energy of the kidneys is disturbed, it may be expressed in the following dreams: "If the energy of the kidneys is exhausted, this causes ships and boats and drowning men to appear in one's dreams. One dreams of lying in the water and becomes frightened," or "If there is an excess of energy in the kidneys, in dreaming one has the sensation that the back and waist are split apart and can no longer be stretched. If an extreme depletion exists, one dreams of approaching a ravine, plunging into water, or being in the water."

Excess fluids of the body convene and are stored in the bladder. Some excess fluid will be evaporated as sweat or passed out with the feces, but most will descend to the bladder for evacuation. The bladder corresponds with the water phase in the cycle of energy evolution. It is paired with the kidney sphere and shares its general correspondences. If the bladder energy is disturbed, it may express itself in the following dream themes: "If an extreme deficiency of energy in the bladder exists, in dreams one takes walks and excursions."

Diseases of the kidney-bladder network tend to produce the following symptoms: sexual disorders, irregular menstruation, deterioration of the bones, lumbago, weak extremities, impaired hearing, forgetfulness, frequent urination (especially at night), incontinence, and water retention.

. . . .

CAUSES OF DISHARMONY AND DIS-EASE

TWO FACTORS ARE NECESSARY FOR ILLNESS TO MANIFEST: A disease-causing influence and a receptive host. A receptive host is a body that is unprotected and weak enough to allow the influence to damage it. Causes of disharmony are either external or internal.

External causes are usually atmospheric factors that attack a person from the exterior. These climatic pathogens are associated with a particular season: spring is the season for wind, summer for heat and fire, Indian summer for dampness, fall for dryness, and winter for coldness. Each climatic pathogen has an affinity for one of the five-element organ networks. Each organ network is particularly vulnerable to disease during its corresponding season according to the five phases of energy evolution.

I had a sixty-four-year-old patient with the metal constitutional archetype. This element corresponds to the lung–large intestine network and autumn, and the patient would develop bronchitis every fall that sometimes was so severe that, despite the consistent use of antibiotics, it turned into pneumonia on three separate occasions. I worked on strengthening the metal element organ network, which included her respiratory and immune systems, with acupuncture and herbs. I also targeted her earth element. Earth is the source for the metal element, which involves the digestive system. After changing her diet, teaching her simple mind-body metal-element exercises, and putting her in a grief support group to help with the recent loss of her husband, she has remained free of respiratory problems for the past three years.

Although the types of pathogenic factors I've mentioned are prevalent in specific seasons, they exist in all seasons. This brings up the question of whether Wellness Medicine recognizes the existence of infectious microorganisms like bacteria, viruses, and fungi and their roles in illness. The answer is yes. But instead of chasing down the tens and thousands of different strains of microbes with specific treatments, our approach is to treat the body's reaction to any invading aggressor. By categorizing the body responses based on the yin-yang energetic polarity and the five-element organ network model, the balance can be restored in a predictable fashion because all phenomena, even microbes, are governed by the same universal law.

Characteristics of a wind attack involve fever and chills, body aches, headache, congestion, and a sudden onset of the condition. Heat invasion creates fever, red face or body rash, thirst, scant and dark urine, and agitation. Cold penetrates and causes chills, paleness, abdominal and joint pain, back pain, frequent and clear urination, loose stools, and fatigue. Dampness seeps and leaves one feeling heavy, swollen, easily tired, and short of breath, with stiff body and joints, loss of appetite, nausea, and diarrhea. Dryness pervades and leads to parched eyes, nostrils, mouth, throat, and skin, dry cough, thirst, and dry stools. Summer heat is season-specific and often attacks without warning, causing fever, irritability, nausea, diarrhea, appetite drop, heaviness, and, in extreme cases, delirium.

Internal causes of illness are primarily related to emotional damage. Emotional damage weakens the organ whose energy is responsible for generating the emotion, which in turn causes imbalance and disorder in the other organs within the five-element organ network. Emotional stress can cause stagnation of energy flow, leading to functional imbalance and ultimately physical breakdown. Many cancer conditions may have their origin in a psychoemotional imbalance. On a typical day, I work with a number of oncologists to help cancer patients cope with their chemotherapy and radiation treatments. I have observed that many of these patients possess the type C personality: They are emotionally depressed and anxious, and they have difficulty letting go of negative experiences and memories. Wellness Medicine considers emotional well-being an essential indicator of health.

Other causes of illness include faulty diet, excessive exertion, toxins, traumatic injuries, animal- and insect-borne diseases (parasitic), hereditary factors, mechanical or radiation damage, and epidemics. Any disturbance of the natural balance of the body, if allowed to continue, will create a state of ill health, ultimately shortening the natural life span.

. . . .

A HEALING PARTNERSHIP

"A SUPERIOR PHYSICIAN TREATS A PATIENT BEFORE HE IS SICK. A mediocre physician treats a patient as the illness has just begun. An inferior physician treats an illness after it has manifested," says the Yellow Emperor.

I want to make it clear that I do not advise you to exclude Western medicine from your health program. Even if you understand the benefits of a preventive approach to health and you prefer to use Wellness Medicine most of the time, I recommend that you still have regular Western medical checkups. By taking regular health inventories, you can discover most problems at a beginning stage, but there is no replacement for good medical expertise. It is important to put together a team of health care practitioners whose personal character and philosophy of healing you respect and have confidence in. Your team may include an exercise coach or trainer, a Wellness Medicine practitioner, an open-minded medical doctor, a nutrition expert, a psychospiritual counselor or teacher, and a community of family members and friends who support you in your quest for health and wellness.

Health care is based around an individual, so your practitioners should be professionals who are sensitive to your needs, can personalize your care, and are capable of establishing a long-term rapport with you. Don't forget that this person is your partner in health; he or she is there for you, and you want to cultivate that relationship effectively. In the West most people don't think about seeing a doctor until they are sick. Well, that is too late. The Chinese philosophy is to develop a relationship with your doctor in which you work together regularly so that you never get to the point where you require drastic medical care. That is simply good health policy.

In ancient China doctors did not get paid when patients got sick. Doctors were paid regularly to maintain the health of their patients. Don't wait until you are ill to establish a relationship with your practitioner. Preventive care and health maintenance are also sound financial policy for the individual and for society. The majority of people spend more money on their health care in the last two weeks of their life than during their whole lifetime. Often society ends up footing the bill. Find a practitioner, form a long-term relationship, and tell him or her that you want to be informed and learn how to maintain health and wellness so that you can take a proactive, preventive approach to your health care. Tell your practitioner, "When I have questions I want to be able to call you and get your advice over the phone, or when I have a problem I need to be able to come in quickly so that we can treat an imbalance or a problem when it's still small." Prevention is truly the best medicine.

CHAPTER 2

SYMPTOMS AND SIGNS
How to Take Your Complete Health Inventory

The secret of health for both mind and body is not to
mourn for the past, nor to worry about the future, but
to live the present moment wisely and earnestly.

—*THE BUDDHA*

IF YOUR GOAL IS OPTIMAL HEALTH AND WELL-BEING, then you must start with an understanding of the present state of your health. A physical examination with your medical doctor is a good place to begin. However, since that is often a once-a-year visit, what you do to keep track of your health the rest of the year is just as important, if not more so.

Before you start anything, whether a project, a trip, or an exercise program, you need a vision, a big-picture idea of the outcome and how it fits into your life's mission. If it doesn't fit, then you must change course. By taking an inventory of your life, you will become aware of where you are in the journey of life. Too often people allow the currents of life to sweep them away—far from where they intended to go. Or they become complacent and refuse to remove obstacles to their life goals.

Self-awareness is essential for reaching your full health and wellness potential. Awareness means attending to and becoming mindful of all things, within and outside of yourself. Are you aware of your body temperature, breathing pattern, and physical sensations at any given moment? Probably not! Most of us are not. These are unconscious functions that we take for granted. You are breathing, talking, moving, thinking, and sensing during waking hours. It's precisely how you breathe, talk, move, think, and sense that define the quality of your life. Becoming conscious of such important acts is critical to living optimally. This will require a little practice, but once you become conscious of these things it is effortless.

Becoming fully aware can be difficult in the midst of endless distractions, but awareness is an ability that every child is born with. Observe how a baby responds to every sound and light stimulus, every touch, the emotions of other people, and the changes inside his or her body: hunger, discomfort, hot, cold, and energy. The baby will cry to communicate needs and dislikes and laugh when happy and content. As that child becomes an adult, some innate awareness is lost and it will be replaced by social etiquette, intellectual learning, and worries about how to fit in. The results of this external conditioning become apparent as we grow older, causing innate awareness to give way to busy mental chatter. However, with practice, you can restore awareness and become fully conscious of your life.

. . . .

CRITICAL QUESTIONS FOR SELF-ASSESSMENT

I SUGGEST TO MY PATIENTS AND STUDENTS—and to you—that the first thing to do upon waking is take a look in the mirror and ask, "Who am I and how do I want to be today?" This might sound tedious. Why would you want to know who you are before you start your day? If you're not aware of the direction of your life, the world's currents will carry you along and you may end up where you do not want to be. It's easy to keep behaving in a certain way because that's what you've been doing for a long time—but to expect a different outcome without a change in behavior is insane. By being conscious of what needs to change, and knowing how to implement that change, you can move toward fulfilling your vision.

The answer to your inner query is very personal, and, of course, it varies from person to person. Here are my daily reflections, which I've refined over time, but which have remained fairly constant over the last twenty years. Each time I ask myself the question I choose my reply consciously.

Q: Who am I?

A: I am a child of the Universal Divine and Mother Earth, a person of love, compassion, and integrity, an instrument of constructive change and a student of Truth.

Q: How do I want to be today?

A: Today I want to be connected in spirit to that of the Universal Divine. I want to be clear in my mind so that I make the correct decisions. I want to be healthy and energized in all that I do. I want to be filled with love in my heart toward my fellow brothers and sisters, to be a good steward of Mother Earth, and I want to be the best that I can be in expressing the essence of my being.

. . . .

A SIMPLE AWARENESS EXERCISE

HERE IS A SIMPLE MEDITATIVE EXERCISE to help you sharpen your awareness. Close your eyes and listen intently to your breath. Is your breathing fast or slow, shallow or deep, rhythmic or irregular? Do you feel your lungs and abdomen expand and contract as you breathe? Does the air feel dry or moist? Is there congestion in your nose, throat, or chest? Do you hear rattling of mucus as you take every breath in? All you are doing is observing your breath, without judgment or correction. Once you are conscious of it, move on to the next segment.

Expand that awareness to your entire body. Keep your eyes closed. Sense and feel every part of your body, starting from your head, and down to your toes. Is there discomfort or pain anywhere? How about pressure and tightness? Can you feel your digestion? Is there movement within your abdomen? Do you feel weakness anywhere? Does your posture feel aligned? Can you feel your heart pounding or pulsating? Are you aware of any tingling, numbness, or burning? Do your hands and feet feel cold? Can you feel the flow of energy and blood throughout your body? Observe and make notes, but do not form an opinion. Once you accomplish the survey of your body, move on to the final segment of the practice.

Expand your awareness to your surroundings. Keep your eyes closed, even when trying to sense the lighting. What is the temperature on your skin and in the environment? What about lighting—does it seem cloudy or sunny outside? What do you hear? Are there subtle sounds beyond those generated by people and animals? Can you make out any smell? Do you feel the airflow or draft? Where is it coming from? What does the clothing on your skin feel like? Can your skin freely breathe? Do you detect electromagnetic fields from appliances and other subtle energies in your immediate environs?

Conclude your awareness meditation by writing down what you observed. With regular practice this exercise should take no more than five minutes. It will help you sharpen your sense of perception, which is vital for any successful wellness-maintenance and self-healing program. Next we'll use our five senses to learn about ourselves and what symptoms and signs may mean in terms of our health. In some situations you'll be alerted by visual cues, and you'll be able to take measures immediately. But the value of self-inspection lies in detecting subtle imbalances and dealing with them preventively through diet, lifestyle, and other restorative principles. Taking care of things while they're small will help you avoid big problems.

VISUAL INSPECTION

Your body speaks a unique language to communicate the imbalances within it. Over the past 5,000 years Chinese medicine has mastered the art and science of reading the body's language. A picture tells a thousand words, and your face, tongue, ears, hands, and feet reflect many processes within your internal systems.

The five-element network is reflected in zones on the face. The forehead corresponds to the fire element, the nose to the earth element,

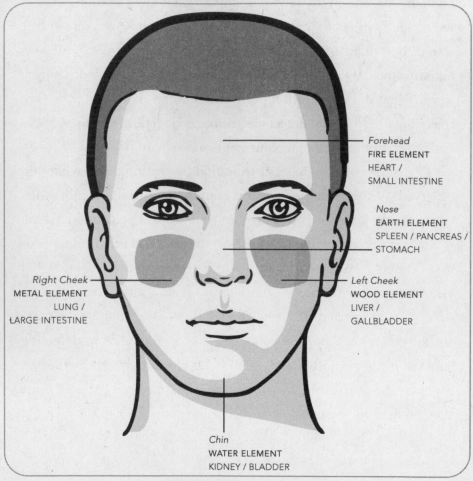

THE WHOLE FACE WITH ELEMENT ZONES

the chin to the water element, the right cheek to the metal element, and the left cheek to the wood element.

THE FOREHEAD

When inspecting your forehead, look for redness or small blood vessels that appear as discoloration. Since the heart–small intestine network corresponds to the fire element, discoloration could indicate a heart problem. The fire element also encompasses the mind-spirit connection, so another possible cause of the discoloration could be a recent emotionally charged experience. Someone who has recently suffered from a broken heart will show discoloration in this area. People who are regularly disturbed emotionally will have a constant furl between the eyebrows.

A heart attack can usually be foretold by reading signs in this area. The signs could be subtle, but look for a blue-green hue on the forehead. I had a patient who was robust and in his thirties. He exercised often but was under a lot of stress at work. During a routine office visit, I noticed a slight purplish hue between his eyebrows. I asked him if he had bruised himself there. He said no. I checked his pulse, and noticed that it was irregular. So I sent him off for an electrocardiogram and a stress test the next day. It turned out that he had blockages in his coronary arteries, which is unusual for someone of his age. If you observe similar changes in your forehead that are accompanied by palpitations, dizziness, shortness of breath, and tingling or pain in your left arm, call your cardiologist for an examination of your cardiovascular system.

THE NOSE

If you wake up and discover a pimple or redness on the tip or sides of your nose, it can point to an imbalance in the earth element or spleen-pancreas-stomach network. Examine what you ate the night before and several days earlier. Most likely you've had too much spicy, deep-fried, fatty, or rich foods, and possibly chocolate. As a result, you may suffer from indigestion, constipation, or diarrhea. In other words, your body is unhappy and it is telling you so. Perhaps a pimple seems like a minor problem. But imagine having a pimple on your liver as a result of your dietary indiscretion!

Broken capillaries or redness on the bridge of your nose can indicate abuse of alcohol and excessive worry and stress, which taxes your earth-element network. This was the case with a patient of mine whose nose would turn red when she drank alcohol or ate chocolate for relief from her stressful executive job in the entertainment industry. I could always tell what she had eaten, and she hated that. I would advise her to manage her stress better, through meditation and other stress-reducing techniques so that she wouldn't need alcohol or sweets to calm her nerves.

CHIN

The chin area reveals the water element and its corresponding kidney-bladder organ network, which includes the hormonal system and its glands. Blemishes, discoloration, or dark patches around the chin and mouth may signify problems within the organ network. Recurring outbreaks of acne around the chin or mouth could signify a hormonal imbalance—most often excess estrogen or testosterone, especially when coupled with irregular menstruation in women or prostate symptoms in men.

The philtrum—the ditch-looking area above the lips—directly relates to a woman's uterus and ovaries and to a man's prostate and genitals. For women, if there are lines going across the philtrum horizontally, or if blemishes and discoloration appear, it may mean infertility due to problems with the uterus or ovaries such as endometriosis or fibroid cysts. One of my patients suddenly developed acne and blemishes over her philtrum area that left scars. I became concerned and referred her to a gynecologist for an ultrasound of her ovaries and uterus. Sure enough, she had cysts on both of her ovaries.

People who possess a small chin have a genetic predisposition to weakness in the kidney-bladder network. This doesn't mean that the person will develop kidney disease, but we can use this information to alert us to the predisposition and make a change in behavior to help prevent the development of a condition. One patient, a fifty-year-old woman with a little chin and a slightly dark, ashen facial complexion, especially around her mouth and lower face, had symptoms of constant urination, but always in small amounts. She took several courses of antibiotics even though she didn't test positive for bacteria in her urine. I suspected a kidney-function problem, so I sent her for a kidney test. Her protein levels were elevated, and there were other signs of kidney failure. Kidney dialysis is automatically indicated in her case, but I worked with her nephrologist on a program that included a low-protein diet, mind-body energy enhancement exercises, and acupuncture along with kidney-supportive herbs. After about nine months, her kidney function improved and she was able to avoid kidney dialysis.

RIGHT CHEEK

Your right cheek is framed by your right eye above, the ear to the right, the nose to the left, and the level of the lowest point of your nose below. The right cheek corresponds to the metal element, or the lung–large intestine network. Look for discoloration, blemishes and skin problems in this area. Just before a cold comes on you may experience a slight outbreak of acne, an eczema patch, or slight redness on the right cheek. This may indicate the onset of upper-respiratory or lung illness.

People who have respiratory allergies or asthma will also tend to have a slight rash, reddish scaly eczema, or a slightly blue-green hue along the right cheek—showing too much heat or inflammation in the respiratory system, or a lack of oxygen from bronchial constriction. One of my many pediatric patients who suffered from allergic asthma always displayed an eczemalike patch right before a flare-up. It was a useful sign to look out for. I instructed her mother to treat her right away with herbs for the allergies to avert an asthma attack. She is now healthy, no longer suffering from asthma.

LEFT CHEEK

Your left cheek is framed by your left eye above, the ear to the left, the nose to the right, and the level of the lowest point of your nose below. The left cheek corresponds to your wood element, or the liver–gallbladder network. Broken capillaries and redness—especially right up next to the bridge of your nose—indicate liver heat, inflammation, or congestion. Bulging veins, redness, and rash sometimes signal high blood pressure and pent-up anger. Yellowish deposits under the left eye may indicate gallstones or high triglycerides or high cholesterol, which are processed by the liver-gallbladder network. Since the liver-gallbladder network includes the nervous system, depression can also show up in the wood-element zone of the face.

Years ago I worked closely with a group of psychiatrists who used analysis, art therapy, and Eastern medical modalities like acupuncture and herbal therapy with their patients, and they referred many bipolar patients to my office. When these patients were in a manic episode, their left cheek area right below the left eye would become slightly reddish, and when they were in a depressive mode, this same area would have a slightly bluish-green tinge.

THE TONGUE

The tongue is one of the most important diagnostic areas in ancient medical traditions. In Chinese medicine the tongue is a map of the internal body. Hidden health problems can be revealed by inspecting your tongue. Like the face, the tongue is divided into five element zones that correspond to internal organ networks. The tip is parallel to the fire element; behind the tip and covering a band-shaped area across the tongue, the metal element; both right and left sides, the wood element; the center and toward the back, the earth element; and the back of the tongue, the water element.

A tongue that reflects optimal health should be pink and muscular without tooth marking or discoloration, and have very little coating. Look for color, shape, and coating changes in specific zones. When the color becomes deeper—going from pale to scarlet to purple—it indicates increasing heat in the body. Heat may mean inflammation, in-

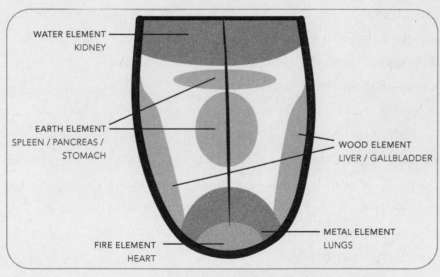

WATER ELEMENT
KIDNEY

EARTH ELEMENT
SPLEEN / PANCREAS /
STOMACH

WOOD ELEMENT
LIVER / GALLBLADDER

METAL ELEMENT
LUNGS

FIRE ELEMENT
HEART

TONGUE WITH ELEMENT ZONES

fection, or hyperactivity of the organ network. For example, the fire-element zone, which corresponds to the heart–small intestine network, and which includes both the emotional and the physical heart, is located at the tip of the tongue. Stress and anxiety will show up as red color and red dots on the tip of the tongue because the spirit resides in the heart network. Increasing heat signs mean hyperactivity in the heart network due to stress and tension.

When the tongue's color becomes lighter—from pink to pale to paper white—it indicates cold, which can mean anemia, pathogenic cold factor, or low energy and function of the corresponding organ network. Many of my patients with low immune-system function, sometimes the result of chemotherapy or chronic fatigue syndrome, exhibit a pale tongue, indicating low energy and functional state.

The thickness and color of the coating, or a lack of coating, can indicate certain problems. When the coating turns from its normal thin and white to a thick, white, yellow, brown, or even black, infection or inflammation is deepening and the toxins from the infection are building up rapidly. Sometimes you may see a "geographic" tongue, meaning that it looks like some spots were scraped out from a particular area. This may mean depletion of essence in the organ network that corresponds to the peeled part of the tongue.

Teeth markings on the sides of the tongue usually indicate stagnation of the energy in the liver network, as the sides of the tongue correspond to the wood element. You may also notice a bluish-green or purplish hue or spots in that same wood-element zone. Dark spots may indicate more serious problems—on more than several occasions I've noticed purple spots in the wood zone in patients suffering from low energy, discomfort, distension around the lower ribs, and swelling in the abdomen. I immediately sent each of them to see a hepatologist (a liver specialist), who, unfortunately, confirmed either liver cancer or cirrhosis in seven out of ten cases.

The bandlike area across the tongue and just behind the tip is the metal-element zone, which corresponds to the respiratory and immune systems. When this area turns reddish, or when red pin-sized dots show up, it usually means a respiratory infection is on its way or is settling into the body. Paleness of the metal zone may reflect a weakened immune system. In rare fungal infections of the lungs, a brownish-black coating over the metal element zone may appear—this is the case with several of my patients who suffer from lesions in their lungs.

Gastroesophageal reflux disease (GERD), which keeps many people awake at night, may be indicated by redness and a yellowish coating in the center of the tongue. This area is the earth element zone, and it is related to the spleen-pancreas-stomach network, so problems of the digestive system most often show up here. Subtle changes in this area may indicate digestive problems that have not surfaced yet—observe this area and take prophylactic steps if necessary.

The back of the tongue reflects many of the body's functions but it is predominantly the domain of the water element, or kidney-bladder network, which includes the hormonal system and sexual glands. The two large, elevated papilla on the back of the tongue are normal—they are part of the taste buds. What you should look for is color and coating. I can usually tell if a female patient is going to get a bladder infection when I see a thick yellow coating at the back-center of the tongue. I tell her to immediately start drinking eight to twelve glasses of water and take 5,000 milligrams of vitamin C a day, and drink cranberry juice or take its extract—a regimen that will typically prevent a bladder infection. Often those who don't follow this preventive treatment call me a couple of days later reporting an infection.

EARS

If you look carefully, you'll see that the ear is an image of an inverted fetus. The human ear provides a perfect map of the body. The head is at the lobe, the body curves around toward the top of the ear, and the spine is along the inner curve. The indentations or cavities inside represent the organ systems. The legs and feet correspond to the protruding upper cartilage of the ear. Because of this level of detail, the ear allows you to detect subtle abnormalities in your body's functioning.

The ear is unique in that it is involved in both health inspection as well as in treatment. In the practice of acupuncture, needles are inserted into zones on the ear that correspond to the diseased or imbalanced organ network or body parts. Similarly, you can perform acupressure by stimulating the acupoints on the ear with a rubber tip used to stimulate the gums, taping a magnetic pellet to the appropriate place, or pressing with your fingertip or fingernail. Simple ear acupressure can give immediate results. For instance, if you suffer from lower back pain, find the tender spot for the lower back by pressing

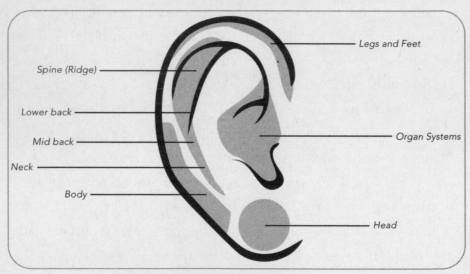

EAR WITH ELEMENT ZONES

along the cartilage that represents the spine. Stretch and pull apart the acupoint on the cartilage with the thumb and index fingers of both hands while bending and stretching your lower back—you may be surprised at how well this works.

Take note of any markings, lines, cysts or pimples, and discoloration on the ear map and then inspect the areas of the body that correspond to any areas of disturbance on the ear. For centuries health practitioners have observed that lines or wrinkles across the earlobe are signs of heart disease, or they may indicate that a person is prone to stroke, since the lobe corresponds to the head.

EYES

The eyes are windows to your soul. By looking observantly into your own eyes, as well as into those of others, you can assess the clarity of the spirit of the person. You can also learn to detect early warning signs of disease by looking straight into your own eyes. Variation in the color of the iris and pupil from person to person is normal, but you want to

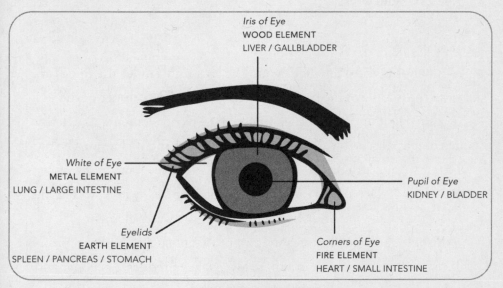

EYE WITH ELEMENT ZONES

look for changes from what is normal for you. For example, if the color of your iris were to go from blue to brown, that would signify potential problems with your liver.

The five element zones of the eyes are as follows: the corners of the eyes relate to the fire element, the whites of the eyes to the metal element, the iris to the wood element, the pupil to the water element, and the eyelids to the earth element. In Chinese medicine swollen or reddish eyelids, for example, indicate earth-element imbalance—digestive problems. Redness or irritation at the corners of the eyes may reflect stress to the heart—the fire element. When the whites of the eyes are irritated and red, it may mean trouble in the respiratory and pulmonary systems. If the whites are yellow, this may indicate jaundice, a sign of liver or gallbladder disorder, which requires immediate medical attention. Any changes within the iris may spell trouble for the liver, and dark circles under the eyes may mean hormonal imbalance, sinus allergies—or simply a need for sleep. A change in the size of the pupils is significant. It may indicate extreme adrenal exhaustion, shock or fright, or kidney disease.

HANDS

Your hands reveal a lot about you. The area right under the third finger to the middle of the palm is the fire element. The upper portion of the palm right under the index finger is the wood element. The fleshy area of the palm below the thumb is the metal element. The area below the fourth and fifth fingers, including the side of the hand in the upper two thirds of the palm, is the earth element. The fleshy inch-wide zone below the earth zone and above the wrist is the water element.

People suffering from respiratory problems such as asthma, bronchitis, and sinus infections almost always have redness, peeling, and itchiness in the metal-element zone. Digestive problems will be re-

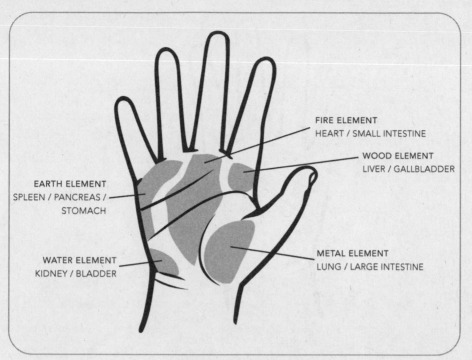

HANDS WITH ELEMENT ZONES

flected in the earth zone, sometimes as swollen or sunken features. People with hepatitis or cirrhosis often have redness in the earth zone, as this heat or inflammation can transfer to the spleen-pancreas-stomach network. Purplish color or hardening of the skin in the fire-element zone can occur in people with heart disease. Hormonal imbalance or kidney-bladder network problems can be revealed through swelling or a purplish hue in the water zone.

FINGERS

Sometimes you may feel pain or discomfort in a finger with no apparent reason. That is when it is important to know which organ system each finger corresponds to. The thumb corresponds to the metal element, the index finger the wood element, the middle finger the fire element, the ring finger the water element, and the pinky the earth element.

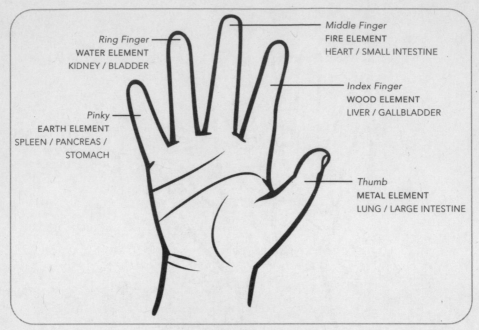

FINGERS WITH ELEMENT ZONES

When inspecting your fingers, look for changes to the texture and color of the skin, swelling or nodules forming on the joints, and veins or broken capillaries that suddenly appear. Also inspect the nails to note any lines, markings, or unusual changes. Dry skin patches, increasing redness, and veins and capillaries reflect heat or hyperactivity in the corresponding organ network. Swelling or nodules usually point to blockage of energy flow. Ridges and markings on nails typically indicate weakness and deficiency of the matching organ.

I often notice itchy eczema patches on the pinkies of patients with digestive-function disorders. And when a patient I'd known for several years suddenly developed nodules on his middle finger, even though he did not have any symptoms I sent him for a cardiac workup. The examination revealed a severe mitral valve defect.

Another patient came to me complaining of darkening and pigment spots on his hands, most noticeably on his ring fingers. Since the ring finger corresponds to the water element or kidney-bladder network (including the hormonal system), I sent him to an endocrinologist, who diagnosed him with Addison's disease, a condition involving the adrenal gland—part of the hormonal system.

FEET

The map of the foot may be familiar to people who are familiar with of reflexology—the practice of stimulating zones on the feet, hands, and ears for beneficial effects on general health and specific parts of the body. The origin of reflexology is uncertain, but we do know that it has been part of the acupuncture health system for several millennia. Just as the body is a microcosm reflecting the inner workings of the natural law, various body parts are their own complete microcosm. I've dis-

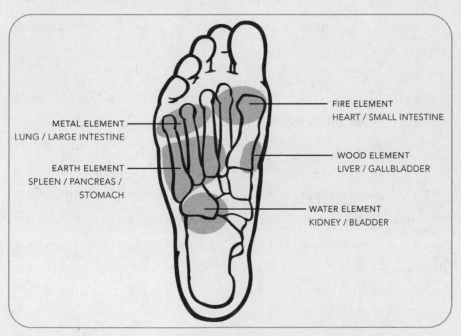

FOOT WITH ELEMENT ZONES

cussed how to read your body's functioning through outward signs on your face, tongue, and hands. The foot is no different, and it can aid you in your process of self-discovery.

The ball of the foot below the toes correlates to the fire and metal element, the arch the wood element, opposite the arch the earth element, and above the heel pad at the edge of the indentation the water element. By noticing changes in color, skin texture, and blood vessels, as well as tenderness from finger pressure, you can discover subtle functional changes within your body.

One patient complained to me about terrible pain on the inside arch and outside edge of her right foot. Countless X-rays and CT scans came up with nothing, and orthotic inserts did not offer any relief for her. I remembered that she had mentioned a family history of diabetes, so I suggested that she ought to rule out problems of the pancreas and digestive organs, since her pain spanned the earth-element zone. Tests confirmed the beginning stage of diabetes and probable peripheral neuropathy as a result.

This chapter represents the cumulative wisdom of five thousand years of Chinese medicine. With a little practice, you can begin to better understand your state of health and what imbalances may be affecting you. Once you identify an imbalance, take corrective measures so that it does not progress to a disease state. That is the fundamental principle of Wellness Medicine. The following chapters will reveal how to enhance the quality of your life with the five principles of self-healing—diet, herbs and supplements, exercise and acupressure, lifestyle and environment, and emotional and spiritual balance.

Please keep in mind that there are many ways in which your body alerts you to imbalances. As you learn this visual method, you'll want to be able to confirm your findings from one body part with observations from others, such as the eyes, tongue, and nails. When all the signs and symptoms add up, you can be fairly certain of your discovery, at which point I suggest you either use Part 2 of this book to deal with minor imbalances naturally or consult with your health care practitioner.

CHAPTER 3

LET FOOD BE YOUR MEDICINE

The Power of Nutritional Healing

The source and preservation of health come from the five flavors of food in the diet. When the body is imbalanced, the physician should use dietetics to harmonize and fortify. The five grains are used to nourish, the five fruits to assist, the five animals to fortify, the five vegetables to fulfill. Combining the energetic properties of these in one's diet can reinforce the essence and energy. One should utilize the methods of dietetics as an indispensable tool to nourish and sustain one's health, and treat illness.

—*THE YELLOW EMPEROR'S CLASSIC OF MEDICINE*

WHAT YOU EAT PROBABLY AFFECTS YOUR HEALTH more than anything else you do. Countless studies have confirmed the healing powers of food—ordinary foods that we eat every day and extraordinary foods that possess powerful compounds that prevent disease and improve organ functioning. In the Chinese medical tradition, diet and nutrition are the cornerstones of healing. Over several millennia, the knowledge of nutritional healing has accumulated and has been passed down through generations, creating the vast tradition of folk medicine. And thanks to the huge amounts of research conducted on food and its healing properties in recent years, we can further verify the usefulness of food in self-healing. As the medical system in the West moves further down biochemical and technological paths, we would be better served by advice from Hippocrates, the founding father of Western medicine: "Let food be your medicine and medicine be your food."

Western nutrition tends to be mechanical and biochemical, concerned with adequate units of protein, carbohydrates, fats, vitamins, and minerals. The U.S. Department of Agriculture's Food Guide Pyramid has been revised several times over the years to keep consumers educated about what makes up a healthy diet. The pyramid was recently revamped into the Food Guide Rainbow to reflect the importance of vegetables and fruits, beans and legumes, and nuts and seeds. The new Food Guide replaced the one-size-fits-all version with a more individualized approach to improving diet and lifestyle. The new symbol is a rainbow-colored pyramid called MyPyramid, which represents an all-new "interactive food guidance system."

The pyramid emphasizes four areas:

1. Variety—eat a variety of healthy foods.

2. Proportion—eat more fruits, vegetables, whole grains, and fat-free or low-fat dairy products, and reduce intake of foods high in saturated or trans fats, sugar, cholesterol, salt, and alcohol.

3. Moderation—choose portion sizes appropriately.

4. Activity—be physically active every day.

Prehistoric humans determined which foods were healthy and unhealthy based on their reactions—as well as the reactions of others—to what they put in their mouths. If they ate something and fell ill soon afterward, the food was deemed poisonous. Once in a while a symptom or some kind of physical suffering was relieved after eating a certain food. That food was noted as healthy, and even therapeutic. Over time patterns emerged and were combined into principles governing healthy diet and nutrition. In ancient China, the yin-yang principle of energetic polarity has proven to be an accurate observation of the universal law. Health and wellness depend on the balance between these two energetic extremes. As we've seen, everything in the universe can be categorized as possessing yin or yang characteristics.

. . . .

THE ENERGETIC PROPERTIES OF FOODS AND PERSONALIZED NUTRITION

DIET AND NUTRITION ARE ESSENTIAL AND FUNDAMENTAL to promoting wellness and correcting disharmonies within one's being. Individualization and balance are the key concepts. The one-size-fits-all diet fads that come and go sow confusion among consumers and neglect each person's individual needs. Selection of foods should be based on the energetic qualities of the foods, such as warming, cooling, drying, or lubricating. Thus you would seek to warm the coolness, cool the heat, dry the dampness, and lubricate the dryness by what you choose to eat.

By understanding your own needs, you can choose the appropriate foods to bring about a balanced state of health. For instance, if you are an excess type who exhibits conditions of heat in the body, like overheating easily, dry mouth, and red face, cooling foods like cucumber, watermelon, and peppermint may be your cup of tea. If you are a deficient type who tends toward coldness—if you get chilled easily, are often tired, and run to the bathroom frequently—warming foods such as ginger, roasted chestnut, and fenugreek may be appropriate for you. In this way health is achieved through balance and personalization.

All foods have inherent healing qualities. On the basis of these qualities, foods are broadly categorized into hot and warming, cold and cooling, and neutral, which is neither hot nor cold. Generally, animal products like poultry, other meat, eggs, and dairy are warming, while vegetables, fruits, and liquids are cooling. Whole grains, beans, legumes, deep-sea fish, and most nuts and seeds are neutral. There are, however, exceptions to the rule. For example, cherries are warming even though they're a fruit, and pork is cooling even though it's an animal product. Neutral-property foods are appropriate for all people except those who have allergies to certain foods. People who are of the excess or hot type will benefit from eating fewer animal products, while those of the deficient or cold type will benefit from adding animal products to their diet. Interestingly, warming and cooling foods correlate with acidic and alkaline foods, as we shall explore next.

· ·

THE ACID AND ALKALINE BALANCING ACT

THE ACID-ALKALINE (OR ACID-BASE) BALANCE of the human body is critical for healthy functioning, and pH is a measurement of the acid to alkaline ratio. The scale goes from 1.0—extremely acidic—to 14.0—extremely alkaline. Human blood pH should be slightly alkaline, at about 7.3 to 7.4. Values above or below this range can lead to discomfort and disease. If blood pH moves below 6.5 or above 8, cells and tissues stop functioning, which can lead to death if the abnormal pH is persistent over time. Consequently, the body is constantly attempting to balance its pH. When this balance is compromised, many problems can occur. Research shows that a prolonged acidic environment can give rise to inflammation and cancer and can lead to premature aging from free radical damage. For example, Norwegian scientists have confirmed that acidic pH can induce metastatic cancer growth of human melanoma cells.

A diet high in acidic foods including animal products, caffeine, sugar, alcohol, and processed foods exerts pressure on your body's balancing systems as it strains to maintain pH neutrality. The process of counterbalancing the acidity can deplete the body of alkaline minerals such as potassium, magnesium, and calcium, making the person prone to chronic and degenerative disease. Minerals are borrowed from vital organs and bones to neutralize the acid. Because of this strain, the body can suffer severe and prolonged damage, leading to an unhealthy condition that may go undetected for years.

In general, it's best to favor alkaline foods such as vegetables, fruits, nuts and seeds, some whole grains such as millet, quinoa, and amaranth, and to eat a smaller proportion of acidic foods such as meat, dairy, sugar, alcohol, and caffeine. Heavy meat eaters tend to be too acidic, and their bodies become overactive, while vegetarians tend toward being too alkaline, rendering their bodies underactive. A balanced diet is essential for functional equilibrium.

. . . .

THE BALANCING SCALE OF YIN-YANG, ALKALINE-ACIDIC

SO HOW DO YOU FIGURE OUT WHAT YOUR NEEDS ARE and what your diet should be? First, you must discover whether your body is in underdrive or overdrive, alkaline or acidic—yin or yang, respectively. The table below will allow you to figure out your symptom pattern. Health is reflected in the middle zone, called the balanced optimal performance (BOP) zone. To the left is the yin, or underdrive or alkaline zone, to the right is the yang, or overdrive or acidic zone.

Our bodies perform best in the midrange between yin and yang—the BOP zone. If you end up to the right of the BOP, you're in the yang or acidic zone. Many studies show that acidic mediums can promote cancerous growth. Not surprisingly, cancer is a phenomenon of excessive or abnormal cells, or overgrowth of cells, so you have to move away from the side of overdrive or yang.

What if you find yourself to the left of the BOP zone, on the yin or alkaline zone? The yin zone represents a weakening of your body functions—in other words, underperformance, which may predispose you to colds and flu, lowered metabolism (and, therefore, overweight), anemia, and lower-than-normal bone marrow function. These conditions may stimulate slow-growing fibroids or cysts that over time may turn cancerous. The bottom line is to avoid extremes and maintain yourself within the BOP zone.

SYMPTOM PATTERNS OF
THE THREE HEALTH ZONES

YIN/ALKALINE/ COOL	BALANCED OPTIMAL PERFORMANCE (BOP) ZONE	YANG/ACIDIC/ HOT
Tends to be chilled	Normal temperature	Tends to be warm
Prefers hot beverages	No preference	Prefers cold beverages
Low energy, fatigues easily	Normal energy	High energy, hyperactive
Tends to be more introverted	Good disposition	Tends to be more extroverted
Slow metabolism	Normal metabolism	High metabolism
Retains water, gains weight easily	Normal fluid exchange	Dehydrates, hard to maintain weight
Pale complexion	Healthy color	Reddish complexion
Frequent or loose bowel movements	Regular bowel movements	Infrequent or hard bowel movements
Frequent, clear urination	Regular urination	Scant, dark urination
Tends to be depressed or anxious	Healthy moods	Tends to be manic or agitated

You may find that you have symptoms from both the yin and yang zones, but see which one you fit into predominantly. Of course, you may find out that you're already in the BOP zone.

THE ENERGY PROPERTIES OF FOODS

THE KEY PRINCIPLE OF RESTORING YOURSELF to the BOP zone is to counter your imbalances by eating more foods with the opposite properties.

A female patient of mine determined that she was in the yang zone, with symptoms of being easily agitated, thirsty for cold drinks, and constipated. She decided to change her diet to include more foods from the yin zone, with cooling properties. She increased her consumption of vegetables, fruits, juice, tea, seaweed, and microalgae, as well as BOP-zone foods. She decreased her consumption of yang or warming foods, such as meats, sweets, spices, eggs, and dairy products until her symptom pattern returned to the BOP zone. Sure enough, within two weeks she felt calmer and was no longer constipated.

Another female patient determined that she had been manifesting the yin zone symptom pattern. This wasn't a surprise, since she subsisted on salads, fruits, some occasional pasta, and fish. In order to correct her imbalance, she increased her consumption of foods with warming properties in proportion to her consumption of fruits and vegetables by adding chicken, turkey, and eggs, along with spices such as ginger, fennel, basil, and coriander, as well as some BOP-zone foods such as beans, legumes, nuts, and seeds. Contrary to her worries about

COOLING	NEUTRAL	WARMING
Vegetables and herbs	Whole grains	Meat, poultry, and fish
Fruits, juices, and green and black teas	Beans and legumes	Natural sweeteners, salt, spices, vinegar, and coffee
Seaweed and microalgae	Nuts and seeds	Eggs and dairy

gaining weight, she lost the water weight she had been carrying around and felt much more energetic and spry.

One of my male patients found himself in the BOP zone, so his challenge was to make sure he ate balanced proportions from all three zones. He noticed that he was leaning a little too heavily into the warming foods, found himself getting irritable, and developed recurring little canker sores in his mouth. When he slightly adjusted his diet to include more yin, or cooling, foods, his canker sores disappeared and he felt more relaxed.

. . . .

COLORFUL FOODS

MANY STUDIES SHOW THAT THE DIFFERENT PIGMENTS in the skins of fruits and vegetables are potent antioxidants critical for maintaining health, preventing cancer, and protecting against toxins from the environment. The natural colors of foods correspond to the elements of the five-element energy evolution and their associated organ networks discussed in Chapter 1. White foods, such as cauliflower, daikon radish, water chestnuts, cabbage, and turnips, contain isothiocyanates, which support the immune system—part of the lung–large intestine network. Black, purple, and dark red foods, such as blueberries, black currants, blackberries, and beets contain anthocyanins, which support the hormonal system that is part of the kidney-bladder network. Green foods, such as asparagus, spinach, and lentils, provide rich chlorophyll and lutein, which are useful for the nervous system and help with the detoxification function of the liver-gallbladder network. Yellow and orange foods, such as pineapple, summer squash, sweet potatoes, and apricots, are high in carotenoids, which support the digestive system, part of the spleen-pancreas-stomach network. Red foods, such as tomatoes, red peppers, and strawberries, are rich in lycopene, which provides excellent antioxidant support for vascular health and the heart–small intestine network.

. . . .

HEALTHY DIET AND NUTRITION GUIDELINES

EACH PERSON IS UNIQUE, SO A DIET SHOULD ALWAYS be planned according to individual needs. Below are ten basic guidelines that can be followed within the scope of your healthy diet.

1. Eat mindfully. Most people eat too quickly, putting an unnecessary burden on their digestive systems. Your frame of mind is of utmost importance at mealtime; relax and slowly chew your food for optimal digestion and assimilation. The dinner table is not the place to discuss the day's problems. Chewing is a major part of digestion—remember, your stomach does not have teeth. The digestive process, particularly the digestion of starches, begins in the mouth, where enzymes are produced to help break down and absorb nutrients. Foods that are difficult to thoroughly masticate, such as sesame seeds, should be ground before eating. Chew each bite of food twenty times and savor the flavor with joy, repose, and gratefulness.

2. Take care with food preparation. The best ways to prepare foods so that nutrients stay intact (or, at least, are minimally lost) are steaming, stir-frying in water, stewing, and baking. Even the best quality oils become carcinogenic when heated. So if oil is desired, drizzle and stir it into the food after turning off the heat. The best utensils for cooking are glass, earthenware, enamel-coated, or stainless steel cookware. Avoid cooking in aluminum, copper, and Teflon-coated pans—these materials can easily leach into the food. Stay away from irradiated foods and avoid using a microwave oven

for cooking whenever possible. (Irradiated foods carry a symbol on their packaging that looks like a flower inside a circle.)

3. Favor whole foods. Foods should be eaten in their wholeness whenever possible. Only peel fruits or vegetables with peels that are hard to digest, like papayas or bananas, or if they are sprayed with pesticides and herbicides. Search out organic foods to avoid the toxic chemical residues of commercially grown produce. Wash nonorganic foods in salt water or with a vegetable and fruit wash to eliminate or neutralize the toxins. Avoid highly processed and refined foods—they're stripped of critical nutrients and then the nutrients are added back into the food after processing.

4. Say no to genetically modified food. GM plants have been genetically manipulated to make them more productive or more resistant to pests, or so the food will contain higher amounts of a certain nutrient. This is similar to the way growth hormones are used to make a chicken lay more eggs or a cow fatten up quickly. It's also similar to an athlete taking steroids— rapid growth is promoted, but there are side effects down the road. It is too early to know the full scope of the impact of eating GM foods—it will take several generations to see how the human body adapts.

5. Eat locally and in season. Your diet should follow the seasons, and you should eat what grows locally. Nature has the perfect plan for providing appropriate foods for each season. The fruits and vegetables that ripen in the summer, like watermelon, collard greens, and zucchini, tend to be on the cooling side to counter the heat of the season. In winter you'll tend toward a warming diet, including leeks, onions, and turnips. And by eating locally produced foods you are lessening global warming by not buying foods that have been transported many miles to get to your dinner table.

6. Support your digestive system. Try to stay away from cold, icy foods and beverages. Body temperature is around 98.6 degrees, and ice cream or cold beverages with ice are often around 30 degrees or lower. Imagine run-

ning outside naked in the near-freezing temperature. How do you think your body would react? You could get sick and catch pneumonia! Likewise, the shock your digestive tract experiences from the sudden drop in temperature from cold foods may cause gastric juice imbalance, decreased blood flow through your gut, and spasm and pain of the bowels, to name a only a few side effects. Try to eat your food at or above the ambient body temperature of 98.6 degrees.

7. Eat regular meals. Your body functions best when fed at regular intervals. Eat breakfast before 9:00 A.M., lunch before 1:00 P.M., and dinner before 7:00 P.M. You may want to snack between meals to keep your metabolism going. Nuts, seeds, dried fruits, and vegetables with healthy low-fat dips like hummus or black bean dip are good snacks to help you maintain your energy level. Eating smaller meals more frequently is what I call just-in-time nutrition—eat just enough to propel you for the next three to four hours so that you don't store more than half of a big meal as fat. And don't eat right before bedtime unless you want your stomach to be working all night long!

8. Eat to live. You have the power to choose what you put into your mouth. Ask whether your food choices will contribute to your health and well-being or cause future problems and suffering. It's easy to eat that awfully tempting ice cream sundae, but it's difficult to work it off by exercising for an hour. Many people live to eat instead of eating to live—they eat lavishly and decadently, falsely fulfilling their bellies in place of their hearts. Eating an abundance of fruits and vegetables to provide your body with more age-reversing antioxidants is an excellent example of eating to live.

9. Find sweetness in life. Many people lack happiness and sweetness in their lives, so they turn to food to fill the empty space within. Eating poorly as a response to feeling depressed and anxious is highly destructive to your health, and can be life threatening. The average American consumes more than 200 pounds of sugar each year. Besides being addictive, sugar and ar-

tificial sweeteners can negatively affect your behavior and personality, and overconsumption increases your risk for inflammation and degeneration. Rather than looking to food for sweetness, seek sweetness from your life by being kind to yourself, by forming meaningful relationships, and by being grateful for what you have.

10. Eat less, live longer. Eating less is generally better for your health, unless you are underweight or suffering from a medical condition such as anorexia. When you overeat, you stress your digestive and other organ systems, and you consume precious energy and produce more waste products and toxins. Many studies show that less food—calorie restriction—increases life span in animals. For example, excess animal protein increases the risks of developing cancer and kidney disease; excess fat leads to obesity and a higher threat of heart disease and stroke. So enjoy your food, but a little at a time. However, make sure to eat a minimum of 1,600 calories a day in normal circumstances.

All foods possess healing properties. Nature is abundant with substances that restore health and well-being. Cranberries, for instance, contain antioxidants including catechins, anthocyanins, and triterpenoids, and they have traditionally been used for preventing and treating urinary frequency as well as urinary tract infections. Studies show that the hippuric acid in cranberries inhibits the growth and attachment of bacteria such as *E. coli* to the bladder. Other studies show that cranberries improve dental health by helping prevent gum inflammation and tooth decay and heal stomach ulcers by inhibiting *H. pylori*, a bacteria responsible for weakening the protective lining of the stomach.

I recommend that patients with a history of bladder or urinary tract infections consume cranberries or their juice on a preventive basis. At the onset of infection, as a home remedy I recommend four to six glasses of cranberry juice a day, along with vitamin C and lots of water.

Often the home remedy will do the job if it is put into action right at the start of the infection. If the infection persists, you should always contact your physician for medical treatment in order to prevent a kidney infection from developing.

Eating well and eating for your unique needs are the bases for good health. Arming yourself with knowledge of healing foods is the first step toward taking responsibility for and participating in self-healing. In the following pages you'll find many nutritional home remedies to help you get started. Always practice self-healing responsibly by working in conjunction with your healing team of doctors, teachers, and trainers. To learn more about healing foods, I recommend that you refer to my book *The Tao of Nutrition*. Happy eating!

CHAPTER 4

MOTHER NATURE'S GENIUS

The Healing Properties of Herbs and Supplements

The art of healing comes from nature, not from the physician. Therefore the physician must start from nature, with an open mind.

—*PARACELSUS*

HERBS HAVE BEEN PART OF EVERY CULTURE AND MEDICAL TRADITION since the earliest humans walked on earth. They've been used to treat everything from colds to ulcers, from parasites to insomnia. They have been part of our diets, including cooking herbs and spices such as rosemary, turmeric, garlic, and ginger. Herbs have been part of most people's diet and nutritional regimen for maintaining health and treating illness until as recently as a hundred years ago. Around that time technology enabled us to identify micronutrients, such as vitamin and minerals, in our foods, laying the foundation for the science of nutrition. Today holistic nutrition addresses the health and healing needs of an individual by using nutritional supplements, which are often extracted from fruits, vegetables, and herbs. In many ways herbs and supplements act as whole foods to support the body's natural regenerative and healing processes. Certain herbs, however, are targeted healing agents used to correct more extreme imbalances.

. . . .

CHINA'S HERBAL TRADITION

HUGE VOLUMES OF MATERIA MEDICA (books about healing plants and substances) have been compiled and disseminated by practitioners of the medical arts, ranging from the asu priests of ancient Mesopotamia to the philosopher-physicians of China, from the Vedic doctors of India to the physicians of ancient Egypt and Greece and the medicine men of the Americas. Today the most complete system of herbal medicine— one that has been in continuous use for several millennia—comes from China, where the most recent government-published edition of Materia Medica contains more than 10,000 entries of natural healing substances.

The herbal medicine of China evolved out of a philosophy that emphasized preventing disease and delaying the onset of aging and dying. China's first book on herbs—quite possibly the world's first—*The Divine Farmer's Materia Medica,* was written over 5,000 years ago by Shen Nong, the father of Chinese agriculture and herbal medicine. It was written to help treat illness, assist in the pursuit of longevity and immortality, and help prevent disease. More than 360 herbs are included in the book, divided into three grades or qualities. The tonic herbs are the edible herbs that promote health, longevity, and spiritual well-being. Fascinating legends about people attaining immortality by consuming tonic herbs are still told today in China. The medicinal herbs help correct the body's imbalances and alleviate sickness. The potent medicinal-grade herbs are used for more serious conditions and are restricted to master healers.

The earliest philosopher-physicians of China were the Taoists; their object in life was the pursuit of spiritual immortality. This was accomplished through self-cultivation, which included upholding one's physical body in optimal health, maintaining a clear and calm mind, cultivating an enlightened spirit, and living a life of peace and contentment by following the Tao, the Natural Way. However plain and ordinary they appeared, the ancient Taoists understood the workings of the universe and possessed extraordinary powers.

. . . .

SECRETS OF OPTIMAL HEALTH

UPHOLDING THE PHYSICAL BODY IN OPTIMAL HEALTH was the prerequisite to an enlightened spirit. The body is the vehicle for the external fulfillment of one's spirit, and it provides nourishment and connection to the mind and the spirit. Herbal supplements have long been essential to self-cultivation. Using tonic herbs, the early Taoists were able to endure arduous martial arts training, sustain themselves during harsh weather in the high mountains, and keep their minds clear and sharp through long periods of intense meditation and fasting. They were vital and potent even in their old age, and most remarkably, they never seemed to age. This was possible largely because of the nutritive values of tonic herbs. It was one of their secrets.

Tonic herbs were used for nourishing the organs, balancing the hormones for women, detoxifying the body of accumulated toxins, beautifying and promoting youthful appearance, rejuvenating sexual energy, and enhancing various meditations and energy practices. A number of these formulas were passed down over the years and are variously referred to as elixirs, superior herbs, or simply tonic herbs. At this point I must reveal that my family has benefitted from a collection of tonic herb formulas that were passed down from our long tradition of healing and self-cultivation. We share these tonic herbs with friends through our family company, Tao of Wellness. I help the company select the best herbs and the best extraction processes to produce the best products. The company is totally committed to manufacturing quality herbal supplements. Of course, if you think my relationship with the company biases my opinion, you can find a number of other companies in the United States that produce tonic herbs.

· ·

THE AMAZING HUMAN BODY

TO AUGMENT THE BODY'S MYSTICAL POWER OF ENDURANCE, we must understand the principles behind the healing practices of the people who pursued immortality. The human body is constructed with the same complexity and intricacy as the universe. Its delicate systems function in synchrony and with amazing precision. Yet it is also fragile and requires constant care and fine-tuning. It reacts to and constantly attempts to adapt to thousands of factors and elements that we contact daily in our life. Most of the time the body self-regulates, but sometimes it does not, and imbalance or illness is the result. Often powerful built-in mechanisms balance the body. However, it cannot perform optimally under the conditions of repeated stress and poor nutrition that are so often a part of our high-pressure style of living. The body requires appropriate conditions and nourishment, which can be obtained through proper living and supplementing our diet with tonic herbs.

I divide the tonic herbs into three categories, based on the unique actions of detoxifying, balancing, or regenerating. I consider them a critical part of an illness prevention strategy.

· ·

TONIC HERBS

YOUR BODY, LIKE YOUR CAR, IS AN EFFICIENT MACHINE that performs consistently only when it is given proper care. A car needs a periodic change of oil, coolant, and the various filters that eliminate waste products that would otherwise degrade its performance—or worse, cause it to break down. The human body is unique. It has all the necessary elimination systems, including the liver, lymphatic system, skin, bowels, and urinary tract. However, these built-in systems can get clogged by chemicals and toxins.

Some of these toxins are the preservatives and additives that are found in the foods you eat, chlorine and other contaminants in the water supply, ozone in smog, formaldehyde in carpets and furniture, pesticides in fruits and vegetables, hormones and antibiotics in dairy and meat, and the diverse chemicals in the workplace and home. It is no wonder that allergies, autoimmune disorders, and cancer are on the rise. I address the topic of environmental health in Chapter 6.

You can avoid chemically enhanced foods by eating only organically grown, natural products. You can drink purified water and breathe purified air. You can avoid enclosed spaces and live away from problem areas like the neighborhood dry cleaner or factories. But even after taking these precautions, harmful chemicals and agents still manage to get into your body when you bathe with city water, get behind the wheel of a car, or simply put on a pair of dyed jeans.

No one is immune to the destructive side effects of our chemical inventions. Your body will process and eliminate some of the hordes of chemicals that enter it. The rest are simply stored in the liver, lungs, kidneys, fat cells, intestines, bloodstream, and skin. Many chronic illnesses result from the accumulation of waste and toxins in the body. Eat organic foods and take tonic herbs to cleanse and detoxify the body on a regular basis to prevent illness or a disruption of the body's functions, and to maintain optimal health.

. . . .

HERBS FOR CLEANSING

THE FIRST TYPE OF TONIC HERBS ARE THOSE that cleanse and detoxify. These herbs help support your liver, lymphatic system, bowels, urinary tract, and skin by cleansing and preventing a buildup of toxins and wastes in the body. To maintain optimum wellness, it is essential to cleanse and eliminate environmental toxins, as they increasingly are the culprit in cancer and other degenerative and chronic diseases. Some tonic herbs known for their cleansing and detoxifying actions are:

Chrysanthemum flower (*Flos chrysanthemi*). Traditionally used to cleanse the liver, brighten vision, disperse wind, clear heat, and neutralize toxins. Studies show that chrysanthemum can lower blood pressure and cholesterol and balance blood sugar.

Citrus peel (*Pericarpium citri*). Includes the ripened peel from orange, tangerine, and lemon. Citrus peel contains beneficial compounds, such as polymethoxylated flavones and d-Limonene, which have been found to lower cholesterol, balance blood sugar, and activate liver detoxification.

Dandelion (*Herba teraxaci*). Studies have shown that dandelion root enhances the flow of bile, improving conditions such as liver congestion, bile duct inflammation, hepatitis, gallstones, and jaundice.

Hawthorn berry (*Fructus crataegi*). A well-known cardiovascular tonic, hawthorn has been used in China to normalize heart function in coronary artery disease and congestive heart failure. Studies show that it helps the body maintain healthy cholesterol and blood pressure. Potent antioxidants such as anthocyanidin, proanthocyanidin, and rutin in hawthorn berry are thought to be responsible for its anti-inflammatory and anti-clotting properties. It is used to cleanse the blood of plaque and other toxins.

Milk thistle (*Herba silybum*). Extensive research has shown that silymarin (the major component of milk thistle extract) exerts both protective and restorative effects on the liver and can stimulate the growth of new liver cells to replace old damaged cells.

Mulberry leaf (*Folium mori*). Traditionally used to release heat and toxins from the skin and the lymphatic system, mulberry leaf has also been found to be useful in expelling impurities from the urinary tract and reducing triglycerides.

Seaweed (*Laminaria sargassum*). The algin in seaweed absorbs toxins from the digestive system, improving digestion, stimulating kidney function, increasing circulation, and purifying the blood. Seaweed can absorb and remove drugs, chemicals, heavy metals, and radioactive strontium from the body. Some experts claim that seaweed's active ingredient, sodium alginate, binds these toxins in the gastrointestinal tract, preventing their absorption into the body. It also reduces cholesterol levels through the retardation of bile acid absorption.

Turmeric (*Radix curcuma*). A common spice, turmeric accelerates the detoxification process in the whole body by increasing bile production and release, which is one of the ways that the body eliminates toxins like heavy metals and other chemicals. It also appears to possess potent anti-inflammatory and anticancer properties and it helps to improve circulation and prevent blood clotting. The blood-thinning drug Coumadin originated from turmeric.

. . . .

HERBS FOR BALANCING

THE SECOND TYPE OF TONIC HERBS BALANCE the body's functions. Restoring balance or equilibrium is what your body constantly attempts to do, but sometimes it does not succeed. Besides the variety of toxins that invade your body, many factors affect the normal functioning of your organs, hormonal glands, and body systems. Drinking caffeinated beverages or smoking cigarettes, for example, can overstimulate the adrenal and thyroid glands and in the long run can cause a decline of the functions of these glands. The result is obesity and fatigue.

Your body can also fall into imbalance when you eat too much sugar and refined starchy foods. This overstimulates the pancreas, as it attempts to produce enough insulin to keep up with the level of blood sugar. You may develop low blood sugar or insulin-resistant diabetes later on as a result of this kind of abuse. Lack of proper rest and sleep can decrease the effectiveness of your immune system, resulting in increased risk for heart disease and ineffectual immunity. Health is maintained by staying in the optimum wellness range of functioning. Illness comes from the seesaw motion of your life, and tonic herbs help to balance the various functions within your body. Balancing tonic herbs help keep the five-element network in a state of equilibrium, and include the following:

Asian cornelian (*Fructus corni*). Considered an excellent kidney and adrenal tonic, Asian cornelian supports healthy functioning of the hormonal and urinary systems and prevents the loss of the body's essence that is said to be stored in the kidney network.

Astragalus. Astragalus is considered an adaptogen, an herb that tends to normalize body functions and restore metabolic balance after physically and emotionally stressful situations have altered those functions. It helps the body to adapt and return to a sense of well-being. It is also a tonic for energy, heart, and circulation. As an adaptogen, it modulates the immune system—it increases immune function during declines and decreases it when it is too high.

Codonopsis. Balances the earth element network, which encompasses the digestive system and the regulation of sugar and energy metabolism. It is traditionally used to strengthen the spleen-pancreas-stomach organ network and boost energy production.

Ginkgo biloba. This herb balances the fire-element network, which includes the cardiovascular and brain systems. It improves blood and oxygen flow to the brain and to the extremities and has been most effective in treating senility, dementia, depression, anxiety, forgetfulness, inability to concentrate, and attention deficit disorder in adults. According to studies, ginkgo also may reduce the risk of heart attack.

Honeysuckle (*Flos lonicera*). A lung and immune tonic, honeysuckle balances and supports the metal element functions. Studies show that it inhibits a wide range of bacterial and viral organisms. Therefore it is an excellent tonic for preventing colds and the flu.

Mint (*Herba mentha*). Considered one of the most versatile herbs, mint (including peppermint, spearmint, and other mint-family plants) is a wood element tonic that is used to treat liver congestion, imbalance of the nervous system, and digestive problems.

. . . .

HERBS FOR REGENERATION

THE THIRD TYPE OF TONIC HERBS ARE THOSE that strengthen, revitalize, and regenerate energy and function. Enhancing performance is a necessity in our ever-demanding lives. Progress in modern life has its costs, but it is good to remember that change is not always positive. As we speed along in our intellectual and technological pursuits, we are forced to rapidly adapt to many changes. The balancing act between home, work, and pleasure causes strain and degeneration and ushers in the aging process prematurely. Tonic herbs can increase vitality, energy, and stamina; enhance concentration and memory; and provide essential nourishment to counteract stress. Tonic herbs that nurture and regenerate include:

Chinese wild yam (*Radix dioscorea*) Traditionally used as a tonic for the kidney-bladder and spleen-pancreas-stomach organ networks and to improve hormonal and digestive functions, wild yam has been found to be rich in DHEA, the mother hormone to estrogen, progesterone, and testosterone. Wild yam is used to stabilize blood sugar, relieve inflammation, and relax muscle spasms.

Cordyceps. A mushroom with energizing properties that has been prized in the East for thousands of years but was in relatively short supply until modern advances in growing techniques made it more widely available. Cordyceps helps increase cellular energy metabolism, boosts adrenal functions to adapt to stress, modulates immune function, increases capillary circulation, and improves oxygen utilization. No wonder Chinese Olympic athletes rely on it for their performance edge.

Dong quai (*Radix angelica*). Throughout China and Asia, angelica root, or dong quai, has been helping to maintain women's health for thousands of years. It is traditionally used to regulate menstrual periods, enhance fertility, build blood, strengthen bones, and maintain healthy hair, skin, and nails. It also relieves hot flashes and other symptoms related to menopausal changes. Studies have shown that dong quai also can increase immune function and reduce levels of damaging free radicals in the bloodstream.

Ginseng (*Panax ginseng*). The most famous of the energy tonics, ginseng has been prized and used for thousands of years to increase physical and mental endurance, reduce cholesterol, and increase energy. It is commonly taken to enhance physical performance, prolong life, and increase sexual potency. Many studies have confirmed its ability to normalize blood pressure, improve blood circulation, and prevent heart disease.

Goji berry (*fructus lycium*)—Also known as lycium berry or wolfberry, goji is a delicious fruit native to China that has long been known for its tonic effects, especially on vision and the brain. Goji berry contains polysaccharides, which stimulate the immune system and signal the pituitary to secrete human growth hormone. Goji also has the highest concentration of carotenoids, especially beta-carotene, of any plant in the world and is thus a powerful antioxidant. The berry is traditionally used together with other Chinese tonic herbs to increase sexual potency and fertility.

Schizandra berry (*Fructus schisandra*). A prized berry that has been used to rejuvenate and revitalize the senses, schizandra contains several vitamins and flavonoids that possess antioxidant and immune-boosting properties. It is an energy tonic that enhances both physical endurance and mental concentration and at the same time soothes the nerves, taking the edge off anxiety. As a beauty treatment, schizandra is said to promote radiant skin tone. It also has been used as an adjunct support for immune function in patients undergoing chemotherapy and helps to protect the liver and kidneys.

MEDICINAL HERBS

MEDICINAL HERBS ARE PLANTS AND NATURAL SUBSTANCES that help correct the body's imbalances and alleviate sickness. Of all the prescription drugs in use today, about 25 percent are derived from herbs. The difference between herbs and drugs is that herbs are whole, while drugs are isolates. Nature created plants—and everything else—with all of their parts for a good reason: balance. This wholeness makes it possible for potentially undesirable chemicals to be neutralized by others, and for beneficial chemicals to be synergistically enhanced by other similar chemicals—all within a single herb. A drug tends to be an isolated, active chemical that is concentrated for its singular action. But this also makes drugs more concentrated in toxicity; they eventually achieve their results, but at the expense of side effects to the rest of the body.

There is a place for both drugs and herbs in medicine. Drugs with their powerful, targeted properties are indispensable for attacking pathogens and cancerous cells, and for the life-saving relief from asthma attacks and anaphylactic shock, for example. But when it comes to chronic conditions and everyday afflictions, the body needs repair and restoration. Herbs are well suited to these tasks, with their gentler properties devoid of serious side effects. There has been much research into the active ingredients of herbs and how they work. In some herbs, the action comes from to one or two compounds, but in many cases, the beneficial properties are derived from many components.

Learning about herbs and their healing properties is an essential part of any self-healing program. For many minor ailments and symptoms, health food stores and natural pharmacies carry a wide variety of products you can use to obtain relief. In Chinese medicine, however, herbs are rarely used singly; rather, they are used in formulations consisting of a dozen or so herbs to maximize beneficial effects and to neutralize unwanted responses. The skill it takes to masterfully put together a synergistic formula for a particular person and condition requires years of training and should only be done with a licensed practitioner. If a trained herbalist isn't available, go with classical and preformulated products instead of attempting to put one together for yourself or your family. This is why you should assemble a knowledgeable healing team to advise you on your health needs. Medicinal herbs include:

Chinese red sage (*Radix salvia*). Traditionally used to balance heart and vascular functions, Chinese red sage has been found to increase the force of the heartbeat, while slowing the heart rate. The active ingredient, tanshinone, works as a vasodilator, causing blood vessels to relax and increasing blood circulation, reducing the risk of arteriosclerosis, stroke, and heart attack. It has also been shown to inhibit bacterial growth, decrease fever, and relieve inflammation.

Gentian (*Radix gentiana*). A bitter herb long used for its digestive benefits, gentian stimulates the digestive juices and increases pancreatic activity and the production of bile. In Chinese medicine it is a liver cleanser and it drains damp heat—a condition usually associated with infection and inflammation of the digestive tract. Gentian has also been used to expel worms and treat malaria and is thought to be more effective than quinine. It is used in China to treat herpes and other sexually transmitted diseases.

Horse chestnut (*Semen Aesculus hippocastanum*). A favorite weed for horses to munch on (hence its name), horse chestnut is a traditional remedy and preventive against varicose veins, spider veins, and broken capillaries. One of the most common circulatory problems encountered as we age is the weakening of our blood vessels, particularly the veins, resulting in conditions such as varicose veins. Horse chestnut tones and strengthens the muscular walls of the veins and prevents vein enlargement.

Saw palmetto (*Fructus serenoa*). Known for easing prostate conditions, saw palmetto balances testosterone levels, reduces inflammation, and provides an abundance of essential fatty acids, according to studies. It can also be helpful for menopausal women when hormonal changes result in increased body hair. It is administered to men to increase the function of the testicles and relieve irritation in mucous membranes, particularly in the urinary tract and prostate.

Valerian root (*Radix valeriana*). Often called nature's tranquilizer, valerian has been used to regulate the nervous system and relieve tension, irritability, nervous exhaustion, stress, anxiety, and hysteria for centuries. As a sedative, valerian relieves sleeplessness without the morning-after grogginess often associated with prescription sleep medications and is nonaddictive. Valerian is also a natural pain reliever that reduces sensitivity of the nerves.

White willow bark (*Cortex salicea*). Contains salicin, a compound found in aspirin—in fact, aspirin was originally discovered in and extracted from white willow bark. The analgesic actions of white willow bark may be slower acting than synthetic aspirin, but the results last longer. Besides its pain-relieving properties, white willow bark is an anticoagulant, which helps prevent the formation of blood clots and the thickening of blood that can lead to heart attacks and strokes. A major advantage of using willow bark over its pharmaceutical cousin, aspirin, is that it does not cause gastric upset and erode the stomach lining. As an anti-inflammatory, white willow bark has been used to relieve the painful inflammation of joints.

. . . .

POTENT MEDICINAL HERBS

THE POTENT MEDICINAL HERBS ARE NATURAL SUBSTANCES used for more serious conditions. Herbs are powerful healing agents, especially those in the potent category, which is why these herbs are restricted to use by knowledgeable and licensed practitioners. Licensed acupuncturists in the United States are trained in the use of potent Chinese herbs. Occasionally the media reports dangers associated with herbs. Are herbs safe compared to pharmaceutical drugs? Let's put the statistics in perspective. Fewer than fifty deaths each year in this country are attributed to medicinal herbs. These deaths are usually due to improper use or atypically high doses of an herb or two. By comparison, more than 100 people die each year in this country from allergic reaction to peanuts, shellfish, and other foods. And several studies published in the *Journal of the American Medical Association* showed that pharmaceutical side effects kill 140,000 Americans a year and seriously injure 2.2 million more, making drug side effects the nation's fifth leading cause of death.

I list only two well-known potent medicinal herbs here to illustrate the actions of this class of herbs. Consult with an expert if you want to use any potent herbs in your health care program.

Euphorbia (*Radix euphorbia*). Traditionally used by doctors of Chinese medicine, euphorbia is a cathartic diuretic and laxative, meaning it expels water from the chest and abdomen and reduces swelling and nodules from extremities through the urinary tract and the bowels. Clinical studies have shown euphorbia to be effective in dilating peripheral blood vessels and reducing ascitis, or water retention, in nephritis or kidney disease and in liver cirrhosis patients.

Ma huang (herbal ephedra). An herb in use for 5,000 years in China for asthma, which has generated controversy in recent years due to deaths from heart problems resulting from college kids using it as a stimulant in very high doses—doses much higher than any trained practitioner would recommend. The FDA has taken the herb off the market but allows its use by licensed acupuncturists or doctors of Chinese medicine. This is an example of a potent herb that should be used by trained professionals only. When prescribed appropriately, ma huang is excellent for asthma and cough because of its bronchial dilating action. It contains ephedrine and pseudoephedrine, compounds found in over-the-counter decongestant and allergy drugs.

NUTRITIONAL SUPPLEMENTS

BEFORE I BEGIN DISCUSSING NUTRITIONAL SUPPLEMENTS, I want to make it clear that eating a varied and balanced diet is the first and foremost step in making sure that you get plenty of nutrients. Only then do I suggest supplementing with vitamins as insurance against possible deficiencies arising from eating foods grown in nutrient-depleted soil, a stressful change or demanding lifestyle, or recovery from illness. Children, pregnant women, athletes, the elderly, and people who are dieting or fasting naturally will require micronutrients to meet their unique or extra demands. It is inexcusable, though, to have a poor diet and to rely on nutritional supplements to keep you out of trouble.

Micronutrients such as the vitamins and minerals in our foods are important for maintaining health. Vitamins are called micronutrients because you don't need high quantities of them for normal functioning. However, even a minor deficiency may lead to serious health problems. For example, a deficiency in folic acid during pregnancy can lead to neural tube defect—a serious birth defect—even though the required daily amount is only 0.4 milligram and can be obtained easily by eating 1 1/2 cups of dark, leafy green vegetables a day. Many studies also confirm the role of folic acid in cancer prevention.

Nutritional supplements can be used like the herbs discussed earlier in this chapter—they both support the body's natural regenerative and healing processes. Micronutrients can be categorized broadly as either nourishing or therapeutic. Nourishing supplements are used to cleanse, balance, and regenerate the body and its functions. There are many books and resources to help you learn about vitamins and their beneficial actions—see the resources section at the end of the book. Therapeutic supplements, on the other hand, are used in a different context to assist in your healing process—even if they are also in the nourishing category. I advise you to consult a knowledgeable nutrition professional who can tailor a supplement program to your specific health and healing needs.

Whenever possible, use supplements that are extracted from whole foods like fruits, vegetables, and grains, which have the best bioavailability, meaning the highest absorption by your digestive system. The best way to take vitamins and minerals is as a powdered or liquid concentrate, or as extracts made from bee pollen, barley, wheat grass, kelp, spirulina, chlorophyll, brewer's yeast, bone meal, wheat germ, flaxseed oil, and fish oils. Avoid taking megadoses or any dose larger than the Recommended Daily Allowance (RDA) of any nutrient, no matter how good it may be for your health. Remember that supplements are, well, exactly that—supplements. They're not intended to replace a well-rounded diet.

. . . .

NOURISHING SUPPLEMENTS

NOURISHING SUPPLEMENTS INCLUDE BASIC MICRONUTRIENTS as well as macronutrients—larger compounds that our bodies need for optimal performance. Wellness depends on your body having all nutritional building blocks available for use at all times. Taking the right supplements will ensure that your body's metabolism operates at its peak, regenerating cells and repairing structures while eliminating wastes and toxins and maintaining balance. Antioxidant nutrients, for example, may help prevent aging damage caused by free radicals—destructive oxygen molecules that are the by-products of environmental toxins, poor diet and lifestyle, and disease. Following is a partial list of nourishing supplements and their beneficial properties.

Alpha-lipoic acid (ALA). Works in cellular energy production as well as with the B vitamins. When the body uses up vitamins C and E during times of stress, ALA converts the by-products into new antioxidant compounds, thus "recycling" the vitamins.

Antioxidant or antirust nutrients are supplements that prevent oxidation within your body, a process similar to rust forming on metal, or the browning of an apple. Oxidative stress, as the internal rusting is called, directly contributes to aging, the decline of bodily functions, and the breakdown of structure. Studies show that the many benefits of antioxidants include prevention of heart disease, cancer, and degenerative diseases. ·

Bioflavonoids. Benefits skin, hair, and blood vessels; often referred to as flavonoids.

Coenzyme Q_{10}. Also called ubiquinone, it is an antioxidant produced by the body for muscle metabolism. It is essential for preventing muscle pain and damage while using statin drugs to reduce cholesterol.

Glutathione. Composed of three amino acids: glycine, glutamic acid, and cysteine. It has potent antioxidant powers and helps recycle other antioxidants such as vitamins C and E; it protects against cancer, detoxifies, regulates immune cells, and is antiviral.

Polyphenols. Antioxidants that are mostly found in green tea, which is an excellent source of epigallocatechin gallate, a natural compound that shows great promise in anticancer research.

Selenium. A component of the enzyme glutathione peroxidase, a powerful antioxidant found in nearly every cell of the body. It has also been found to prevent cancer.

Vitamin A and beta-carotene. Required for bone formation, gastrointestinal and eye health, and in assisting the immune system and skin.

Vitamin C. Required for the manufacture of collagen in the body, assists immune function, and helps boost the effectiveness of other antioxidants in the body.

Vitamin E. Especially helpful in preventing the oxidation of fats, and assists in the utility of oxygen and selenium.

Zinc. Has antioxidant properties, helps with vitamin A absorption, and promotes hormonal health.

. . . .

THERAPEUTIC SUPPLEMENTS

THERAPEUTIC SUPPLEMENTS ARE USED TO FACILITATE the healing process and many are widely available in health food and vitamin stores. However, since the dosing of these nutrients varies according to the condition and constitutional needs of each person, it is best to work with a licensed health care professional to tailor a supplement program to your health and healing needs. Following are some therapeutic supplements and their uses.

Chromium. Possesses properties to help stabilize blood sugar, making it useful in controlling diabetes and hypoglycemia (low blood sugar).

Glucosamine and chondroitin. Extracted from shellfish, these nutrients have been found to support joint and cartilage health and consequently are often recommended for arthritis sufferers.

L-carnitine. An amino acid produced by your liver, L-carnitine helps reduce triglycerides and increase good cholesterol, and is useful for reversing and preventing heart disease. It also helps regulate fat metabolism and promotes fat loss, so it is essential for any weight-loss program.

Melatonin. A powerful antioxidant hormone produced by the pineal gland. It is important for normal sleep patterns and as a result is recommended for jet lag and certain types of insomnia.

Niacin (B_3). Helps dilate capillaries and promotes blood flow to the tiny blood vessels in the inner ear. As a result, studies show some promise for using niacin to improve minor hearing loss and tinnitus (ringing in the ears). Wellness medicine practitioners have also been using niacin to help lower cholesterol because studies show that it lowers overall cholesterol and raises HDL, the good cholesterol.

Phosphatidylserine (PS). A compound made by the body from the amino acid serine. PS's role in reversing age-related dementia and memory loss is well documented in Europe. It has been found to decrease the stress response and increase the release of neurotransmitters in the brain that facilitate thought, reasoning, and concentration.

SAMe (S-adenosyl methionine). Produced from methionine, an amino acid that plays a role in the production of feel-good neurotransmitters such as dopamine and serotonin. It has been used successfully in Europe to help treat depression.

Mother Nature has given us an abundance of plants and natural substances with healing properties. They are available to you to explore for your health and wellness needs. I firmly believe that there is an herb for every disease on earth—we are only limited by not having discovered them all. Think of all the undiscovered herbs in the Amazon rain forest. Who knows what lies beneath the surface of the sea? There is much that awaits to be uncovered, and yet we are already blessed with many herbs—over 10,000 Chinese herbs alone—for our use. At the same time, nutritional science is our new frontier. It is advancing with exciting discoveries, which will eventually bear out my belief. We will continue to marvel at Mother Nature's genius.

CHAPTER 5

THE RIVERS WITHIN

Keep Your Vital Energy Flowing with Physical Activity, Mind-Body Exercise, and Acupressure

Lack of activity destroys the good condition of every human being, while movement and methodical physical exercise save it and preserve it.

—*PLATO*

MOVEMENT IS THE UNCHANGING LAW OF NATURE. We experience cosmic movement through the ceaseless circling of the planets within our solar system. The seasons come and go, the months wax and wane, day dawns and night draws near. Within your body, even while you lie still, blood circulation, intestinal peristalsis, and nerve impulses continue unabated in order to maintain normal functions. The abilities to work, play, communicate, create, and procreate all depend on movement. Whether fluid or energy, blockages within your being lead to disorder and disease. The inactive body is a residence for depression and toxins. Physical movement, mind-body exercise, and acupuncture assist the body in maintaining and restoring healthy flow.

Physical movement or exercise is one of the most important elements in preserving health and promoting wellness. But despite its well-known benefits, exercise may be the most universally despised endeavor, with many people subscribing to the following exercise program, written by an unknown author: "Too many people confine their exercise to jumping to conclusions, running up bills, stretching the truth, bending over backward, lying down on the job, sidestepping responsibility, and pushing their luck."

If we were designed to lie down or sit all the time, we would look more like invertebrates. The key to getting off the couch is to find exercise in everyday activities and to have fun in the physical movements you choose to do. Walk instead of drive, bicycle for short errands, take stairs rather than the elevator, park the car farther from your destination, vacuum and clean your house, and enjoy gardening. If you do any of these activities regularly, you already are doing some exercise.

How about getting some fun exercise? There are aerobic exercises like skipping as you walk down the street, or running up the stairs, jumping rope, jumping on a trampoline, dancing, skating, hiking the hills, jogging, cycling, swimming, cross-country skiing, and rowing. If these don't appeal to you, try a sport like tennis, basketball, soccer, hockey, badminton, or Ping-Pong. The varieties are endless, but the important thing is to be active every day.

Movement is essential for proper metabolism and energy circulation. Our cardiovascular and lymphatic circulatory systems rely on movement to help with the circulation of blood and the expelling of cellular waste. The movement of muscles, joints, and tendons promotes renewal and circulation and extends your range of motion, preventing arthritic buildup and stagnation. Moderate load-bearing exercise is essential for bone density and muscle strength, which is especially important as we age. Cardiovascular exercise increases heart rate and provides stimulation for the heart muscles, maintaining proper rigor and endurance. Exercise also helps us burn off excess blood sugar, preventing it from getting stored as body fat.

THE HEALTH BENEFITS OF EXERCISE

Perhaps having fun by itself won't persuade you to exercise. Research also shows that exercise may encourage the brain to work at optimum capacity by causing nerve cells to multiply, strengthening their interconnections, and protecting them from damage. It also directly assists in learning and the healing of neurological diseases. If you're still not convinced, with exercise you can also:

• Improve the look and feel of your skin as a result of increased blood flow.

• Boost your energy and aerobic capacity so you won't tire as easily.

- Increase your metabolism, burn fat, and maintain a healthy weight.

- Elevate your good (HDL) cholesterol, which protects you from heart disease.

- Increase muscle tone and strength and improve your endurance.

- Enhance your sex life by promoting better circulation and hormonal stimulation.

- Decrease or normalize your blood pressure.

- Balance your blood sugar and decrease insulin resistance, which can prevent diabetes.

- Strengthen your bones, cartilage, and ligaments and lower the risk of osteoporosis.

- Improve your sleep by restoring normal body rhythms and reducing stress hormone levels.

- Lower your risk for heart disease, stroke, cancer, depression, diabetes, and other chronic degenerative diseases.

- Become happier, sexier, and more vivacious.

BEWARE THE WEEKEND WARRIOR

HOW YOU APPROACH EXERCISE MAY DETERMINE the benefits and enjoyment that you'll get from it. I have a number of patients who are weekend warriors—people who don't exercise much during the week but go to the extreme on weekends. They'll engage in vigorous physical activities like mountain biking, basketball, or high-impact aerobics. And they'll usually end up in my office with injuries. There is nothing wrong with these types of athletic activities, but when they are done infrequently they often cause injuries. It isn't necessary to work out to the extreme or to get your pulse rate up to the maximum to get the health and weight-loss benefits of exercise. On the contrary, many studies show that regular, moderate exercise does more for your health and waistline than periodic intense workouts. When you exercise to the extreme, not only are you more prone to injuries but you also put unnecessary wear and tear on your body. And that is exactly the opposite of the point of exercise.

I've found that many people who exercise way too hard frequently suffer from lactic acidosis—a state in which the body is full of the waste products of excessive muscle use, causing aching in your muscles, rapid breathing, and fatigue. The tendency to go into lactic acidosis is increased by age, nutritional deficiency, obesity, hormonal imbalance, and disease. Moreover, when exercising beyond a healthy heart rate, your body switches from burning fat to burning carbohydrates for energy. The old maxim of "no pain, no gain" is destructive to many people's health—the wear and tear of physical strain takes its toll.

. . . .

FINDING YOUR OPTIMUM EXERCISE ZONE

WHAT, THEN, IS A HEALTHY RANGE FOR HEART RATE and workout intensity? The answer is simple and logical: If you strain to breathe rapidly during your physical training and feel achy and tired afterward, you've gone beyond the limit of what is healthy for you. A healthy range of heart rate during exercise for the average person is between 90 and120 beats per minute. For more athletic people the range is higher. A sports medicine specialist or trainer can help you establish what is ideal for you individually. When you are in the optimum zone, exercise should make you feel energized and happy afterward, motivating you to repeat the experience over and over and over again.

From my clinical experience and research, I am convinced that it is best to exercise four times or more a week for thirty minutes at a time. It can be as simple as a brisk walk around your neighborhood, or the Merry-Go-Round Circle Walk that I describe in Part 2 of this book. If you suffer from a physically debilitating condition, are recovering from an illness, or are just terribly out of shape, start your exercise program gently and gradually. You may want to exercise only five minutes a day to start with, but do it every day. Then incrementally increase the time on a weekly basis—say, five additional minutes per week. By the sixth week you'll be up to thirty minutes a day.

. . . .

MIND-BODY EXERCISES

IT MAY COME AS A SURPRISE TO YOU that gentle, slower, and deliberate movements are just as beneficial for your health, if not better than, abrupt, fast-paced, and forceful exercises. This is particularly true as part of a self-healing program, but it is also important as you get older. Gentle, deliberate movements engage your mind, breathing, and body motion as one. Unique to China are the gentler kind of movement arts that promote energy, balance of function, and a calm mind. I call them mind-body exercises, and they include tai chi, qi gong, and Dao In Qi Gong. Certain dance forms fall into this category as well. These exercises have traditionally been associated with health and longevity. Many recent studies have confirmed their balancing action on blood pressure, blood sugar, cholesterol, equilibrium, and other organ functions. Mind-body exercise works through a system of energy communication within the body. By deliberately activating the flow of energy and removing blockages, communication is restored and organ functions return to their optimal level.

In order for you to be physically, mentally, and spiritually well, it is essential that your internal energies flow in an unimpeded and harmonious manner. What does this mean? Under ideal conditions, a person's internal energies course throughout his or her being in much the same way as the planets and other heavenly bodies course through the vast body of the cosmos. In both cases, the movements are determined by universal natural laws. When you experience stress during the course of daily life, your subconscious mind will direct extra energy to certain areas of the body to handle the stress. Over time your body becomes habituated to energizing those areas and neglecting others, and the normal course of energy circulation becomes distorted and unbalanced. In this case, the movements no longer follow natural law. This distortion results in personal disharmony, manifesting as physical and mental diseases.

. . . .

THE CIRCULARITY OF ALL NATURAL MOVEMENT

THE NATURAL MOVEMENT OF EVERYTHING IN THE UNIVERSE follows a circular pattern. The earth spins on its axis as it orbits the sun. The sun, in turn, orbits the galactic center of the Milky Way. And the Milky Way follows a circular pattern as it courses through the universe. Life itself consists of cycles, and the energies of the human organism also circulate through their microcosmic energy network. The movements of tai chi are a series of circles that reflect this eternal cosmic law.

Everything in nature follows a cyclical process of growth and evolution. All things grow and develop and, after their peak has been reached, revert to their source to regenerate again and again. The movement of evolution is not a linear process. Anything that continues in a straight line must eventually run out of power and come to an end. The multiuniverse is able to continue its process of evolution eternally because it reverts to its source for regeneration before reaching the absolute end of its impetus. You could say that the energy is recycled.

This is an essential principle of tai chi—in the movements you never extend your body or energy completely so you are left with energy in reserve. You go only to a certain point and then draw inward again to the center to gather your energy. The movement is repeated, the force is recharged, and the energy is recycled at the same time. This is called the law of reversion. In this way tai chi expresses the principle of perpetual self-regeneration.

. . . .

TAI CHI AND QI GONG FOR HEALTH AND HEALING

ACCORDING TO HUA-CHING NI, AN EMINENT AUTHORITY ON TAI CHI, qi gong, and other Taoist healing arts, who also happens to be my father and teacher, "When practicing tai chi or gi gong, first the mind, afterward the body. The abdomen is relaxed, the energy is gathered into the bones, the spirit is at ease, and the body is quiet. At every moment be totally conscious."

The ancient masters developed a system of physical movements that are based on the natural motion of the heavenly bodies. By moving the body in this fashion, we guide the internal energies to flow according to the same natural laws that keep the planets on course and the galaxies propelling through space in harmony. By practicing these mind-body exercises, you can unblock and relieve energy congestion in certain parts of the body and gradually eliminate the stress that has accumulated over the course of time. You may also redirect the flow of vitality so that every muscle, nerve, and organ is nourished and toned. Through the calmness and relaxation generated by tai chi and qi gong, the vitality that has been locked within a tense and imbalanced body is released and allowed to restore and sustain natural health.

Often when we are engaged in a physical activity our minds are engaged in an unrelated activity. Through the consistent practice of tai chi, qi gong, and other mind-body exercises, we can strengthen and integrate our physical and mental functions. People generally either engage in mental activity and are oblivious to their bodies, or they engage in physical activity but their minds are wandering and not aware of what the body is doing. In this way the body and mind, which are essentially one inseparable system, are split.

Consciousness directly influences the energy flow and the general state of energy. When this split is created and the body and mind do not function as one unit, the ability to realize our full potential is greatly impaired. Nerve synapses atrophy from lack of use and vast areas of the brain lie dormant. Input from the external environment is inaccurately or incompletely transmitted to the brain, which in turn relays faulty messages as a response. As a result, the nervous system doesn't fully develop and the awareness of reality, both internal and external, is distorted.

THE PRACTICE OF MINDFULNESS IN MOVEMENT

THE PRACTICE OF TAI CHI AND QI GONG trains the mind to follow every detail of the body's actions. Rather than literally scattering energy through unaware physical activity, you are able to gather energy into your being. The peaceful mental atmosphere created by tai chi and qi gong movements allows negative thought patterns to dissolve and to be replaced by positive, life-affirming attitudes.

The human body is like a tree—if energy circulates to all parts of the tree, the entire tree is full of life. However, if one part of the tree does not receive its supply of energy, then that part withers. In the human body, the energy must always be regenerated and it must be able to circulate freely to all parts of the body. In ordinary exercise, circulation is stimulated but energy is also burned up and lost in perspiration. Thus you may generate energy but you also lose energy. In tai chi and qi gong the body is allowed to blossom in perfect condition without perspiring. Your muscle tissue will be neither flaccid nor rigid but full of energy like a ripe plum.

Ordinary exercise and sports may produce quick and shallow breathing, which causes more oxygen to enter the system, but they may strain the heart and lungs when performed to extreme intensity. In tai chi and qi gong the heart is relaxed and the breathing is deep and full, which enables even more oxygen to enter the bloodstream, using the full capacity of the lungs. The rhythmic movements of these mind-body exercises produce friction between the organs, causing gentle warmth, which strengthens and fortifies them.

The expanding and contracting movements of tai chi invigorate and tone the stomach and intestines, promoting good digestion, and strengthen the entire respiratory system by using the full capacity of the lungs. The deep and rhythmic breathing that is an intrinsic part of tai chi movements allows the diaphragm to massage the internal organs and aids the circulation of fresh blood to the heart. It also promotes proper functioning of the endocrine system, which restores the chemical balance of the body, improving metabolism.

. . . .

BODY-MIND INTEGRATION

TAI CHI AND QI GONG ARE THE INTEGRATION of yin and yang energy polarities. The polarization of the primal energy as it alternates between yin and yang is not a divisive or separating process but is always integrated by the power of undivided oneness. If it were a division rather than an integrated movement, the multi-universe would inevitably come to an end. The principle of undivided oneness applies in tai chi and qi gong movement as well as in the reality of daily life. For example, when we walk, each leg cooperates with the other, and both are governed by the oneness of the person who is walking.

All movement may be explained in terms of yin and yang. For example, leftward movement is yang, rightward movement is yin. Upward movement is yang, downward movement is yin. Inhalation is yang, exhalation is yin, and so forth. The movements of tai chi are a continual sequence of yin and yang movements. If there is an upward movement, then there is a downward movement to balance it. If there is a movement to the left, then there is a movement to the right to give it symmetry. Inhalation and exhalation are also coordinated with each movement so that yin and yang, which are sometimes also called the negative and positive vibrational polarities of the human energy system, are always balanced.

. . . .

GENTLE RHYTHMIC MOVEMENTS

ANOTHER UNIVERSAL PRINCIPLE REVEALED in tai chi and qi gong is the idea that sudden movement causes energy to stagnate, while gentle, rhythmic movement brings about its flowing. Sudden movement must always stop quickly—there is inevitably a pause or inhibition of energy flow. A similar principle is that hasty action ultimately results in slowness because it quickly exhausts our energy, while gentle rhythmic movement can be continued with great endurance. So, for example, those who are violent can afford only one show of force at a time, and, in reality, are weak, and those who move in a gentle rhythm can keep going continually and prove to be the strongest. Or, if you try to run all the way to a distant place you become exhausted before reaching your destination, but if you walk at a comfortable pace, you will still get there, without using up all your energy. Or to put it in another way, you can spend all your energy at once running a hundred-yard dash or pace yourself and spread the energy over the twenty-six miles of a marathon. As any marathon runner will tell you, your rhythm is critical to pacing your energy. This is a fundamental principle of these exercises too, and it indicates the "constant virtue," or constant quality, inherent in gentle rhythmic movement.

. . . .

TYPES OF TAI CHI AND QI GONG FOR HEALTH AND SELF-HEALING

TAI CHI IS A CONTINUOUS, choreographed set of movements practiced in its entirety each time, while qi gong usually consists of sets of short movements that aren't connected and are practiced repetitively in sections. Generally, qi gong is easier to learn than tai chi, and its benefits are more immediate and targeted. There are several popular styles of tai chi and many styles of qi gong. The differences between styles have to do with the family tradition they come from, their therapeutic actions, and their intent—some are geared toward martial arts, while others are healing and spiritually oriented.

Throughout this book I suggest the practice of three types of qi gong: Eight Treasures, Self-Healing, and Dao In. Eight Treasures Qi Gong is unique to my family, having been passed down for many generations. It consists of thirty-two movements divided into eight sections. Each section is designed to strengthen and promote self-healing in a particular organ network. Self-Healing Qi Gong consists of five movement sections, each targeting an organ network for balance and preventive health. Dao In Qi Gong is a set of floor exercises similar to yoga in that it involves stretching, breathing, and strengthening postures that have healing properties. Refer to the Resources section for more information about Eight Treasures, Self-Healing, and Dao In Qi Gong.

. . . .

ACUPUNCTURE—AWAKENING AND ACCESSING THE RIVERS OF ENERGY WITHIN

BY UNDERSTANDING THAT GENTLE RHYTHMIC MOVEMENTS like tai chi, qi gong, and other mind-body exercises are tools for self-healing based on movement of energy within your being, you can come to appreciate the art of acupuncture. It seems incredible, but the ancient masters used their clear and unimpeded vision and recognition to compile knowledge of the energy circulation in the channel system of the human body. Even for someone who is not interested in spiritual evolution, it is valuable to understand the principles of energy within the body in order to maintain our equilibrium and health, both physically and mentally.

Acupuncture, a facet of Chinese medicine, is a precise science dealing with the processing, storage, distribution, and functioning of vital energy within the human organism and the relationship of this energy with the cosmos. Acupuncture affects the circulation of energy within the human being on an extremely subtle level. The ancient Chinese physicians discovered that there is a subtle energy manifestation circulating throughout the organs and flesh that ultimately permeates every tissue and cell of the body. The name given to this energy is *chi*, or *qi*, which has been translated as "vital energy" or "life force." Human beings are the embodiment of all the energies of the universe, including the energies of the sun, moon, and stars as well as the various energies of the earth.

As a small universe of the larger cosmos, our being mirrors that of the natural world surrounding us. To understand the channels that carry energy within our body, we merely have to look to the melting snow packs that originated from evaporation and condensation from the seas. Snow melts, springs feed alpine lakes high up in the mountains, and the water courses its way from brooks to streams and into rivers. As it makes its way downward to ultimately rejoin with the sea, it nourishes the land that it traverses, giving rise to vegetation and living creatures. Water, then, embodies the potent symbol of life force on our planet. Likewise, what flows within the channels of our body is the life force that provides nourishment and function to our entire organism.

. . . .

HOW ACUPUNCTURE WORKS

THE ENERGIES OF THE HUMAN ORGANISM have distinct and established pathways, definite directions of flow and characteristic behavior as definite as any other circulation within the body, such as the circulation of blood and lymph through their respective systems. This claim has been validated in recent years by studies of the acupuncture meridians. The ancient physicians observed that illness often produced painful areas upon the skin, and that the pain would disappear when a cure was accomplished. They also noticed that stimulation or sedation of various points on the body would produce an effect on the functioning of the internal organs. Thus stimulation of a point below the knee might affect the face, while stimulating another point on the thumb would affect the lungs or throat.

After countless years of observation and experience in treatment and response, a systematic order of these sensitive points was formulated. These sensitive points were classified into twelve main groups and two minor groups. All the points of a specific group could be connected by a line, which was considered the path the energy of the body followed as it circulated throughout the organism. These observations were correlated and refined over thousands of years, and from the results, it was deduced that lines of energy transmission existed that not only connected all of the organs of the body but also connected the external to the internal.

Modern science has begun to peer into the inner workings of acupuncture. We've discovered that all the parts of the body, including all its cells and molecules, form a continuous interconnected semiconductor electronic network. Each element of the organism, even the minutest part, is immersed in and generates a constant stream of vibratory information. This information records and feeds back all the events throughout the body. Whole health relates to complete connectedness. Past physical and emotional strains damage the links, causing the body's defenses and repair systems to become weakened, and illness is often the result. Acupuncture reestablishes and balances the electronic circuitry that in turn enhances the body's self-healing mechanism.

In 1997, the National Institutes of Health released an efficacy statement endorsing acupuncture for a variety of conditions, including postoperative pain, dental pain, tennis elbow, carpal tunnel syndrome, and nausea. In the same year, the Food and Drug Administration (FDA) reclassified the acupuncture needle from "experimental" to "medical device" status, recognizing that the acupuncture needle is a safe and effective medical instrument. There has been a wealth of research on acupuncture—a recent search of PubMed, a service of the National Library of Medicine and National Institutes of Health, found 11,778 research articles on acupuncture alone. Many studies have found that acupuncture can induce the release of endorphins in the brain, countering the destructive effects of stress hormones in addition to providing pain relief. Acupuncture can also increase the body's production of natural corticosteroids, bringing on a reduction in inflammation and promoting self-healing. And acupuncture has been found to affect the autonomic nervous system—the part of the nervous system that automatically maintains life-sustaining functions including digestion, circulation, and respiration without conscious intervention—via mechanisms at the hypothalamic and brain stem levels, helping to promote homeostasis, or functional stability, in the body. In other words, acupuncture encourages self-regulation that leads to health and balance.

CONDITIONS THAT CAN BE TREATED WITH ACUPUNCTURE AND ACUPRESSURE

THE WORLD HEALTH ORGANIZATION HAS CITED more than forty conditions that acupuncture can treat, including addiction, asthma, common cold, ulcer, sciatica, migraine, paralysis, sinusitis, headache, depression, facial pain, neck pain, knee pain, lower back pain, arthritis, insomnia, diabetes, PMS, prostatitis, colitis, and urinary tract infections. Many studies show that acupuncture is effective in conditions ranging from environmental illness due to radiation, pesticide poisoning, exposure to toxic compounds, and air pollution to infertility, menopause, and premature aging.

Some conditions respond dramatically to acupuncture. For instance, researchers have found it to be effective for a variety of osteoarthritis and rheumatoid arthritis conditions, bringing relief to 80 percent of those who suffer from arthritis. Some studies show that getting acupuncture during in vitro fertilization increased pregnancy rates by over 40 percent. Because acupuncture promotes homeostasis—the automatic self-regulating system of controls that maintains the internal environment of living things and regulates the balance between the internal and the external in the body—it can significantly increase your sense of well-being. Acupuncture should be an essential part of your health and wellness program.

Can't find a practitioner of acupuncture in your area? Don't worry, because you can enjoy the health benefits of acupuncture at home by using finger pressure, or acupressure, on the same acupoints. Simply refer to the acupressure recommendations in Part 2 of this book. To learn more about acupuncture and acupressure, log on to www.acupuncture.com.

THE CHANNELS AND ACUPOINTS

AS I'VE MENTIONED MANY TIMES, the human body is a microcosm of the universe. Like a miniature universe, the cyclical and constant movement and transformation of fluids, molecules, cells, chemicals, and energies within the body characterize life. Chi, or life force, traverses the body within tributaries and canals that we call channels. The twelve main channels each correspond to a particular organ, and like the self-sustaining universe, the energy flows perpetually, filling the empty and draining the excess from parts of the body regulated by an intrinsic balancing mechanism. The channels play an important role in the healthy functioning of human life.

The direction of energy flow is highly important. In the human body in general and under normal circumstances, yang energy flows upward and yin energy flows downward. The front of the body corresponds to yin, the back to yang. So the yin channels flow toward the front side of the body to meet in the chest, and the yang channels move toward the back of the body. All of the channels are connected and polarized so that the energy circulates in a continuous and constant pattern.

Cutting-edge studies show that the channel system is extended into the interiors of every cell in the body through the cytoskeleton or the nervous system of the cell, and even into the nuclei that contain the genetic material. The channels are simply the transmission lines in the continuous molecular fabric of the body. The organ systems use the channels as an invisible network of communication. They are not based on a nerve, vessel, or lymphatic circulation path but are distinct pathways through which bioelectric energy and information are transported. They generally run symmetrically along both sides of the body.

The channels also have internal pathways, a subject too complex to go into here.

. . . .

THE TWELVE MAIN CHANNELS

1. Lung Channel (LU)—Starts at the front of the shoulders and runs down the insides of the arms to the ends of the thumbs.

2. Large Intestine Channel (LI)—Starts from the end of the index fingers and runs up the outside of the arms, to the top of the shoulders, up the sides of the neck, and crosses over the upper lip to the opposite side just along the sides of the nostrils.

3. Stomach Channel (ST)—Starts just below the eyes, runs down the cheeks, down the front of the neck, down the chest through the nipples, abdomen, front of the thighs, knees, and shins to the lateral ends of the second toes.

4. Spleen Channel (SP)—Starts from the medial side of the big toes, up the insides of the ankles, up the insides of the lower legs, knees, and thighs, over the lower abdomen, and up to the sides of the rib cage.

5. Heart Channel (H)—Starts in the armpits and runs down the inner sides of the arms to the ends of the pinkie fingers.

6. Small Intestine Channel (SI)—Starts from the pinkie finger, runs up the outside of the arms, crisscrosses through the shoulder blades, up the sides of the neck and the sides of the face to the front of the ears.

7. Bladder (Urinary Bladder) Channel (UB)—Starts at the inside corners of the eyes, runs up the corners of the eyebrows straight over the head, down to the base of the skull, the base of the neck, down along the band of muscles along the spine to the buttocks, down the backs of the thighs, the backs of the knees, the backs of the calves, to the outsides of the ankles and the feet and ends at the outside of the small toes.

8. Kidney Channel (KID)—Starts from a point in the center of the soles of the feet, runs up the insides of the feet to the insides of the ankles, up the insides of the calves, the knees, and the lower back, through the body to the lower abdomen, up alongside the navel and the center of the chest, and ends at the collarbone.

9. Pericardium Channel (P)—Starts near the outsides of the nipples, runs down the inside middle of the arms, and down to the ends of the middle fingers.

10. Triple Warmer or Triple Heater (San Jiao) Channel (SJ)—Starts from the ring fingers on the sides next to the pinkie fingers, runs up along the outside center of the arms, up the shoulders to the ears, around the back of the ears, and to the outside of the eyebrows.

11. Gallbladder Channel (GB)—Starts from the outside corners of the eyes, runs in front of the ears, up the sides of the head, up and down in an arc on the sides of the head, and comes down to the shoulders, down the sides of the body to the fronts of the armpits, zigzags across the rib cage and the sides of the abdomen and buttocks, down the outside center of the thighs and calves, and down to between the pinkie toes and fourth toes.

12. Liver Channel (L)—Starts from between the big toes and second toes, runs up the insides of the ankles, calves, and thighs, through the genitals and up to the liver in the lower chest.

Each of the channels follows its specific course of circulation, so the free flow and sufficiency of qi or its opposite—blockage or deficiency—will show up in the twelve channels. The twelve main channels connect with the organs, and disorders of the organs will be reflected in their corresponding channels. It is possible, therefore, to determine which channel is affected by studying the location and characteristics of a disorder's symptoms and signs.

The main blockage manifestations of the twelve channels are described as follows:

1. The Lung Channel—Cough, asthma, coughing up blood, congested and sore throat, sensation of fullness in the chest, and pain in the collarbone, shoulder, back, and insides of the arms.

2. Large Intestine Channel—Nosebleed, watery nasal discharge, toothache, congested and sore throat, pain in the neck or front part of the shoulders and upper arms, noisy intestines, abdominal pain, diarrhea, constipation, dysentery.

3. Stomach Channel—Noisy intestines, abdominal distension, stomach pain, vomiting, excess hunger, nosebleed, Bell's palsy, congested and sore throat, fever, mental disturbance, pain in the chest, abdomen, and outer part of leg.

4. Spleen Channel—Belching, vomiting, stomach pain, abdominal distension, loose stools, jaundice, sluggishness and general malaise, stiffness and pain at the back of the tongue, swelling and coldness in the inner thighs and knees.

5. Heart Channel—Chest pain, palpitations, rib pain, insomnia, night sweats, dryness of the throat, thirst, pain in the insides of the upper arms, feverishness in the palms.

6. Small Intestine Channel—Deafness, yellow in the whites of the eyes, sore throat, swelling of the cheeks, distension and pain in the lower abdomen, frequent urination, pain along the back and outer parts of the shoulders and arms.

7. Bladder (Urinary Bladder) Channel—Retention of urine, bedwetting, mental disturbance, malaria, teary eyes, nasal stuffiness or runny nose, nosebleed, headache, pain in the nape of the neck, upper and lower back, buttocks, and backs of the lower extremities.

8. Kidney Channel—Bedwetting, frequent urination, nocturnal emissions, impotence, irregular menstruation, asthma, dryness of the tongue, congested and sore throat, swelling, lower back pain, pain along the spinal column and inner thighs, weakness of the legs, feverish sensation in the soles of the feet.

9. Pericardium Channel—Chest pain, palpitations, mental restlessness, stifling feeling in the chest, flushed face, swelling under the arm, mental disturbance, spasm of the arms, feverishness in the palms.

10. Triple Warmer (San Jiao) Channel—Abdominal distension, bedwetting, difficulty urinating, deafness, ear ringing, pain in the outer corners of the eyes, swelling of the cheeks, congested and sore throat, pain in the backs of the ears, shoulders, and outer parts of the arms and elbows.

11. Gallbladder Channel—Headache, pain in the outer corners of the eyes, pain in the jaw, blurring of vision, bitter taste in the mouth, swelling and pain in the collarbone, pain in the armpits, pain along the outer parts of the chest, ribs, thighs, and calves.

12. Liver Channel—Low back pain, fullness in the chest, pain in the lower abdomen, hernia, headache on top of the scalp, dryness of the throat, hiccups, bedwetting, difficulty urinating, mental disturbances.

.   .   .   .

THE EIGHT EXTRAORDINARY CHANNELS

THE EIGHT EXTRAORDINARY CHANNELS can be viewed as a regulating mechanism or reservoir for the twelve channels. When there is an excess or deficiency of energy along the twelve main channels, the eight extraordinary channels start to function. They store excess energy or provide stored energy from the kidney network, which includes the hormonal system. This "give and take" reservoir process is a self-regulating function but can be activated and accessed through certain acupoints called control points, where energy converges. You can also regard them as automatic valves, so when you stimulate a control point with an acupuncture needle or finger pressure, your body's self-regulation mechanism kicks in and initiates the repair and regeneration.

The eight extraordinary channels have their own distinct pathways; they borrow points by crisscrossing the twelve main channels, all except the Governing (DU) and Conception (REN) channels, which have their own distinct points.

The pathways of the eight extraordinary channels are described as follows:

1. Governing (DU) Channel—Originates from the inside of the lower abdomen. Descending, it emerges at the perineum, the area between the external genitals and the rectum, and then ascends along the interior of the spinal column to the nape, where it enters the brain, ascends to the top of the head, and comes down the forehead to below the nose.

2. Conception (REN) Channel—Originates from the lower abdomen and emerges from the perineum. It runs to the pubic region and ascends the front midline to the throat. Running farther upward, it curves around the lips, passes through the cheeks, and enters the region below the eyes.

3. Vitality (Chong Mai) Channel—Originates from the lower abdomen, descends and emerges from the perineum, then ascends and runs inside the vertebral column, while its superficial portion passes above the genitals, where it splits into two and coincides with the kidney channel, running up to the throat and curving around the lips.

4. Belt (Dai Mai) Channel—Starts below the lowest rib. Running obliquely downward, it runs transversely around the waist like a belt.

5. Yang Connecting (Yang Qiao) Channel—Starts from the sides of the heels. Ascending along the legs, it goes along the lateral aspects of the thighs. From there it winds over to the shoulders and ascends along the neck to the corners of the mouth. Then it enters the inner corner of the eyes to communicate with the Yin Connecting (Yin Qiao) channel. It then runs farther upward along the urinary bladder channel to the forehead, where it meets the Gallbladder Channel.

6. Yin Connecting (Yin Qiao) Channel—Starts from the insides of the feet in front of the ankle bones and ascends along the calves and thighs to the external genitalia. From there it ascends up the chest to the collarbone. Running farther upward alongside the Adam's apple and then along the cheekbones, it reaches the inner corners of the eyes and communicates with the Yang Connecting (Yang Qiao) channel.

7. Yang Regulating (Yang Wei) Channel—Begins at the sides of the feet. Ascending to the external ankle bones, it runs upward along the gallbladder channel, passing through the hip region and farther upward to below the ribs and the posterior armpits to the shoulders. From there it ascends to the forehead and then turns backward to the back of the neck, where it communicates with the Governing (DU) channel.

8. Yin Regulating (Yin Wei) Channel—Starts from the insides of the legs and ascends along the thighs to the abdomen to communicate with the spleen

channel. Then it runs along the chest and communicates with the Conception (REN) channel at the neck.

. . . .

ACUPOINTS FOR HEALTH AND WELL-BEING

THE EIGHT CONTROL OR CONFLUENT POINTS are used to activate the eight extraordinary channels at locations where they communicate with the twelve main channels. When symptoms are experienced, stimulation of the corresponding control points will help activate self-balancing and healing. Their locations are described below.

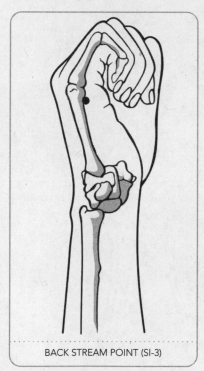

BACK STREAM POINT (SI-3)

1. SI-3 (Back Stream point)—Activates the Governing (DU) channel. When a loose fist is made, the point is found in the depression at the end of the crease below the base of the little finger.

Indications: Headache with stiff neck, redness in the eye, deafness, epilepsy, malaria, fever, night sweats, psychosis, nosebleed, paralysis of the upper extremities, high blood pressure, hysteria, rib pain, low back pain, nerve pain in the legs, jaundice, fullness in the chest, hand tremors, and spasm of elbows, arms, and fingers.

2. LU-7 (Branching Crevice point)—Activates the Conception (REN) channel. On the side of the forearm just above the bony prominence, about one and a half thumb-

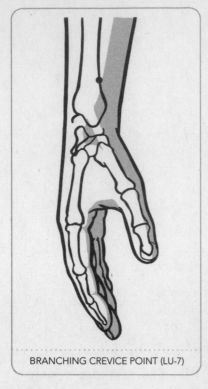

BRANCHING CREVICE POINT (LU-7)

widths above the inside crease of the wrist at the base of the thumb.

Indications: Cough, sore throat, facial paralysis, headache, neck stiffness, toothache, wrist weakness, asthma, acute swelling of the extremities, hot palms or heat in palms, trigeminal neuralgia, hives, facial spasms, radial neuralgia, pain in the elbows, malaria, chills in the back, lack of energy, epilepsy, phlegm obstructing the throat, vomiting of phlegm, swelling of the shoulders, rheumatism of the shoulders, sensation of heat with sweating on the chest and back, sensation of cold in the chest and back.

3. SP-4 (Heredity point)—Activates the Vitality (Chong Mai) channel. On the inside of the foot, above the middle arch, in the depression below and in front of the bone extending back from the big toe.

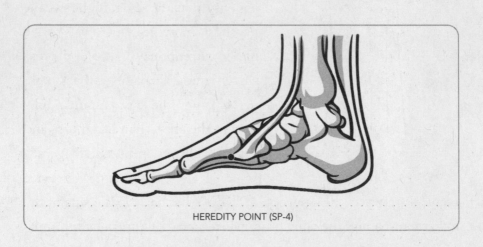

HEREDITY POINT (SP-4)

Indications: Vomiting, diarrhea, poor digestion and appetite, abdominal or stomach pain, dysentery, noisy intestines, epilepsy, swelling, facial swelling, endometriosis, irregular menstruation, menstrual cramps, tidal fever, fever with abundant sweating, thirst, chest pain, discomfort in the heart region, sighing often, high blood pressure, pain or paralysis of the big toe and bottom of foot, rest of foot, and ankles.

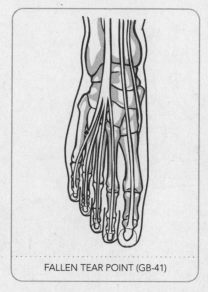

FALLEN TEAR POINT (GB-41)

4. GB-41 (Fallen Tear point)—Activates the Belt (Dai Mai) channel. About one inch toward the ankle from the junction of the two smallest toes (in the depression behind the small tendon and between the bones).

Indications: Conjunctivitis, dizziness, blurry vision, pain in the sides of the ribs, breast infection, swelling and pain of the tops of the feet, irregular menses, headache, vertigo, dizziness, shortness of breath, ear ringing, deafness, arthritis, chest pain with chills, excess sweating, pain in the collarbone, pain and coldness in the hips, extremities, and calves.

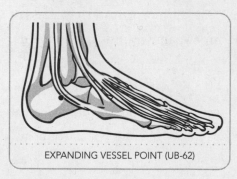

EXPANDING VESSEL POINT (UB-62)

5. UB-62 (Expanding Vessel point)—Activates the Yang Connecting (Yang Qiao) channel. In the depression directly below the tip of the anklebone on the outside of the leg (opposite KID-6).

Indications: Headache, dizziness, vertigo, Ménière's disease, pain in the low back and legs, epilepsy, psychosis, tinnitus, stroke, insomnia, painful menses, foot swelling, arthritis of the lower extremities, palpitations, fever and chills, meningitis, high blood pressure, eye pain, nosebleed, swelling of the neck and armpits, paralysis, tiredness.

6. KID-6 (Illuminate the Sea point)—Activates the Yin Connecting (Yin Qiao) channel. In the indentation directly below the inner tip of the anklebone (opposite UB-62).

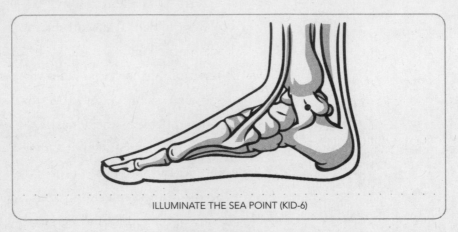

ILLUMINATE THE SEA POINT (KID-6)

Indications: Dry sore throat, irregular menses, uterine prolapse, vaginal discharge, itchy vulva, frequent urination, urinary retention, constipation, foot and leg, epilepsy, psychosis, insomnia or sleepy all the time, hernia, eye pain, vision problems, menstrual cramps, fever, asthma, loss of appetite, bedwetting, dark urine, pain and weakness of the extremities, postpartum abdominal pain, cramps in the hands, headache.

7. SJ-5 (External Gate point)—Activates the Yang Regulating (Yang Wei) channel. Two thumb widths away from the crease of the wrist on the outside forearm, halfway between the bones (opposite P-6).

Indications: Headache, ear ringing, deafness, pain in the fingers, pain in the elbows and arms, hand tremors, fever, common cold, pain

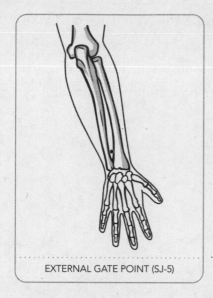

EXTERNAL GATE POINT (SJ-5)

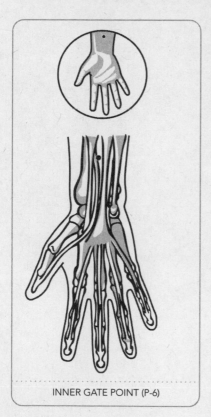

INNER GATE POINT (P-6)

in the cheeks, mumps, pain in the ribs, constipation, swollen throat, bedwetting, stiff neck, paralysis, inflammation of the eyes, teary eyes, cataracts.

8. P-6 (Inner Gate point)—Activates the Yin Regulating (Yin Wei) channel. Two thumb widths away from the crease of the wrist on the inside forearm, between the two tendons (opposite SJ-5).

Indications: Chest pain and fullness, palpitations, epilepsy, vomiting, contracture and pain of the elbows and arms, malaria, fever, delirium, stomach pain, psychosis, hiccups, stroke, jaundice, postpartum vertigo, asthma, shock and emotional trauma, migraine headache, hyperthyroidism, swollen and painful throat, postoperative pain, hemorrhoids, rheumatic heart disease.

By stimulating these and other acupoints with your fingers, you will discover their healing actions and experience the magic of your body's self-healing capabilities.

In summary, whether it's through enjoyable physical exercise, playful sports, or serene tai chi, with mind-body movement you are activating and circulating the vital substances of your being—energy and fluids—that sustain health, vitality, and life itself. The life force can be further stimulated in the energy network of the body through acupuncture and the simple self-healing art of acupressure. Learn to turn on your body's powerful healing capabilities and your body will thank you for it.

CHAPTER 6

THE RHYTHMS OF EVERYDAY LIFE

Live in Harmony at Home, at Work, and with the Environment

The next major advances in health of the American people will come from the assumption of individual responsibility for one's own health and a necessary change in lifestyle for the majority of Americans.

—*JOHN H. KNOWLES, FORMER PRESIDENT,*
ROCKEFELLER FOUNDATION

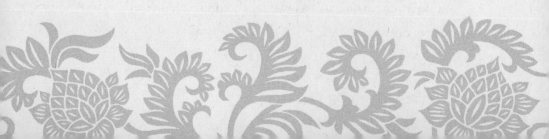

IT IS IMPOSSIBLE TO ESTABLISH CLARITY AND ORDER IN OUR BEING unless our internal energies are in a state of harmony and balance. By using the same cosmic principles that assure the harmonious functioning of the universe, we can nurture our vital energy and establish the internal balance necessary for a happy life. The principles treasured by ancient and modern sages are simplicity, equilibrium, harmony, and quietude. These principles allow our energy to evolve and function normally. By personifying these cosmic principles, we come to realize that we embody the entire universe. Microcosm and macrocosm become one.

We must regulate daily life so that there is a balance between rest and activity, and so that one activity is not engaged in to the exclusion of others. And we all must contend with the by-products of modern science and technological progress—damage to our health and lives from pollution and toxins. Not only have we made our environment unhealthy for ourselves, but we've also made it harder for other organisms to thrive. Since the Industrial Revolution, hundreds of thousands of species have vanished from our planet. And if we don't heed the warning signs, we may eventually extinguish ourselves. That wouldn't do much for your health and wellness goals.

The ecology of our planet is resilient, similar to the human body, if we tread gently and follow the natural law. But our constant assault on the environment—with pesticides and dioxins in our soil and water, for example—threatens not just other creatures but also our own health. For instance, paper products are not naturally white. White paper is bleached with chemicals that leave behind residues of dioxin, a known carcinogen. Such residues are found in coffee filters, paper towels, toilet paper, napkins, facial tissues, diapers, and lunch bags. When it enters the landfill as waste, dioxin leaches into the soil, contaminating groundwater.

Likewise, pesticides and herbicides in produce and antibiotics in meat, poultry, and dairy show up in such diverse places as the water supply, breast milk, and urine. They cause degenerative changes, hormonal and immune-system disorders, and cancer in people and animals. Using unbleached paper products and eating organic produce and animal products are good for both you and the environment.

Our homes should be our sanctuaries, places that nurture our health and soothe our spirits. In the same way, our workplaces should nurture our creativity and help us express our individual gifts and talents. Nowadays, however, the synthetic materials found in buildings, furniture, carpets, furnishings, and electronic devices emit volatile organic compounds (VOCs) into our living and working environments. These toxic gases include formaldehyde from carpets and furniture, benzene from wall coverings, and xylene from computer screens. Such indoor air pollutants aggravate allergies and fatigue; in severe cases they can lead to cancer and birth defects. But Mother Nature can come to the rescue: Plants are our best air purifiers, producing oxygen and eliminating VOCs at the same time. Most effective are indoor palms, English ivy, ficuses, peace lilies, and chrysanthemums. So fill your home with houseplants and bring fresh air indoors!

Energy and blood traverse miles of meridians and vessels within our bodies. Disease, according to Chinese medicine, is the result of stagnation and blockage in either energy or blood. In our living and working environments, too, energy can stagnate, creating disharmony and disrupting health. Arrange your furniture to promote natural movement throughout your home, with special attention to corners, which tend to become stagnation points and collect dust. Proper flow also includes good airflow and cross-ventilation to clear away stale indoor air.

· ·

SUBTLE ENERGY FIELDS

FENG SHUI, OR GEOMANCY, IS THE STUDY OF ENERGY MERIDIANS that crisscross the Earth and the practice of aligning with them. The planet is like a large, magnetized ball with positive and negative charges circulating across its latitudes. Its electromagnetic impact on us is subtle yet profound. Arranging your surroundings in harmony with the earth's energy meridians will bring health, while violating this energy web can result in imbalance and illness. Feng shui is the knowledge of the location of subtle energy rays in the physical universe and their relation to human life. Subtle energy radiations influence our marriages, health, financial situations, and all other aspects of life—whether we harmonize with the subtle energy or violate it.

By applying the knowledge of feng shui, we may skillfully proceed with our lives, choosing appropriate and favorable times and locations to engage in business or to establish a residence. Discovering and using the subtle energy in the universe is a gift that is accessible to everyone. If we are equipped with the knowledge and special techniques, we can make use of the subtle energy just as we use the physical power inherent in air, water, sunshine, and mineral wealth in the form of, say, coal, oil, gas, wind, electricity, or solar or atomic power.

A number of my patients suffer from chronic insomnia, but one case in particular stands out as an example of subtle but powerful energetic influences in the living environment. This female patient lives in a beautiful townhouse with an open loft space over the living room. When she first moved in, she slept in a small bedroom off to the back corner. A few friends from New York convinced her to sleep in the loft space. At first she had no trouble sleeping, but as the years wore on, she began to suffer from insomnia, tossing and turning all night long. She showed up at my office seeking relief.

After a few acupuncture treatments and some herbal remedies, there was no appreciable difference in her sleep, so I asked about her bedroom arrangement. That was when I realized that the open and spacious qualities of the loft, with lots of light and no drapes or walls, might be the culprit. When you are asleep at night, you need to feel safe, protected, and ensconced in a cocoonlike atmosphere. Otherwise the spirit and sensory organs will remain awake to "guard" you from danger and the things that go bump in the night. Soon after I suggested that she try sleeping in the small bedroom, her chronic insomnia went away and has not returned. I have other patients with similar stories. As an aside, the spacious, open loft would be a perfect creative space for an artist or writer, or as a home office, because of the abundance of energy flow.

Feng shui is based on the same principles of natural law—polarity and the five-element energy evolution—that apply to everything in our universe. As I discuss below, the five elements correspond to a direction, color, or aspect of your life, and by nurturing and balancing the energetic expressions of each element, you can maximize positive influences and minimize negative outcomes, both in health and in life. Your home is a structure that conducts energy in the same way that your body does. Your entire being mirrors the energy of your home. You are a microcosm of your immediate habitat. Cluttering up your home is like experiencing a blockage of energy and blood flow in your body—you will soon experience the unpleasant effects of the energy imbalance in your health or other aspects of your life.

THE FIVE ELEMENTS IN YOUR HOME AND WORK SPACES

ALLOW ABUNDANT LIGHT TO PERMEATE AND AIR TO FLOW unimpeded in the southern direction of your house and workplace. This direction is the fire element, which is experienced through the color red, and it represents your passion, fame, or rank in the world, and the cardiovascular system of your body. By placing candles, a fireplace, light sources, or electronic appliances in this area of your space, you can promote the fire energy and its healthy expression in your life.

The northern direction correlates to the water element. A little pond or trickling stream placed in this direction inside or outside your home or office will accentuate the water energy. Or you can simply place a tabletop waterfall in the northern part of your house. This expresses your willpower, relationships, and career. As we've seen, the water element also represents the kidney-bladder network and the hormonal system relating to reproductive health.

The eastern direction represents the wood element. Plant or place trees and green foliage in and around your house or office—but make sure they are well taken care of, as dead plants do not help you. The wood element represents growth and flexibility in your personality, the prosperity of your family, and your health, especially that of your liver-gallbladder network and nervous system.

The western direction represents the metal element, so place something solid and grounded here, like a rock, crystals, or glass furnishings. The color of the metal element is white, clear, or shiny metallic. You can also place rocks in the western section of your garden to help enhance metal energy, which corresponds to your lung–large intestine network and immune system. The metal element speaks of the ability to express yourself, your intelligence, and a sense of righteousness. It also symbolizes monetary wealth, children, and offspring.

FIVE ELEMENTS IN YOUR HOME AND WORK SPACES

NORTH : WATER
WILLPOWER,
RELATIONSHIPS, CAREER

KIDNEY-BLADDER NETWORK /
REPRODUCTIVE HEALTH

Place in this area:

- A little pond or trickling stream
- Tabletop waterfall

WEST : METAL
SELF-EXPRESSION, RIGHTEOUSNESS,
INTELLIGENCE, CHILDREN, WEALTH

LUNG–LARGE INTESTINE NETWORK /
IMMUNE SYSTEM

Place in this area:

- Solid and grounded items like rocks, crystals, or glass furnishings
- White, clear, or shiny metallic
- Place rocks in the western section of your garden

CENTER : EARTH
GENEROSITY,
COMPASSION

SPLEEN-PANCREAS-STOMACH
NETWORK / DIGESTIVE SYSTEM

This area should be:

- Peaceful and spacious
- A gathering point for people
- Filled with comfortable furniture

EAST : WOOD
PERSONALITY GROWTH,
FAMILY, HEALTH

LIVER NETWORK / NERVOUS SYSTEM

Place in this area:

- Trees and green foliage plants (but make sure that these are well taken care of since dead plants do not help you)

SOUTH : FIRE
PASSION, FAME

HEART–SMALL INTESTINE NETWORK /
CARDIOVASCULAR SYSTEM

Place in this area:

- Abundant light
- Unimpeded airflow
- Red
- Candles, fireplace, light source, or electronic appliance

The center of your house or workplace should be a place of peace and spaciousness. It is ideal to preserve the middle of your house as a gathering point because it correlates with the earth element. Earth energy is expressed through generosity, compassion, and care for others, as well as an abundance of materials. By placing inviting and comfortable furniture here, you encourage the congregation of people, and in doing so you strengthen the earth element, which also relates to your digestive system.

A patient came to see me with indigestion and heartburn, which began around the time he moved into a new house. At first he thought his symptoms were a result of stress from the move, so he took antacids and he saw a gastrointestinal specialist, who diagnosed him with GERD, or acid reflux, and put him on more antacids. A year later he was still suffering from bloating, flatulence, and heartburn despite taking the medications. I changed his diet to make it more alkaline by increasing his intake of vegetables and fruits and eliminating red meat, alcohol, coffee, tea, sugar, tomatoes, citrus fruits, vinegar, and spicy foods. He also underwent acupuncture treatments, herbal therapy, and stress-management training, and I put him on digestive enzymes to help him with his digestive function.

After about three months, his symptoms improved by about 75 percent. However, his condition stubbornly persisted. During a reevaluation visit he was accompanied by his woman friend, and I asked him about his home environment. His friend complained that although the move was over a year ago, he still had unpacked boxes stacked in the family room, which sits in the middle of the house. There wasn't much furniture in the family room, so they would gather with friends in the kitchen. Immediately I knew that the clutter of the boxes had created an energetic blockage in his earth-element area, which relates directly to the spleen-pancreas-stomach network—the root of his digestive problems. The following weekend he unpacked the boxes and went out to buy comfortable couches and tables. It may seem coincidental, but a couple of weeks later his symptoms vanished. His follow-up gastric examination confirmed no presence of inflammation.

. . . .

COSMIC ENVIRONMENTAL INFLUENCES

COSMIC INFLUENCES SUCH AS THE SEASONS and atmospheric factors can have a profound impact on your health. For example, viruses and seasonal mood disorders are most common during the winter, and asthma and lung ailments peak during the fall. By understanding the rhythms of nature and how they affect your health, you can become proactive in adapting to them and thus prevent illness. This is what it means to be in harmony with your environment.

Harmonizing ourselves with the changes in our personal environment and living according to natural law are essential to maintaining good health. You should engage in activities that are in harmony with the energies of the season, and conduct every aspect of your life accordingly. *The Yellow Emperor's Classic of Medicine* recognized the seasonal influences on health and illness nearly five millennia ago.

. . . .

THE FOUR SEASONS

DURING THE THREE MONTHS OF SPRING all living things begin to germinate and grow. At this time, nature is enveloped in a vivacious atmosphere, and all things are alive. Go to bed when night comes and get up early. Wear your hair and garments loose and take walks. Your mental and physical activities can be like the weather—active and alive, open and unsuppressed. If we go against this principle, the liver energy (which includes the nervous system), could be damaged, and our adaptability to the energy of summer will be weakened.

During the three months of summer the energy from the sky pours down and the energy from the earth rises. From this interaction of sky and earth, all plants mature, and animals, flowers, and fruits appear abundantly. Go to bed later at night and get up early. Don't neglect the sunlight. Try not to get angry easily, and maintain a lively and pleasant spirit and a calm and peaceful mind—so that your spirit is full, like all things in nature. Do not block the pores of the skin—allow yourself to perspire freely, evaporating not only your sweat but also your emotions and desires. All things should follow the principle of going outward; this is the way of nurturing growth in summer. If we go against this rule, we damage the heart energy, which corresponds to the fire element and the season of summer. When fall comes, fevers will arise easily, so that we will not be able to cope with the harvesting energy of fall. The season of summer is followed by late summer, which correlates to the earth element. Imbalance may include disorders of the spleen energy and the digestive system.

During the three months of autumn all things are ripe and ready for harvest. The weather is cool and plants look solitary. Go to bed earlier and get up at dawn. Keep calm and peaceful. Only by conserving our spirit, keeping calm, and practicing breathing exercises can we cope with the changing weather. But it is by this weather that the lung energy can be purified. This is how to nurture our energy in the fall. Going against this rule will damage the lung energy, and when winter comes the system won't digest food properly, and will show itself in the bowel movements. The "storage" quality of winter energy will be compromised.

During the three months of winter all living things should return home and be conserved. Water is turned into ice and the ground is cracked by coldness. Nature shows an overall condition of hidden yang energy. Go to bed early and get up only when the sun is in the sky. Our emotions shouldn't be too strong, as when we are truly content. Avoid coldness, and linger around warmth. Avoid excessive perspiration and the resulting escape of yang energy with sweat. This is the way to nurture storage. If we go against this rule, weakness and coldness in the extremities will occur when spring comes and our adaptability to the growth energy of spring will be weakened.

· ·

THE CIRCADIAN RHYTHMS AND
A HARMONIOUS LIFESTYLE

ALL OF THE MANIFESTATIONS IN THE UNIVERSE adhere to the cosmic cycle of energy rotation. As it circles, the energy undergoes stages of transformation. For the purposes of description, the great sages of ancient times divided this universal circle into twelve distinct sections and developed a system of twelve time-energy units that apply to all yearly and daily cycles.

The energetic channel system in the human body closely mirrors the energy network of the universe. Each acupuncture channel experiences a waxing and waning of energy during the twenty-four-hour cycle. The peak of this flow lasts two hours for each channel. For example, energy is fullest in the stomach between 7:00 and 9:00 A.M., which explains why breakfast is the most important meal of the day. Below I list the peak hours for each organ network and its energy channel within the body. This ancient human bioenergetic clock preceded the discovery of the circadian rhythm in the West by some two thousand years, and it remains critical in acupuncture therapy. Sometimes acupuncture is applied during the maximum organ hours in order to remedy the imbalance of particular organs.

Everything in the universe has a time to be born, grow, ripen, mature, and finally a time to fall, become latent, and be reborn again. Human civilization has a life span, from its inception to the height of its development. When the peak of prosperity is reached, then it must decline and again come to rest. The circle will continue and a new culture will be born—similar to the cycle of the four seasons.

Like the yearly revolution of the earth, the life of a human being follows its own circle of energy rotation. The potential life span of a human being is 120 years. The first quarter of a person's life is like springtime, a time to grow and cultivate oneself. The second quarter corresponds with summer and is a time to develop and prosper. The third quarter of the cycle is the autumn of one's life, a time to harvest and enjoy the fruits of one's development. The winter quarter is a time to come back to quietness, to cultivate the vital root of life and to restore one's energy. You should engage in activities that are appropriate for the season of your life. For example, when it is the spring of your life, you should be active; when it is autumn, you should accept that it is autumn and develop a mellowness of personality. The best policy is to follow what is natural, and to keep yourself in a natural condition without becoming disturbed by the styles and fads of the external world.

The cyclical changes that occur in us on a daily basis also follow the energy rotation of the universe. The cycles known as circadian

BIOENERGETIC CLOCK

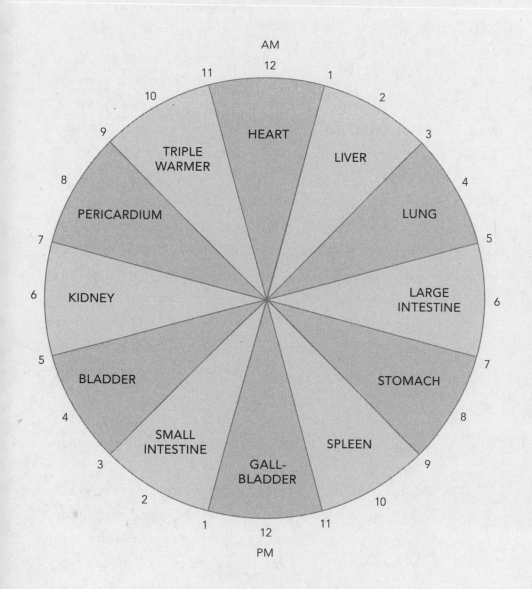

rhythm—which govern your body's natural cycles, and regulate appetite, sleep, and mood—are controlled for the most part by light, according to research over the last two decades. Your body is less like a machine and more like an orchestra—and its conductor is the circadian rhythm. Research into the circadian rhythm has spawned a new field called chronobiology, which studies the internal human clock and the biochemical changes that recur in daily, weekly, and monthly periods. Chronomedicine is a medical subspecialty that focuses on disorders that come from the disturbance of the human biological clock, like the common experience of jet lag.

Chinese medicine practioners have long believed that respect for nature's cycles brings health, and violation of its rhythms leads to disease. Biochemical changes occur when humans transgress the natural behavior patterns associated with the division of night and day. I have had several patients who worked nights and slept during the day for ten or more years. Among them the men all have some form of heart disease—arrhythmia or coronary artery blockage—and the women all have fibrocystic breast disease and two had breast cancer. Studies show shift workers on night duty and others with unpredictable working hours have a 30 percent higher risk of heart attack than day workers with set hours. Mice forced to live on a night-shift schedule show a life span 11 percent shorter than average.

Adequate and quality sleep, then, is critical to staying in synchrony with our biological clock. Our bodies run on biological rhythms and function best with consistent routines. To ensure restful sleep every night, form your own routines and rituals that help you go to sleep—and stay asleep. In my previous book, *Secrets of Longevity*, I suggested the following: hot baths, foot massage, journaling, meditation, aromatherapy, relaxing music, reading spiritual books, praying, and taking an evening stroll. Rituals help calm your mind and allow you to feel peaceful within. Once you find an activity that works, be sure to practice it consistently.

Equally important are how and when you wake up in the morning. This will often determine your well-being for the day. Upon sensing the light at dawn, your adrenal gland releases cortisol, a stimulating hormone that functions as an internal alarm clock. It increases your blood pressure, body temperature, and heart rate. If you miss nature's wake-up call and sleep past, say, 9 A.M., you may be groggy because you've missed your free morning ride, courtesy of the cortisol. On the other hand, if you jump out of bed and force yourself awake, you may overtax your system—so much so that you could suffer a heart attack or stroke. Studies show that strokes and heart attacks most commonly occur between 6 A.M. and noon because of the sudden and dramatic increase in blood pressure and heart rate in the morning. It's better to gradually wake up with soft music, stretches, and self-massage before getting into the shower or driving.

I advise you to try to discover your own internal rhythm. You can find your peaks and valleys by charting them. Keep a log monitoring your energies, activities, and feelings every hour for a week and you'll see a trend. You'll see dips or valleys and you'll see peaks when you perform the best. Working on challenging (or unappealing) projects at your peak will help you a great deal. Likewise, dealing with difficult people at peak times will enable you to have more tolerance—you'll perform better and you'll be less likely to get into a conflict. Leave the simple and easy tasks for the valleys.

Many people find that they get more out of exercise by doing it in the afternoon rather than early in the morning before going to work. Exercising in the afternoon fits better with the circadian rhythm, as your aerobic capacity and muscle strength are at their peak between mid-afternoon and early evening. And by exercising at the same time each day you can establish a pattern, strengthening your performance at that particular time of day. This is called entrainment, and it allows us to override the circadian rhythm to an extent. You can use entrainment to help overcome jet lag, for example. Say you exercise at noon every day. By exercising at noon in a new time zone, your circadian rhythm will adjust to that new time zone more quickly.

Finally, envision how you want to live. Why spend the next thirty years living a lifestyle that you don't enjoy—and that may even be harmful to your well-being? Why not better yourself and your life? A healthy lifestyle is one of the simplest secrets to health and happiness. If you feel emotionally fulfilled, your body will feel it and reflect a state of well-being. Make small changes regularly. Don't expect to make drastic changes overnight, but small improvements over time will help you feel and see the differences in all areas of life—mental, spiritual, and physical. Stay in tune with your internal and external rhythms, and learn to dance to the music of the divine composer. You will then appreciate the life-giving, sustaining, healing force we have all been endowed with.

Because we violate the natural equilibrium of the energy network of our being, we require self-cultivation to bring us back to a state of evenness and balance. Most people develop only the physical aspect of their being, neglecting the spiritual because the pressures of society turn their attention away from the subtle truths of life. Thus their lives manifest imbalance and disharmony. The Integral Way—an esoteric spiritual tradition of China that dates back to the Yellow Emperor—works to refine gross physical energy to the more subtle level of spiritual energy so that we may once again connect our being with the Subtle Origin of the universe. Following the Integral Way, this is the goal of one's life, sometimes called embodying or realizing the universe within your body. It isn't just an idea or a theory—it has been experienced by generation after generation of achieved ones.

CHAPTER 7

THE YIN AND YANG OF THE MIND

Why Emotional Balance, Intellectual Stimulation, and Spiritual Growth Are Essential for Optimal Wellness

The human body experiences a powerful gravitational pull in the direction of hope. That is why the patient's hopes are the physician's secret weapon. They are the hidden ingredients in any prescription.

—*NORMAN COUSINS*

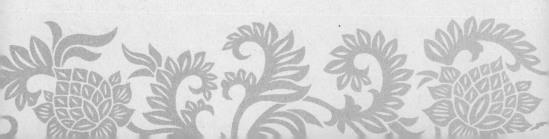

WELLNESS MEDICINE RECOGNIZES THAT THE BODY, MIND, AND SPIRIT function as one inseparable unit. Feelings, for instance, can be both the cause and the result of physiological changes. Researchers have confirmed that joy and laughter elicit positive immune responses. In this case, emotions cause physical change. On the other hand, patients suffering from hepatitis can exhibit periodic outbursts of rage—an example of emotional changes resulting from physical illness. What about the spirit? How does it influence your well-being? Studies show that people who believe in a higher power and pray for recovery from illness—either for themselves or for others—have an overwhelmingly positive response. Learning how to manage your emotions, instruct your mind, and attune your spirit is essential for optimal wellness.

. . . .

EMOTIONS

HUMAN LIFE IS SUPPORTED BY VARIOUS ENERGIES. We obtain our energy from the food we eat as well as from the physical and subtle universal environment. The energy outside of our bodies is called universal energy, and even though this external energy is generally not under our direct control, we can depend on the normal course of nature and live within the order of the universal law. The energy growing inside of us may be called our individual energy, and it is guided by the individual to a certain extent. This energy manifests as physical energy, emotional energy, mental energy, and spiritual energy. Depending on each person's disposition, these energies may manifest positively and in a focused, creative way, or negatively and in destructive ways.

In many emotional states, especially those involving strong negative emotions, the energy is almost as palpable as physical energy.

Emotion lies on the margin between body and mind, and is a transferable and transmissible medium. We can be influenced emotionally by other people and by our environment, and in less perceptible ways by chemical changes in our bodies and by the subtle universal energy cycles. For example, at family gatherings during the holidays, emotions from the past often come up between members of the family. The abundance of sugar and alcohol, coupled with insufficient daylight in the middle of winter, further heightens emotional reactions and displays.

Joy, anger, sorrow, happiness, worry, anxiety, frustration, love, and hate are the elements of emotion. If any one of these is extreme, it will destroy the normalcy of the entire being. Likewise rain, snow, frost, fog, heat, cold, and wind are the changing faces of atmospheric energy. If any one weather pattern becomes extreme, it will upset the balance of the seasons and possibly bring on natural disaster. When each emotion is manifested in accordance with the circumstance, it is normal and appropriate, but if one overreacts, it can produce sickness and destruction.

. . . .

EMOTIONS AND THE FIVE-ELEMENT NETWORK

EMOTIONS ARE CLASSIFIED INTO FIVE PREDOMINANT STATES: joy, rumination, sadness, fear, and anger. These states correspond to the five evolving elements of fire, earth, metal, water, and wood, respectively. The five emotions are generated by the activities of the five organ networks when they are stimulated by external change. Thus the emotions are a manifestation of the energy of the organ networks and may be thought of as the motivating energy of the body.

The continual shift of emotional states is a natural phenomenon. Most children embody this spontaneity, moving through and experiencing a range of feelings in a short period of time without getting stuck. However, dwelling on one particular emotion will disrupt the natural cycles of energy transformation and circulation within the body and throw stress upon the corresponding organ. A child's tantrum is an example of stuck emotions. In adults it could manifest as prolonged sadness and depression. If dwelling on one emotion continued to excess, the stress from imbalance can result in disease.

Anger, the emotion of the liver network, rises so that the energy is strongest in the head and shoulders. The nervous system, which corresponds with the wood element, extends the energy of the liver-gall-bladder network and develops like a tree. The rising motion of the liver's energy can be seen when a person becomes angry, causing blood to rush to the head and the face, and the face to become red. The energy from anger can be used constructively to get through a situation of persistent obstruction with confidence. However, high blood pressure, headaches, and pain in the neck, shoulders, and head may be the consequences of prolonged anger. In severe situations stroke and heart attack may result.

Joy, the emotion of the heart–small intestine network, concentrates energy in the chest, allowing the opening of our hearts to promote acceptance and love. Our indulging in happiness causes the heart energy to become dispersed, though, affecting the functions of the other organ networks as well. Imbalance arising from extreme joy and excitement may present abnormal heartbeat, palpitation, dizziness, tiredness, and, in severe instances, fainting or loss of consciousness. Studies show that people who talk the fastest—usually a sign of overexcitement—have the highest rate of heart disease.

Grief or sadness is the emotion of the lung–large intestine network. Though the heaviest of all emotional energies, sadness produces tears that wash away pain, sorrow, and anguish. In healthy expressions, the tenderness of sadness promotes empathy, caring, and understanding, which bring out the humanity in all of us. One study, at Southampton General Hospital in England, showed that a five-minute episode of feeling genuine care or compassion can enhance the immune system, causing a gradual climb in IgA, your body's natural antibody against colds, flu, and infections. However, when sadness becomes a persistent state, it consumes energy and leaves the body weak and exhausted. Health conditions that may arise from chronic grief include problems of the respiratory system such as asthma, chronic bronchitis, and sinus conditions. Other conditions include immune system imbalances—either as weakness that leaves a person prone to getting colds, or excess that creates inflammation throughout the body.

Fear, the emotion of the kidney-bladder network, concentrates this system's energy downward to the abdomen and the lower extremities. The abdomen is where one's physical essence is stored and can be accessed. Therefore it is not surprising that fear is the greatest motivator of human behavior. Perhaps the subconscious fear of the extinction of our DNA prompts us to search for opportunities to procreate. The fear of pain, sickness, and infirmity keeps people away from bad habits and spurs them to search for health and wellness. The fear of getting a ticket keeps most people from driving recklessly. But fear in excess creates paralysis rather than action, and it is the single biggest obstacle to achieving our full potential. Extreme fear of pain can cause some people to become addicted to substances. And since fear drives energy downward, extreme fear can cause some people to involuntarily move their bowels and pass urine, and in severe cases they become incontinent. Other symptoms of imbalance from fear include pain and weakness in the lower back and legs.

Rumination, the emotion of the spleen-pancreas-stomach network, concentrates energy within the brain. For example, when we continually ponder problems, the most frequent symptom experienced is insomnia. In this case, the energy stays in the brain at night instead of following its normal course of descending to the lower part of the body, which allows us to sleep peacefully.

Shock is connected with the heart–small intestine network, and it means that consciousness is disturbed. In clinical practice the beginning of an illness can often be traced back to a time of intense shock that weakened the system. Witness the cases of hurricane victims and war veterans whose mental or physical illnesses can be traced directly back to the original trauma.

Worry, a variation of the energy of the spleen-pancreas-stomach network, coagulates energy so that the body becomes sluggish. When energy congeals from worry, we become unable to do even the smallest tasks. When the spleen-pancreas-stomach network is unable to transform nutrients and transport waste freely, we become prone to digestive problems.

. . . .

EMOTIONAL BALANCING

WHEN WE'RE UNAWARE OF THE SUBTLE INFLUENCES that affect our moods, it is easy to become dominated by our emotions. We tend, then, to identify completely with our emotions, and they are no longer just a single component of life. This reveals itself in statements such as "I am angry," "I am depressed," and so forth, and will inhibit the ability to spontaneously respond with the appropriate expression in any given situation.

When unaware of our emotional imbalances, we often content ourselves with mental consolations such as "I am entitled to feel however I feel. This is the way I am." Or we may fall into the opposite extreme and suppress our emotions, denying the positive and healthy function of normal emotional reactions. This violates our true nature and occurs frequently in religious traditions or families that discourage healthy emotional development.

A positive emotional life comes from the conscious guiding and directing of our internal energy. Below I describe a three-step process for guiding your feelings in a healthy, constructive way using the positive emotional attributes associated with the five elements and their corresponding organ networks.

The first step is self-awareness. When a feeling arises in reaction to a situation, become aware of the true feeling and acknowledge it. The emphasis is on the true feeling rather than a false, rationalized feeling. For example, I recently had a patient who did not get the promotion she was expecting. Instead of acknowledging her disappointment, sadness, and resentment, she rationalized that maybe she didn't deserve it or that her boss didn't like her. She was depressed and paralyzed by a fear that she was not liked. I pointed out to her that by identifying and acknowledging her true feelings, which were sadness and anger, she could prevent unconscious emotional suppression and then move on to working with these energies.

Step two is association. Connect the emotional energies to the positive qualities associated with each corresponding element. Sadness is associated with the metal element, or the lung–large intestine network. Crying tears of disappointment or releasing anger through singing can relieve sadness quickly. My patient got instant relief from her emotional burden by both crying and singing. Her sadness also allowed her to develop empathy for the pressure her boss was under. Anger, in its healthy form, motivates action: the patient was able to positively harness her anger by implementing a plan of action to improve her odds of getting the next promotion. I also reminded her that her sadness could affect the respiratory and immune systems of the lung–large intestine network and the nervous system of the liver-gallbladder network, and vice versa. I asked her to look out for the sadness transferring to these networks, but also to keep in mind that problems in these areas could make her more vulnerable to sadness and anger.

The third step is transformation. Convert your emotional energy to health-enhancing energy. Through meditation, acupressure, and mind-body exercises like tai chi and qi gong, you can promote the ceaseless circulation of your internal energy and convert emotions into beneficial physical or spiritual energy. To continue with the example above, I taught my patient to activate acupoints along the lung–large intestine and liver-gallbladder energy networks while reciting "I release sadness and anger from my lungs and liver and fill my being with empathy and confidence." This technique can correct any imbalance that the emotions may have caused and transform the emotional energy into productive physical energy. Another method involves practicing qi gong exercises that work to strengthen the metal and wood elements. Ideally the patient will be able to convert her sadness and anger into healing energy for her lung and liver networks.

. . . .

REST AND RELAXATION

EMOTIONAL IMBALANCE OFTEN COMES FROM tiredness and tension. Most parents know when their children are about to have an emotional breakdown—when they are overtired, hungry, or hurried. Unfortunately, adults are often woefully unaware of the impact of low energy and stress on their own emotional lives. Rest and relaxation are essential for renewal and emotional balance. Activities for children such as nap time, quiet time, and story time are designed to help them rest and relax. You, too, can benefit from regular, structured times for rest and relaxation, which will help you restore your physical energy and maintain emotional balance.

It also helps to observe your emotions with a clear and centered mind because emotions reflect the state of your physical and mental energy. A person with balanced energy will manifest appropriate and harmonious emotional reactions.

. . . .

MIND

SINCE BEHAVIOR IS AN EXTENSION OF THE MIND, it is necessary to set the mind in order so that it is filled with positive energy. Carefully choose your thoughts and words and weed out those that are negative in nature. Negative thoughts will attract negative energies of the same frequency, which will manifest in your life as negative experience. In other words: garbage in, garbage out.

Through the study of neurophysiology, we are closer to revealing the inner workings and the potential of our brain-mind connection. Our mind stores experiences and impressions from the past that help define our reality. Programming your mind for health and wellness will help you actualize what you want in life. For example, during flu season, you might be concerned about getting sick. Instead of worrying incessantly and visualizing the agony of being bedridden—and lowering your immunity in the process—be positive by visualizing a protective energetic shield around your body and summoning the energy of the immunity-boosting emotions of joy and laughter.

. . . .

THE YIN AND YANG OF THE MIND

YOUR MIND HAS DISTINCT YIN AND YANG ATTRIBUTES that are opposite yet complementary, similar to the left brain–right brain split. The yin side is like the right brain: intuitive, receptive, patient, kind, cooperative, artistic, and musical. The yang attributes are more like the left brain: logical, aggressive, progressive, discerning, competitive, mathematical, rational, and verbal.

To achieve harmony, it is necessary to balance the yin and yang expressions of your mind. For example, patience, which is a yin or passive virtue, is a good virtue to develop. Progressiveness, a yang or active virtue, is also a desirable virtue to cultivate. Patience and progressiveness must stand in balance within our individual personality. Incomplete virtue can cause problems. Take kindness as an example—without the application of discernment, kindness is only a blind kindness, and it can do a lot of damage, as when parents spoil their children.

Balanced development of the yin and yang aspects of your mind is essential to living a full, complete life. Otherwise you are just a fragment of your potential. The highest principle of mental development is the recognition of your own intrinsic value. When you're aware of your intrinsic value, you are able to restore and maintain a balanced personality, and don't depend on any external evaluation and acceptance. By relying only on what you truly are, you develop the positive elements of your being and eliminate the negative. Self-love and self-respect, then, are fundamental to the development of a healthy mind.

Many people carry around emotional pain from childhood. They felt deprived of love and respect as they were growing up, but now, as adults, we all have a second chance to parent ourselves in a way that promotes love and respect. A new patient of mine had spent twenty years in psychotherapy dealing with her traumatic childhood. She came to me to help her lose weight and control her diabetes. It was clear that she was stuck in a destructive mind-set that kept playing itself out in behaviors like overeating and indulging in sweets. She was constantly blaming her parents and herself.

At one point I suggested that since she hated her parents, she should disown them and take over as her own ideal parents. I asked her what she would say to her child if she fell off her bike while learning how to ride. Would she scold her with remarks like "You are so clumsy, you'll never learn to ride a bike," or would she encourage her with words like "I know you must feel bad—how about we try again when you are ready"?

With some coaching on positive self-talk designed to foster self-worth and self-confidence, she stopped saying to herself, "You are worthless and totally out of control with your eating," and began saying, "I know you felt bad about your diet yesterday—how about snacking on raisins, dried cranberries, and almonds today? You'll feel better and have more energy." Slowly her eating behavior began to change and she stopped putting herself down when she strayed from her program. Over three months she lost twenty-seven pounds, and she is still losing steadily. Her blood sugar levels improved and she was able to work with her medical doctor to reduce her diabetes medication.

Out of awareness of her negative self-talk, she realized that she could empathize with her parents' impatience, inattention, and threats of punishment during her childhood. I encouraged her to continue to work with her therapist on forgiving her parents and on improving her own self-respect and self-love. Already we see progress and increased health.

SPIRIT

SPIRIT IS THE ESSENCE OF OUR BEING. If spirit is the directing energy in our life, then our desires and impulses are balanced and harmonious. They fulfill their natural function as expressions of the positive, creative, and constructive nature of the universe. Why is this important in health and healing? Attuning your spirit is important because all disease and suffering are the consequences of violating the universal law.

Our inner awareness is our spiritual light. All our motives, actions, relationships, and values should be inspired by our own being and guided by our awareness. Spirituality and personal faith are the hidden elixirs of life. Cultivating yourself spiritually, strengthening your connection to the universal divine, or God, no matter what your religious faith, will bring you inner peace and the ability to cope with life's troubles.

We lack tranquility in our lives because we've strayed from our true nature and have lost our knowledge of universal law, which is not outside us but within. After all, we are the embodiment of universal law itself; we are universal law manifesting as human beings. The personalities of those who have reached true self-awareness remain unchanged under any circumstance, and their inner peace enables them to overcome any obstacle.

Our true nature cannot be separated from the nature of the universe—they are one and the same. Through self-discovery, meditation, and spiritual practices you can learn to quiet the ego and allow the spirit to emerge. By being attuned to the cycles of energy evolution and change, you will realize the infinite source of energy for healing and for nurturing life.

THE POWER OF PRAYER

PRAYER IS THE COMMUNICATION OF OUR NEEDS OR DESIRES to a higher power. Through prayer we may affect the subtle energy. As I've said many times now, human nature and the nature of the universe are one and the same. There is no distinction between individual energy and universal energy. To support this claim, I'd like to share a personal example with you.

One spring week while I was in medical school in China, five of my classmates and I set off on a backpacking trip in the mountains. We were young and ill prepared for the weather, and things quickly turned ugly. We were swallowed by a severe snowstorm, a complete whiteout all around. We were stranded, cooped up in our tents with the storm howling outside. This was the first experience of the wilderness for three people in our group, and they took turns having emotional breakdowns.

Our food supply dwindled down to trail mix. Amid the desperation and increasing hopelessness, I began to pray—all night long when I could. I knew that the only way we were going to survive was to keep our spiritual faith strong. At one point on the seventh night I momentarily fell asleep, overcome by fatigue.

I awoke to the sound of utter silence. It seemed so peaceful and eternal that I thought it could be the sound of death. I got up, put on my coat, and went outside. What I saw struck me as a divine image—the clearest night sky I had ever seen. A large, bright, full moon illuminated the mountain ranges around us. I stood in solitude on that mountaintop and I knew that I was one with the divine.

Prayer is a powerful force, but don't rely on it alone for health and healing. The universal divine, or God if you prefer, helps those who help themselves. Get on the path of building a constructive and healthy life and a healthy mind, and cultivate a spiritual connection to the divine. The divine will surely respond.

Study spiritual works, apply your learning to improve your life, engage in prayer and meditation, and express universal love through service to others. This will enrich and add years to your life. How can we practice universal love? Be grateful for the sources and the people that make it possible for you to have what you have—be it food, clothing, shelter, job, education, or a relationship. Practice kindness by looking for opportunities to make someone else feel happy: Sweep the sidewalk in front of your neighbor's house, give up your seat on a bus to an elderly person, bring food to the homeless. Once you begin you'll find many pathways to universal love.

Leading an ordinary, balanced life is a great accomplishment. Radiating your inner harmony and positively influencing those around you is a service both to the world and to yourself. Health and optimum wellness are your ultimate reward.

CHAPTER 8

EAST MEETS WEST

Integrative Medicine in Action:
Joy's Recovery from Cancer

Science can never be a closed book. It is like a tree,
ever growing, ever reaching new heights. Occasionally
the lower branches, no longer giving nourishment to
the tree, slough off. We should not be ashamed to
change our methods; rather we should be ashamed
never to do so.

—CHARLES V. CHAPIN, FORMER PRESIDENT, AMERICAN
PUBLIC HEALTH ASSOCIATION

NOW THAT I'VE DISCUSSED THE PHILOSOPHY AND PRINCIPLES OF self-healing in detail, I'd like to conclude the first part of this book with an example that demonstrates the power of integrative medicine.

My first clinical experience with cancer was during my post-graduate residency at Zhong Shan Hospital, the teaching hospital of Shanghai Medical University. I learned firsthand how chemotherapy and radiation therapy can be used in conjunction with Chinese medicine.

The increased efficacy of using Western and Eastern medicine together in cancer care has been extensively documented in Chinese studies. One study involved 285 people with a variety of cancers that had metastasized to the lymph nodes above the collarbone. The patients were divided into three groups: those who received a single treatment of either chemotherapy, radiation, or Chinese medicine; those who received chemotherapy and Chinese medicine; and those who received radiation and Chinese medicine. The group in which patients received a single treatment produced less than a 25 percent shrinkage of the lymph nodes. The group in which chemotherapy was combined with Chinese medicine showed 55 percent shrinkage, and the group that was given radiation combined with Chinese medicine showed a 75 percent shrinkage.

More important, I witnessed the increased quality of life of patients treated with integrative medicine. I was touched by how integrating the two medical traditions brought humanity back into cancer care and restored faith and peace in cancer patients. What I experienced during my residency in China convinced me that in some ways cancer care in China is ahead of cancer care in the United States because of the effectiveness of the East-West combination treatment.

Upon returning to the United States in the mid-eighties, I began to apply what I learned in Shanghai to my patients who were seeking to get through their cancer therapies alive and in halfway decent shape.

Very quickly several oncologists got wind of my work and began to refer their patients to me while they were undergoing conventional cancer treatments. As more oncologists sent me their patients, the Wellness Community—a community support center for cancer patients—also began to refer patients to me. My cancer patients over the years have included doctors, even oncologists.

There is no question of the value of integrative cancer care. Nearly all the cancer survivors I've treated will tell you that the integrative approach to their treatment was essential in their triumph over their illness and that it improved their overall quality of life. I now want to share a story with you that shows integrative medicine at its best.

. . . .

THE SHOCKING NEWS

JOY CAME TO MY OFFICE ONE OVERCAST WINTER DAY. Her face was pale and her demeanor hesitant. Clutching a peacoat close to her body, she was trembling slightly. I asked her if she needed anything before we began our consultation. She politely declined but then asked for a cup of hot tea. She said that she was referred to me by a friend of hers who had breast cancer two years earlier and who was helped by my treatments while going through her anticancer therapies.

Joy was diagnosed with breast cancer one month before. She was in her mid-forties, and she wasn't ready for this devastating news. She tried to be strong, and she consulted several well-known oncologists, all of whom I've worked with. One oncologist told her that she needed a lumpectomy followed by eight weeks of chemotherapy and six weeks of five-times-per-week radiation. And since her breast cancer was estrogen-receptor positive, the doctor recommended that she take tamoxifen, an estrogen blocker, for five years after her treatments. Another oncologist advised her to get a radical mastectomy. Since she had only one positive lymph node out of twelve, she would need only six chemotherapy treatments and no radiation treatments. A third oncologist thought that since her one lymph node was barely positive, she needed only the six-week radiation treatment and not the chemotherapy. Each doctor wanted her to take tamoxifen for periods of three to five years. Some also suggested that she undergo genetic testing to see if she possessed the breast cancer gene, and if she tested positive, to consider double mastectomy even though her cancer was found only in one breast.

Joy was frightened and confused. She wanted to make the right decision for her kids, for her husband, for her parents, and for herself. She wanted to do everything she could to increase her chances of survival, but she was reluctant to cause unnecessary and potentially permanent damage to her health. She was scared to make the wrong decision, and she wanted to know my opinion. I explained to her that since each of the oncologists was reputable, they likely made their recommendations based on their clinical experience. The more aggressive the treatment method, the more likely that any remaining cancer cells would be permanently destroyed—a sort of insurance policy against recurrence. However, the more aggressive the therapy, the more injury there would be to the body.

. . . .

THE ROLE OF CHINESE MEDICINE IN CANCER CARE

SHE THEN WANTED TO KNOW WHAT I COULD DO to help combat the side effects of the treatments and minimize the damage. I told her that over most of my career in Chinese medicine, I had worked with oncologists to help patients improve their quality of life during and after anticancer treatments. I would use acupuncture to reduce the nausea, vomiting, and other gastric distress that often accompanies chemotherapy. Acupuncture also helps to increase energy and improve mood, sleep, and appetite. I would also advise patients on a diet plan to support the body during chemotherapy and an anticancer diet plan to prevent recurrence.

Further, since research done in China and Japan has confirmed the immune-stimulating properties of certain Chinese herbs, I would also formulate a synergistically combined herbal prescription to help support her immune functions and the production of red and white blood cells by the bone marrow. This herbal formula would also protect nerve endings, lessen fatigue, and improve concentration and memory. I explained that some herbs used in China have well-documented anticancer properties but aren't allowed to be used here without FDA approval. Finally I would teach her, or arrange for her to learn, meditation and qi gong exercises. Tens of thousands of cancer patients in China experience an increased sense of well-being and better control of their health and destiny with mind-body meditation and exercise. Chinese studies show that qi gong and tai chi stimulate the activities of lymphocytes, neutrophils, natural killer cells, and other immune cells that play a role in fighting cancer.

. . . .

CANCER WILL CHANGE YOUR LIFE—FOR THE BETTER

AS WE'VE SEEN, CHINESE MEDICINE doesn't consider the body to be separate from the mind. Physical ailments may have their origin in the

mind, and mental-emotional disorders may stem from physical imbalances. I asked Joy where she thought her cancer came from. At first
she wasn't sure what I meant. She repeated what her oncologists had
told her, which was essentially "unknown." I asked again, emphasiz-
ing that I wanted to know what she herself thought. Her eyes welled up
with tears and then came an outpouring of anger and resentment toward people in her life and her feeling of being helpless and trapped and
unable to do anything to change it. I let her talk for as long as she felt
comfortable sharing.

Afterward I explained to her that according to Chinese medicine,
the seed of cancer is planted by exposure to negativity, be it physical
toxins, a virus, or emotional stress such as the suppression of negative
emotions like anger and sadness, which block energy flow and, in turn,
force the energy to be expressed through the growth of abnormal cells
and tissues. I told her about a visualization meditation and a ritual that
would help release her pent-up feelings, and I suggested a psychotherapist who specializes in patients with cancer. Additionally, I talked
to Joy about cancer being a wake-up call for her to change her life so
that she would no longer be unhappy—cancer is her spirit screaming
that she is unhappy. Cancer can be empowering—it can provide the
courage and the impetus to make changes that people usually don't
make out of fear or apathy—like resolving a long-standing conflict with
another person or pursuing a dream that had become crushed under the
weight of an unfulfilling life.

At the end of her visit, Joy was noticeably more relaxed. Her face
had warmed to a subtle red glow. Since all three oncologists were highly
reputable and qualified, I encouraged her to work with the one she
could best communicate with and connect with. And when she decided on one, I advised her to trust the doctor implicitly and to embrace

his or her protocol 100 percent. She said she would make a final decision within the next week and return to see me the following week.

My parting words were that getting cancer would change her life forever, for the better.

. . . .

SUPPORTIVE STRATEGIES DURING CHEMOTHERAPY AND RADIATION

DURING OUR SECOND VISIT, I mapped out a treatment course for her based on the protocol she'd be undergoing. She decided to have only the cancerous lump removed, followed by chemotherapy and radiation, saving her breast. Her treatment plan with me included weekly acupuncture treatments before her surgery to help her immune system, after surgery to speed her recovery, and during chemotherapy and radiation. I gave her a diet plan to support her vital functions during the anticancer treatments, and I put together a customized formulation of herbs based on a number of criteria, including her age, constitution, the type of chemotherapy agent, and the length of her anticancer treatments.

Over the next nine months, Joy came in for her acupuncture and herbal treatments weekly—sometimes on the day after her chemotherapy, when she was throwing up and had lost her appetite. But consistently she reported that the acupuncture and the herbal therapy immediately made her feel much better. Often she would get off the acupuncture treatment table with a sense of well-being, in a better mood, and with more energy. Joy continued to work throughout her nine-month ordeal even though we discussed the virtue of having some downtime to rest and reevaluate her life. She felt strongly that by continuing to work she would have a reason to get up every day. Her white blood cells remained within normal range most of the time, and during the entire treatment she only had to receive one shot of Neupogen, a drug used to increase white blood cell production in the bone marrow to counter the immune-suppressing side effects of the chemo agents.

Although Joy did have a couple of emotional breakdowns in my office, her energy and outlook stayed strong through both chemotherapy and radiation. She was quite disciplined and followed her diet, acupuncture, and herbal therapies as prescribed. I encouraged her to reevaluate her life and to rediscover her life's purpose and what was important to her. I told her that all disease is simply symptomatic of life out of balance. She began to see a psychotherapist and to attend cancer support groups at the local Wellness Community and at her church.

. . . .

CANCER EMPOWERS POSITIVE CHANGES

ABOUT EIGHT MONTHS AFTER HER DIAGNOSIS, Joy came into my office and declared that she had decided to quit her job. She had come to the realization that her boss was emotionally abusive and that she was not nurturing herself by staying at her job. Since the breast is an organ that provides nourishment for a baby, she reasoned, the problem with her breast was symbolic of the fact that she had stopped nurturing herself a long time ago. This realization empowered her to make a change that she had been afraid to make for many years. Likewise, she began to make changes at home, carving out time for pottery and other interests, which she couldn't find time for before. Her kids became more responsible and engaged in their individual and family chores. Joy became more intimate with her husband, demanding and spending more quality time with him and the family. This is not to say that there weren't painful adjustments for Joy and others in her life, but the changes were well worth it, as evidenced by the increased happiness and fulfillment in her life.

After her second chemotherapy treatment, Joy came in with her head shaved and covered by a wig. That was a very sad day for her. She cried and was afraid that her hair would never come back. I assured her that her hair would come back, and I gave her an herbal hair tonic—a formula passed down through my family's medical lineage—to massage into her scalp daily. To her amazement, by the fifth month her hair began to grow back. One year after her diagnosis and three months after finishing her anticancer treatments, she stopped wearing her wig. Strangely, her hair was thicker and curlier than it had been before. I had never seen her so happy as the day, when her oncologist told her that she was free of cancer.

Around the middle of her treatment course, Joy received a big blow to her confidence. Her sister-in-law back East, who was also battling breast cancer, had died of complications. Joy sat in my treatment room that day, depressed and deflated, feeling that her efforts would be in vain and that she would lose the battle as well. I asked her to focus on herself one day at a time, and to think positively and believe in her innate powers. She had not been diligent in her meditation and qi gong practices up to this point, so I gently reminded her about the power of gaining self-control through these ancient practices. I then gave her an acupuncture treatment specifically to uplift her mood and energy. She left that day feeling more peaceful and positive in her outlook. The acupuncture helped regulate serotonin levels in her brain and released endorphins that elevated her mood instantly.

DEALING WITH INSTANT MENOPAUSE
AND THE LIFE THEREAFTER

AFTER THE NINE-MONTH ANTICANCER TREATMENT COURSE, Joy went on tamoxifen, which caused severe menopausal symptoms. The constant hot flashes, night sweats, frequent headaches, sleeplessness, and moodiness were sometimes unbearable. Joy had experienced artificial menopause earlier during her chemotherapy—her periods had abruptly stopped and the symptoms of menopause had begun. With acupuncture and herbal treatments, we managed to restore her periods. However, with the use of tamoxifen, which inhibited the production of estrogen in Joy's body, menopause was now in full rage. Joy continued to come in for acupuncture and herbal treatments twice monthly, and she kept up her dietary and qi gong practices for relief of her menopausal symptoms and prevention of breast cancer recurrence.

It has been seven years since Joy was first diagnosed with breast cancer. She continues to be cancer-free. She has started her own pottery business. Her kids are in college and she has become closer with her husband. Her relationships with others are more meaningful and she doesn't rush around like she used to. She takes time to smell the roses and to nurture herself. When I spoke to her last she said to me, "I didn't believe it when you first told me that my life would change for the better with cancer. But now I see what you mean. Getting cancer was truly a blessing in disguise for my life." Joy is more happy and fulfilled today, after surviving cancer, because she chose to approach it in a positive way. She used everything available to her to combat her disease. She was the beneficiary of a carefully implemented union of East and West, ancient and modern.

Joy's story is a powerful example of Chinese medicine working with Western medicine to battle a devasting disease. But the potential of integrative medicine goes beyond cancer care. Every day at Tao of Wellness in Santa Monica, California, our acupuncturists work with orthopedists on sports injury and pain management, with rheumatologists on arthritis and autoimmune diseases, with gynecologists on menstrual disorders and menopause, with reproductive endocrinologists on male and female infertility, with neurologists on Parkinson's disease and stroke complications, with endocrinologists on diabetes and thyroid disorders, with cardiologists on cardiac rehabilitation and hypertension, with gastroenterologists on gastric reflux disorder and irritable bowel syndrome, with mental health professionals on depression and anxiety disorders, with pulmonary and immunologists on asthma, allergies, and viral infections—with many kinds of doctors on many different health conditions.

The key to successful collaboration between Eastern and Western medicine is patient-centered focus—working together and doing what each medical tradition does best to serve the health and well-being of the patient. I see a model in which we first use the diagnostic technologies of Western medicine to determine the disease and the cause. Then, as the first line of treatment, we use the noninvasive, side-effect-free approaches of natural medicine like acupuncture, herbal and nutritional therapies, mind-body exercise, and bodywork that are offered by Chinese medicine. Finally, we bring in drugs and surgery and other biotechnological treatments as the situation calls for them. I am happy to see that an increasing number of integrative medicine centers and clinics are now being established, many with close ties to medical schools and teaching hospitals like Stanford, Harvard, Columbia, UCLA, and the Mayo Clinic. To me this represents the emergence of a new medical paradigm of patient-centered and wellness-promoting care.

PART 2

SELF-HEALING REMEDIES
FOR COMMON AILMENTS

ACNE

COMMONLY CALLED PIMPLES OR ZITS and universally disdained by teenagers and adults alike, acne occurs when skin follicles get blocked by the oil or sebum that normally drains to the surface of the skin. Sebum secretions increase with hormonal changes, especially around puberty, pregnancy, and menopause, and when the sebum is blocked it allows bacteria and yeast to grow, causing the skin to become inflamed and eventually resulting in acne.

The severity of the infection defines the characteristics of the acne. Whiteheads are secretions trapped beneath the skin; blackheads are the sebum breaking through the skin, colored black as a result of the body's natural pigment deposits; and cystic acne is characterized by severe pus-filled infections under the skin, which can be painful. Medical conditions like polycystic ovarian syndrome and adrenal or pituitary gland tumors also can cause acne. In severe cases, acne can lead to permanent scars.

I recall a teenage girl who had such severe acne on her back and face that she refused to go to the beach or to swim. She had used antibiotics and all kinds of topical cleansers and creams, as well as the drug Accutane, without success. Her acne hurt her self-image and brought on emotional problems. I treated her with diet and nutrition, topical and internal herbal therapy, and acupuncture. Her condition cleared up substantially after six months of treatment. I saw her mother recently, and she happily reported that her daughter is back to her outgoing self and has quite a social life now. To her credit, she stuck to the diet I recommended.

In Chinese medicine, the skin is controlled by the lungs; acne is commonly a sign of pathogenic heat in the lungs and intestines. So the Chinese approach to treating acne is to cool the heat, cleanse the lungs, detoxify the intestines, and externally heal the condition. Work with your dermatologist to find natural and effective treatments for your condition.

Here are my favorite home remedies.

✳ DIET ✳

• Eat plenty of squash, cucumbers, watermelon, winter melon, celery, carrots, cabbage, beet tops, dandelions, aloe vera, mulberry leaf, carrot tops, lettuce, potatoes, cherries, papaya, pears, persimmons, raspberries, buckwheat, alfalfa sprouts, millet, brown rice, mung beans, lentils, and split peas.

....

• Avoid excess sugar, dairy products, chocolate, caffeine, carbonated beverages, nuts, seeds, shellfish, and fatty, fried, and processed foods.

✳ HOME REMEDIES ✳

• To make a salve, chop 1 cucumber and blend with 2 tablespoons aloe gel. Apply externally, 3 to 5 times a day. Leave it on for 20 minutes, then wash it off. This is one of my favorite self-healing tips for quickly cooling the heat of inflammation.

....

• Apply 2 tablespoons plain organic yogurt to the affected area, 3 to 5 times a day. Leave it on for 20 minutes, then wash off.

....

• Make a tea with dandelion, carrot, and beet tops: Boil 1 bunch each of fresh dandelion greens, carrot tops, and beet tops in 4 cups of water for 20 minutes. Strain, and drink the liquid. Drink 3 cups a day.

....

• Drink 12 ounces lukewarm water mixed with 1 tablespoon honey every morning on an empty stomach to lubricate the intestines. If you don't move your bowels regularly, toxins end up either in the liver or the skin.

....

ACNE

• Boil 1/3 cup fresh or frozen raspberries in 2 cups water until reduced to 1/2 cup. Strain the juice and discard the raspberries. Keep the concentrate in a glass jar in the refrigerator. Use a cotton ball to soak up the juice and wash the affected area with this solution twice a day.

....

• For oozing, infected acne conditions, make a mask by mixing 1/2 cup pearl barley powder (found in Asian markets, online or Eastern medicine practitioners' offices) with just enough aloe vera gel or egg whites to make a paste. Cover the area with the paste, leave it on overnight, and wash it off when you wake up. Do this once a day for a week.

✳ DAILY SUPPLEMENTS ✳

• Taking up to 30 milligrams of zinc a day can help relieve the symptoms of acne.

....

• Vitamin A can help to reduce sebum production. Dosages should not be more than 5,000 IU a day to avoid potential side effects; the usual daily dose is 1,000 to 2,000 milligrams.

....

• Vitamin B_6 can be used to treat acne that worsens before a woman's period or at midcycle and it also helps alleviate PMS mood swings. You may take up to 100 milligrams daily, all month long, to combat PMS-related acne.

✳ HERBAL THERAPY ✳

• Herbs can be found in health food or vitamin stores, online, and at the offices of Chinese medicine practitioners. Herbs should be used according to individual needs; consult with a licensed practitioner for a customized formulation. To learn more about the herbs listed here, go to www.askdrmao.com.

....

• A traditional Chinese herbal remedy consisting of siler, rhubarb, peony, angelica, astragalus, and other herbs is used in China to relieve acne. The formula can be obtained online, in Chinese herbal stores, and acupuncturists' offices, under the name Fang Feng Tong Sheng San.

• You may benefit from a one-week cleansing diet based on our Tao of Wellness Cleansing and Detoxification Program, which includes fresh vegetable juices and broths, herbal therapy, body brushing, Tui Na lymphatic massage, acupuncture, cupping (which uses suction cups to stimulate circulation), far-infrared sauna, and mind-body exercises. Many acupuncturists offer a similar treatment. Log on to taoofwellness.com for more information.

• Tea tree oil applied to acne lesions can be used to help eliminate bacteria and reduce inflammation. Tea tree oil contains a compound called terpinen-4-ol, which is responsible for its antimicrobial activity. A 5 percent tea tree oil solution can be made by mixing 1 part tea tree oil to 19 parts water and using it as a skin cleanser. Oregano oil, which is antimicrobial, can also be used in this manner.

─────────────── ❋ EXERCISE ❋ ───────────────

Cardiovascular exercise, like brisk walking, biking, or running, can help increase circulation and boost skin immunity. Perspiration can help unblock pores and follicles, so sebum can be discharged. Make sure to wash right after exercising to keep the skin clean.

Doing exercises that affect the body's energy channels can help to drain excess heat from the skin. I've taught the following Liver Cleansing Qi Gong sequence to my patients with acne problems, with good results.

Stand with your feet shoulder-width apart in front of a tree. On an inhale, raise your right leg, then exhale and place your right foot on the ground in front of you between your body and the tree.

Inhale, and raise both arms out from the sides until they come together over your head. Exhale, and lower your hands in front of your face. Visualize green light running down your face as your hands move down to your chest.

ACNE

Inhale, and move your hands to the right rib cage over your liver. Exhale, and move your arms down the right side of your abdomen and right leg, as if pushing down and out with your hands. Visualize the green light moving the toxins out of the liver and down the liver meridian on the inside of your right leg and out of the big toe.

The tree is a receptacle of liver energy and is capable of regenerating itself, similar to the way it can absorb toxic carbon dioxide and produce oxygen.

--- ✳ ACUPRESSURE ✳ ---

• Place your left hand on your chest and locate the acupoint Winding Gulch (LI-11), at the end of the skin crease in the right elbow. Apply moderate pressure with your left thumb. Hold for 1 minute. Repeat on the left elbow. Alternate sides for a total of 10 minutes each day. This is traditionally used to clear heat and toxins from the body.

. . . .

• Find the acupoint Inner Court (ST-44), in the web between the second and third toes of your right foot. With your right index finger and thumb, pinch the web between the two toes. Hold for 3 to 5 minutes, then repeat on the left foot.

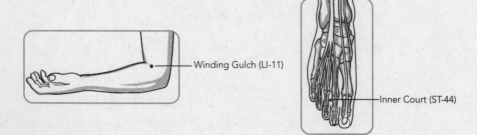

Winding Gulch (LI-11)

Inner Court (ST-44)

--- AVOID ---

• Medications such as birth control pills, steroids, and psychotropic drugs, which can trigger acne or make it worse.

. . . .

• Stress, the use of chemical cosmetic, skin, and hair care products. Extra weight, since being overweight can also make acne worse.

• Resting your chin in your hands, picking and touching your face, pressing a cell phone to your face, or nesting your face in your pillow at night. Also avoid biting your nails, which introduces bacteria to the skin around your mouth.

ALLERGIES

THE HUMAN IMMUNE SYSTEM is designed to identify and combat matter that is foreign to the body. In most circumstances it performs this duty very well, protecting you from bacteria, viruses, and other potentially harmful substances. But throughout the last century, our immune systems have been overwhelmed with chemicals and pesticides, not to mention the stresses of modern life. As a result, our immune systems have become oversensitive.

When the immune system overreacts to a pathogen or particle, it mobilizes with full force, producing severe inflammation and allergic symptoms. Allergies were first identified in Western medical literature at the turn of the twentieth century when doctors began to notice that some people were more sensitive to dust or pollen than others. Today allergies in various forms affect over 50 million Americans, and that number is on the rise. In addition to respiratory symptoms, allergies may show up as eczema, rashes, and digestive disturbances.

In recent years I've seen an increasing number of people who have suddenly developed allergies. I see many allergy sufferers here in Los Angeles, the city with the worst air quality in the nation. But many others fly in from high-allergy areas of the country such as Phoenix, Atlanta, and Virginia seeking treatment. One patient from Phoenix typical of the trend suffered from allergic rhinitis, a type of sinus inflammation, and eczema for over ten years. He had received allergy shots, and he used antihistamines, decongestants, and steroid creams without consistent relief. After eliminating dairy, wheat, and corn from his diet and undergoing a course of acupuncture and herbal therapy, he has been allergy free for the past six years.

In Chinese medicine, the immune system relies heavily on the lung network or respiratory system. The lungs are responsible for managing the defensive energies of the body, which protect you against foreign invaders and nourish the skin. If the lung network is not nourished properly, or if its energy is weak, the immune system becomes debilitated. Nourishment for the lung network comes from the spleen or digestive system, so an appropriate diet is critical for treating allergies. When I treat allergies, I focus on getting the immune system to work properly by restoring balance in the digestive and respiratory systems. Acupuncture, herbal therapy, and specially tailored diets are essential for achieving a healthy functioning immune system.

Here are some recommendations I make to my patients.

✳ DIET ✳

• A wholesome, seasonally balanced diet rich in soluble fiber and complex carbohydrates can help maintain good respiratory health and vitality of defensive qi. Incorporate more whole grains, including quinoa, brown rice, and millet into your diet. Eat more cabbage, beets, beet tops, carrots, and yams. Papaya, cranberries, pears, pineapple, wild cherries, mangoes, and citrus fruits such as grapefruit and limes also help. Green leafy vegetables such as spinach and kale contain essential nutrients for healthy immunity, as does broccoli. Ginger, onions, basil, garlic, bamboo shoots, black mushrooms, dandelions greens, and chrysanthemum flowers help fight inflammation. Vegetables need to be thoroughly washed in running water to remove residues of pesticides and chemicals. Water intake is essential for proper lymphatic drainage, so increase your water intake to 80 ounces a day—that's ten 8-ounce cups. Avoid cold water—drink it either hot or warm.

• Avoid foods that produce mucus and dampness, including dairy products, cold raw foods, greasy foods, and simple sugars such as white sugar and bleached flour. Wheat, chocolate, shellfish, potatoes, tomatoes, and eggplant may overstimulate the immune response and should be eaten in moderation. Soft drinks and most fruit juices have a high content of corn syrup, which produces dampness and mucus.

• Short of performing an exhaustive allergy test, you can try rotating your foods by waiting at least four days before repeating any one food item. For example, if you eat wheat bread on Monday, don't eat it again for at least four days. Eat brown rice on Tuesday, millet on Wednesday, oats on Thursday, and, if you like, eat wheat products again on Friday. This will reduce your body's allergy burden immediately and substantially.

❋ HOME REMEDIES ❋

• One of the key factors in treating allergies is eliminating the substances that overstimulate the immune system. Our homes, cars, and workplaces need to be free of these substances. Dehumidify and aerate your home regularly, and use the air conditioner and central heater sparingly, as they tend to permeate the home with the dust and particles collected in their ducts. Fungal colonies, dust mites, and pollen can collect in the house, so clean the floors regularly, and consider opting for solid wood or stone floors rather than carpet, as carpet collects enormous amounts of dust and bacteria. To prevent mold, use vinegar to disinfect surfaces that tend to get wet or damp.

• Pets shouldn't be allowed free reign in the home. Beds, bedrooms, and couches should be off limits.

ALLERGIES

• Drink green tea and chamomile tea—they both contain natural antihistamines and can help balance the immune system.

. . . .

• Steep 2 slices of fresh ginger in a cup of boiling water for 5 minutes; drink this tea twice a day.

. . . .

• Eating 1 teaspoon of local, unfiltered, and unprocessed honey daily can do wonders for allergies.

—————————————— ✳ DAILY SUPPLEMENTS ✳ ——————————————

• Taking up to 10,000 IU of beta-carotene can help balance the immune system.

. . . .

• Vitamin B$_6$ (30 milligrams), pantothenic acid (300 milligrams), and vitamin's C (1,000 milligrams), D (800 IU), and Vitamin E (800 IU) help maintain a healthy immune system.

. . . .

• Taking 500 milligrams of the enzyme bromelain and of the antioxidant quercetin daily can help modulate histamine release, the function that causes the allergic response.

. . . .

• Selenium (100 micrograms) is useful for reducing inflammation caused by chemical allergies.

. . . .

• Probiotics (3 to 5 billion organisms), with their benefits for intestinal flora, are essential in protecting against allergic reactions.

—————————————— ✳ HERBAL THERAPY ✳ ——————————————

• Herbs can be found in health food or vitamin stores, online, and at the offices of Chinese medicine practitioners. Herbs should be used according to individual needs; consult with a licensed practitioner for a customized formulation. To learn more about the herbs listed here, go to www.askdrmao.com.

. . . .

• Mint, echinacea, licorice, chamomile, rose hips, fenugreek, elderberry, and black cumin help maintain a healthy and balanced immune system.

....

• Magnolia flowers, xanthium, mint, dandelion, Chinese basil, siler root, and schizandra all have allergy-reducing properties.

....

• Our Chinese herbal formula Allergy Tamer is a formula from my family used to relieve allergy symptoms and balance the immune system.

❊ EXERCISE ❊

In addition to strengthening the body against infection and illness, exercise also helps regulate immune function. Simple cardiovascular exercise such as a brisk walk (2 to 3 miles per hour) for 30 minutes a day or a more intense aerobic workout can help improve circulation and strengthen the body.

Massaging the Wind Pond Acupoint (GB-20) is a simple exercise to help harmonize the immune system. Sit at the tip of a sturdy chair with your back erect, spine stretched, and head tilted slightly forward. Keep your legs at a comfortable distance, forming a 90-degree angle.

As you inhale, using your thumbs press and massage the Wind Pond acupoint located in the natural indentation at the base of the skull on both sides of your neck, tilting your head slightly upward.

Exhale, and massage the point as you bend forward at the waist, tilting your head forward. Bend only as far as you comfortably can do so. Continue breathing and massaging for 30 to 60 seconds.

On an exhale, return to the original position while continuing to massage the Wind Pond point.

You can do this exercise anytime during the day—It's great to counter lack of energy and fatigue.

❊ ACUPRESSURE ❊

• For immediate relief from sinus allergies, locate the acupoint Welcome Fragrance (LI-20), on either side of your nose, where your nose and cheek meet. This is traditionally used to open nasal passages. Apply moderate pressure with both index fingers, one on each side of the nose. Take deep, slow breaths and continue pressing for 3 minutes.

• Locate the acupoint Wind Pond, in the natural indentation at the base of your skull on either side of your neck. Press and lift up toward the base of your skull with your thumbs and lean your head back. Use the weight of your head against your thumbs to apply steady pressure. Breathe deeply and slowly and continue pressing for about 5 minutes.

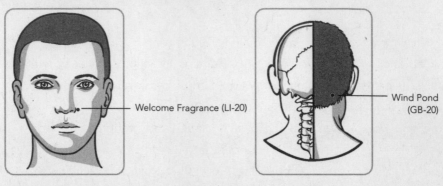

Welcome Fragrance (LI-20)

Wind Pond (GB-20)

— AVOID —

• Extreme temperature and weather fluctuations by dressing and protecting yourself appropriately.

• Exposure to substances and circumstances that cause allergies, including dusty, dirty, and polluted environments. Use a respiratory mask if necessary.

• Stress and exhaustion, as they weaken the immune system. Get plenty of sleep and relaxation.

• Alcohol, smoking, and drugs.

 ARTERIAL PLAQUE

THE RESULT OF PLAQUE FORMATION in the arteries is a hardening of the blood vessels also known as atherosclerosis. This plaque is made up of cholesterol crystals and calcium deposits. Over time arterial plaque causes narrowing of the arteries, impairing blood flow. Accumulation of plaque can also lead to an aneurysm—the bulging and rupturing of a blood vessel, causing internal bleeding. Atherosclerosis is commonplace today, a result of stressful lifestyle combined with poor eating habits.

Unfortunately, because arterial plaque has no outward symptoms and signs, the condition is often discovered too late—with devastating consequences. In the United States in 2004 the first symptom of atherosclerosis experienced by 65 percent of men and 47 percent of women who had it was either heart attack or sudden death. A routine blood test for C-reactive protein (CRP) can reveal inflammation and potential plaque dangers. Metabolic disorders such as diabetes, blood sugar intolerance, high blood cholesterol, stress, obesity, inflammation, and high blood pressure can put you at risk for high levels of arterial plaque.

In Chinese medicine, we examine our patients through tongue and pulse diagnostic techniques. I recall seeing a young man in his late thirties who appeared to be in good health. When I examined his tongue, though, I saw that it was purplish with bulging veins underneath. His pulse was choppy, which indicated obstruction of blood flow. Because of family history—his father died of a heart attack at age forty-five— I sent him to a cardiologist for a full cardiovascular workup. His chest CT scan showed that he had 65 percent occlusion or obstruction in his main coronary artery, the artery that supplies the muscles of the heart. In his case, diet and emotions played key roles in causing the obstruction of energy and blood flow.

In my approach to treating plaque buildup, I activate circulation and work to reduce inflammation with acupuncture, reduce dampness and mucus through diet and nutritional therapy, and reduce plaque and cholesterol with Chinese herbal therapy and exercise.

Effective stress reduction is essential for promoting good cardiovascular health—I recommend meditation and tai chi.

Here are some of my favorite home remedies to help maintain good cardiovascular health and clean arteries. If you experience severe pain in the chest, radiating to the shoulders or down the left arm, or severe shortness of breath, go to the emergency room immediately—these symptoms may signal a cardiac emergency.

❋ DIET ❋

• Eat whole grains containing a fiber-rich bran layer such as whole oats and brown rice—the fiber traps and eliminate cholesterol from your intestines. Eat smaller meals more frequently. Favor green leafy vegetables, whole grains, brown rice, black and white fungus (soak in water, then cook like vegetables), Chinese black dates, peanuts, vinegar, celery, seaweed, cassia seeds (make tea), lotus root, jellyfish (soak in water and cook), chrysanthemums (make tea), hawthorn berries, water chestnuts, mung beans, pearl barley, peach kernels, ginger, soybeans, sprouted vegetables, wheat bran, bananas, watermelon, sunflower seeds, lotus seeds, black sesame seeds, garlic, and green tea. Drink at least six 8-ounce glasses of room temperature water a day.

• Avoid foods with preservatives, additives, and pesticides. Refrain from eating foods that are fried, greasy, and spicy; simple carbohydrates, including sugars and white flour; sodium; and MSG. Alcohol, coffee, and tobacco should be avoided, as should cheese and aged, cured meats.

❋ HOME REMEDIES ❋

• Make a glass of asparagus juice with pulp by blending 4 to 6 fresh asparagus spears and 1 cup water in a blender, and add 1 teaspoon honey. Drink twice a day for 1 month to show cholesterol-lowering effects. The rich supply of B vitamins and the potent antioxidant glutathione in the asparagus helps reduce cholesterol and inflammation.

• Take alternating hot and cold showers to help stimulate circulation. Start slowly with hot and lukewarm showers, alternating every 3 minutes. Over 4 weeks gradually increase the temperature difference to hot and cold.

• Make a tea by steeping 1 tablespoon green tea, 1 tablespoon dried chrysanthemum flowers, and 1 tablespoon ground cinnamon in 3 cups of boiling water for 10 minutes. Strain, and drink at least 3 cups every day to help prevent arterial plaque.

❋ DAILY SUPPLEMENTS ❋

• Taking niacin (300 milligrams) can lower total cholesterol levels by 18 percent on average over 6 months.

• Taking coenzyme Q_{10} (50 milligrams) increases oxygen supply to the heart.

• Taking magnesium citrate (2,000 milligrams) along with calcium (1,000 milligrams) works as a natural calcium blocker, useful for preventing and assisting in the treatment of heart disease.

• Taking fish oil supplements (at least 1,000 milligrams omega-3 essential fatty acids) helps to reduce inflammation in the blood vessels.

❋ HERBAL THERAPY ❋

• Herbs can be found in health food or vitamin stores, online, and at the offices of Chinese medicine practitioners. Herbs should be used according to individual needs; consult with a licensed practitioner for a customized formulation. To learn more about the herbs listed here, go to www.askdrmao.com.

• Salvia, peach kernel, red peony, safflower, ginger, cinnamon, and hawthorn berry can help stimulate circulation in the chest and support healthy cholesterol.

• To support healthy cardiovascular function, you can try my herbal tea beverage Ancient Treasures Tea, which includes hawthorn berry, chrysanthemum, motherwort, and other select Chinese herbs to regulate cholesterol and circulation and promote tranquility. Steep tea bag in boiling water; drink 3 cups a day. Order at www.askdrmao.com.

✳ EXERCISE ✳

Exercise is essential for promoting circulation and strengthening heart function. Thirty minutes of cardiovascular exercise every day will increase blood flow, optimize oxygen supply to the heart, and reduce arterial tension. It's important to get your heart rate above 110 beats per minute to promote blood flow and improve circulation. Exercise also helps reduce cholesterol by increasing HDL—the good cholesterol. Swimming and brisk walking are both good choices.

Energy exercises like tai chi and the Eight Treasures Qi Gong have been found to improve cardiovascular health. In fact, doing an arm swing warm-up to tai chi and the Eight Treasures Qi Gong can make a noticeable difference. Here I describe the arm swing warm-up:

Start with your feet shoulder-width apart. Freely swing your arms from front to back until you reach a point of natural resistance. Now let your arms swing to the front again.

After a couple of minutes of arm swinging, increase the workout by bending your knees and lifting your heels as your arms swing back and forth. Then increase the workout further by jumping off the ground as your arms swing back, as if the momentum of your arms swinging were carrying your body upward, jumping progressively higher each time for 5 minutes. Swing your arms for 10 to 15 minutes, then gradually slow down and stop.

Do this exercise twice a day.

✳ ACUPRESSURE ✳

• For a general acupressure treatment for a healthy heart, locate the acupoint Gate of Spirit (HE-7), on the palm side of your right hand at the end of the wrist crease below the little finger. This is traditionally used to strengthen heart function and calm spirit. Apply moderate pressure with your left thumb. Hold for 5 minutes. Repeat on the left hand.

• Locate the acupoint Great Surge (LIV-3), in the natural indentation on the top of your right foot between the big and first toes. Apply moderate pressure with your right thumb for 5 minutes. Repeat on the left foot. This point is traditionally used to release all types of blockages.

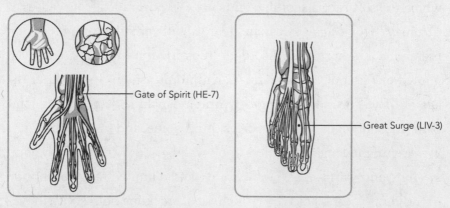

Gate of Spirit (HE-7)

Great Surge (LIV-3)

AVOID

• Sedentary lifestyle and stress, as they increase the risk of heart problems and also cause other disorders such as obesity and diabetes, which worsen cardiovascular problems.

• Cavities and dental plaque—make sure to see your dentist on a regular basis. Poor dental health can contribute to inflammation in the blood vessels, leading to arterial plaque buildup.

• Smoking and exposure to secondhand smoke, as they contribute to hardening of the arteries.

ARTHRITIS

ARTHRITIS

ARTHRITIS IS A CONDITION in which chronic swelling and inflammation damage joints. It is currently the leading cause of disability in people above the age of sixty-five. Of the many forms of arthritic conditions—including rheumatoid, psoriatic, and gout-related arthritis—osteoarthritis (OA) is the most common form, affecting at least 21 million Americans.

Unlike rheumatoid arthritis, in which there is an active inflammatory process occurring at the joints, OA is a degenerative disease in which the soft cartilage of the joints is slowly degraded. The causes of OA may involve aging, wear and tear, genetic predisposition, obesity, metabolic and hormonal disorders, repetitive-use injuries, and even gout. The onset of OA is gradual. Symptoms usually appear after the age of fifty. The most common symptoms include deep, aching joint pain (most often in the back, knees, hips, spine, and fingers) that gets worse with movement, stiffness upon waking and with inactivity, joint swelling and warmth, and inflexibility and a limited range of motion in the joints accompanied by crunching or crackling noises with movement. In severe cases abnormal bony growths, such as bumps on the outermost finger joints, may be present. One of the best preventive measures for OA is exercise and weight loss. Research has shown that with regular moderate exercise, pain and inflexibility can be reduced by at least 25 percent.

Inflammation produced by a faulty immune system can lead to rheumatoid or psoriatic arthritis. The causes of the immune reaction are unknown. However, clinical observations suggest pathogens, environmental toxins, and emotional stress (when coupled with genetic predispositions) as the most likely triggers.

According to Chinese medicine theory there are several disease factors that can cause arthritis. These include cold invading the joints, pathogenic wind disturbing the joints, dampness congealing in the joints, and heat scorching the joints. Chinese medicine categorizes arthritic conditions into four types based on their symptom presentation: cold, wind, damp and heat.

• Cold arthritis symptoms include sharp, stabbing pain in fixed locations and coldness in the joints. The pain is relieved by heat. These individuals usually have a pale complexion.

• Wind arthritis manifests with pain that shifts locations, comes and goes suddenly, and sometimes causes dizziness—behaving much like the wind.

• Damp arthritis symptoms include sluggishness, heavy sensations in the extremities, swelling, obesity, and dull, deep lingering pain.

• Heat arthritis is characterized by red, swollen, painful joints that are warm to the touch, and general disability. These symptoms often occur suddenly.

Sometimes these condition types can be seen together, as in the cases of dampness and heat or dampness and cold.

I work with rheumatologists and orthopedists and have seen many patients with arthritis. My approach focuses on proper differentiation of the type of arthritis according to Chinese medicine and then modulating the immune system—by reducing excess or nourishing deficiency—to support healthy immune function. Acupuncture works well in managing pain and inflammation, while herbal and nutritional therapies nurture the healing process. Tai chi and qi gong exercises help strengthen the joints.

Here are my recommendations according to arthritic type:

———————————————— ✳ DIET ✳ ————————————————
• Diet for cold arthritis should include heat-dispersing foods such as green onions, garlic, bell peppers, mustard greens, ginger, black beans, sesame

seeds, grapes, grapevines, parsnips, spices such as turmeric, fennel, anise, and horseradish, and organic chicken and lamb. Rice wine can also be helpful, but avoid it if you have high blood pressure. Avoid cold foods, raw fruits and vegetables, and exposure to cold environments.

• Diet for wind arthritis should favor scallions, grapes, grapevines, mulberries, mulberry vine tea (garden cuttings), black beans, whole grains, and green leafy vegetables. Nonpoisonous snake meat is a great food remedy for wind arthritis. Snake meat can be found in Asian markets and certain specialty restaurants. Avoid other meat, shellfish, sugars, alcohol, smoking, and other stimulants.

• Damp arthritis sufferers should consume more barley, mung beans, mustard greens, red adzuki beans, millet, brown and sweet rice, cornsilk tea, and bland and diuretic foods. Avoid cold foods, raw fruits and vegetables, dairy products, and exposure to damp environments.

• Heat arthritis requires cooling and heat-reducing foods such as fresh fruits and vegetables, dandelion greens, cabbage, mung beans, winter melon, soybeans, and soybean sprouts. Avoid spicy foods, alcohol, smoking, stress, and warming foods such as green onions. Tomatoes and eggplants may exacerbate the inflammation and should be avoided as well.

✳ HOME REMEDIES ✳

• For cold arthritis, make a tea by boiling 5 3-inch sticks of grapevines and 2 slices of ginger in 3 1/2 cups water for 20 minutes. Strain. Drink the tea 3 times a day for 2 to 4 weeks. Also try boiling 1/2 cup chopped parsnip, 3 grams cinnamon, 1 gram of black pepper, and 3 grams dried ginger in 2 cups of water. Strain. Drink twice a day for 1 month.

• For wind arthritis, boil 1/4 cup chopped scallions in 2 cups of water. Strain. Drink the tea 3 times daily for 1 to 2 weeks. Boil 1 bunch of Chinese parsley in 3 1/2 cups water for 20 minute. Strain.

• For damp arthritis, cook 1/3 cup each of soaked mung beans, pearl barley, and red adzuki beans for 1 hour in 4 cups of water and eat daily for 1 month. Cornsilk tea is also beneficial for damp arthritis. Boil 1 handful of cornsilk in 3 1/2 cups water for 20 minutes. Strain. Drink 3 cups a day.

• For heat arthritis, boil 1 cup each of dandelion greens and peppermint leaves in 3 1/2 cups water for 30 minutes. Strain. Drink 3 times a day. You may also apply a crushed whole dandelion poultice to the affected joints, changing every two hours. Make a poultice by macerating the leaves in a mortar with a pestle until mashed.

• I often recommend an innovative physical treatment involving far-infrared saunas. The far-infrared spectrum of light is often called the "golden light of life," as it mimics the energy frequencies of healthy cells. When the infrared light penetrates deep into the body it stimulates the cells into dumping toxic waste products into the bloodstream, and they are eventually eliminated through sweat. The deep heating also stimulates the cells' regenerative mechanisms and warms the tissues.

———————————— ✳ DAILY SUPPLEMENTS ✳ ————————————

• Taking glucosamine sulfate (1000 milligrams) and chondroitin sulfate (400 milligrams) together has been shown in trials to reduce symptoms of OA, and to help regenerate the affected joints.

• Taking S-adenosyl methionine (SAMe; 1200 milligrams) is a better choice than nonsteroidal anti-inflammatory and pain medications, as it has far fewer side effects.

• Supplementing with Vitamin D (400 IU) can prevent breakdown of cartilage, and Vitamins A (200 IU), E (800 IU), and C (1,000 milligrams) are good sources of antioxidants to prevent further damage to the joints.

• Taking niacinamide (a form of vitamin B₃; 250 to 500 milligrams) can increase range of motion and reduce the need for pain medications.

• Omega-3 fatty acids (1,000 milligrams EPA; 800 milligrams DHA) can help with joint stiffness. Manganese (25 milligrams), bromelain (450 milligrams), and boron (3 milligrams) also provide some benefit.

───────────── ✳ HERBAL THERAPY ✳ ─────────────

• Herbs can be found in health food or vitamin stores, online, and at the offices of Chinese medicine practitioners. Herbs should be used according to individual needs; consult with a licensed practitioner for a customized formulation. To learn more about the herbs listed here, go to www.ask drmao.com.

• White willow bark, black cohosh, sarsaparilla, guaiacum resin, aspen bark, boswellia, and turmeric are useful for arthritic pain management. Taking ginger twice a day can also help alleviate arthritic pain and inflammation.

• Capsaicin cream (derived from hot chiles) is a good topical for relieving the pain and discomfort of arthritis.

• Traditional Chinese herbs used to manage arthritis include pubescent angelica root, siler, gentiana, mulberry, eucommia, achyranthes, cinnamon, cnidium, rehmannia, peony, ginseng, poria, and licorice.

───────────── ✳ EXERCISE ✳ ─────────────

As mentioned above, one of the best preventive measures for degenerative joint and bone disorders is exercise. Exercise can help strengthen the joints and bones and stimulate the body's regeneration mechanisms. When it's difficult to engage in strenuous exercise due to pain, soreness, and inflexibility, I recommend tai chi or qi gong. In my clinic I teach a form known as the Eight Treasures Qi Gong, a 30-minute daily practice that has been clinically shown to strengthen bones and joints and prevent arthritis, and that has been passed down through my family. The entire form can be learned quickly and is far less stressful and strenuous than other types of physical exercises, with much greater benefits, as it emphasizes stretching and the strengthening of joints, tendons, and muscles. Most licensed practitioners of Chinese medicine are able to teach these exercises and can help you learn and practice qi gong or tai chi. Learn the Eight Treasures and other qi gong at chihealth.org.

✳ ACUPRESSURE ✳

• Make a loose fist with your right hand and find the acupoint Back Stream (SI-3), on the outer side (pinkie side) of the right hand just behind and below the knuckle of the pinkie. Press with your left index finger until you feel soreness. Hold for 3 minutes. Repeat on the left hand.

• Find the acupoint Kunlun Mountains (UB-60), between the outer ankle-bone and the Achilles' tendon on your right foot. Pinch it with your thumb and index finger for 3 minutes. Repeat on the left foot.

• Activating both of these points is good for relaxing and strengthening the tendons, joints, and muscles.

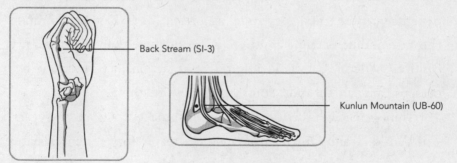

Back Stream (SI-3)

Kunlun Mountain (UB-60)

AVOID

• Smoking and consuming excess alcohol, as doing so can deplete the body of vital nutrients needed for joint health.

• Obesity and inactivity, as they are key risk factors in developing arthritic disorders. Studies show that shedding just 10 percent of total body weight can produce healthful effects.

• Stress, worry, and tension, as they irritate the immune system and can trigger autoimmune reactions that injure tissues.

ASTHMA

ASTHMA IS A CHRONIC LUNG DISORDER in which the walls of the airways become inflamed, often as a result of exposure to environmental triggers. The immune response causes swelling of the bronchial tubes and production of excessive mucus from the bronchial walls, causing the tubes to narrow and blocking the passage of air. Symptoms range from mild wheezing, shortness of breath, chest tightness, and cough to potentially life-threatening conditions in which the prolonged constriction of the airways reduces oxygen supply to the body. An estimated 20 million Americans suffer from asthma and every day 5,000 patients visit the emergency room as a result. It is the most common chronic condition among children, affecting more than one in twenty children. Allergies, chronic respiratory infections, and immune hypersensitivity are the most common causes of asthma.

Chinese medicine has been used for asthma for thousands of years. The World Health Organization includes respiratory system diseases such as asthma and bronchitis on its list of the forty diseases that can benefit from acupuncture. There have been many studies demonstrating how successful acupuncture and Chinese herbs are in the treatment of asthma. In 1993, for example, the Department of Anesthesia and Intensive Care at the University Hospital of Vienna, Austria, conducted a study that showed that after ten weeks of acupuncture treatments, over 70 percent of longstanding asthma patients achieved significant improvement.

I have worked in conjunction with many pulmonary specialists on asthma patients. My treatment plan works to balance the immune system, reduce allergic reactions, eliminate excess mucus, and increase lung capacity. I incorporate Chinese herbs, acupuncture, and specialized qi gong exercises to achieve these results. Below are some of my recommendations. It is important to have regular medical checkups and to be aware of asthma triggers to prevent potentially life-threatening attacks. Do not stop your asthma medications unless supervised by your physician.

 ✳ DIET ✳

• Being overweight or obese can be a contributing factor in developing asthma. A diet rich in complex carbohydrates, low in fat, and moderate in protein is recommended. During remission it is important to nourish the lungs by incorporating into your diet more tomatoes, carrots, green leafy vegetables, green and yellow bell peppers, yams, pumpkin, winter melon, squash, figs, daikon radish, mustard greens, sesame seeds, walnuts, almonds, apricot kernels (eaten raw like nuts), basil, tangerines, litchi fruit, loquats, and honey. Studies show that eating apples regularly can protect against asthma. Drink plenty of warm or room temperature water.

• Reduce or eliminate foods containing arachidonic acids, found in shellfish, meats, and egg yolks, which can trigger asthma. Avoid foods that produce mucus, including dairy products (especially ice cream), wheat, corn, cold and raw foods, watermelon, bananas, salty foods, and soda and other sweet foods containing simple processed sugars.

✳ HOME REMEDIES ✳

• Take hot baths with Epsom salts daily, and take alternating hot and cold showers. Start slowly and gradually increase the change in temperature over time.

• Make a hot mustard chest compress by warming up 1 tablespoon prepared mustard. Apply to your entire chest, then cover with a hot towel for 15 minutes. Repeat 2 to 3 times a day when there is a flare-up.

• Drink 3 cups of honey-vinegar water daily: Combine 1 tablespoon apple cider vinegar and 1 tablespoon raw comb honey with 1 cup of hot water.

• Make a tea by boiling 1 clove of fresh garlic in 3 1/2 cups water for 10 minutes. Strain, and drink 3 cups daily.

❋ DAILY SUPPLEMENTS ❋

• Both EPA (eicosapentaenoic acid; 1000 milligrams) from fish oil and GLA (gamma-linolenic acid; 400 milligrams) from borage or evening primrose oil help to reduce arachidonic acid in the body.

• Supplementing with Vitamin C (1,000 milligrams) can help counter inflammation.

• Quercetin (200 milligrams) acts similarly to many asthma medications, inhibiting the inflammatory response.

• Vitamin B complex, including B_6 and B_{12}, has been shown to act like an antihistamine and to ease childhood asthma.

❋ HERBAL THERAPY ❋

• Herbs can be found in health food or vitamin stores, online, and at the offices of Chinese medicine practitioners. Herbs should be used according to individual needs; consult with a licensed practitioner for a customized formulation. To learn more about the herbs listed here, go to www.ask drmao.com.

- Several Chinese herbs are known bronchodilators, including ginkgo seeds, ephedra, schizonepetae, perilla leaf, white mustard seed, platycodon, and Chinese chive bulbs.

....

- White mustard seeds, perilla seeds, and radish seeds can be used to reduce mucus.

....

- Mullein, magnolia, and albizzia can be used as decongestants and to treat allergic reactions.

✳ EXERCISE ✳

Do not exercise during an asthma attack, as exercising will worsen the situation. Calm and rest are important. Sitting or walking calmly in fresh air can help. During remission, moderate physical exercise like walking can be integrated. For children and adults alike, swimming can help increase lung capacity. I recommend daily qi gong exercises to strengthen the body, open the lungs, and improve lung capacity. Performing the Eight Treasures Qi Gong movements daily for 30 minutes can improve overall health. The second movement of the practice, called Great Bird Spreads Its Wings, is targeted to the lungs. Perform this exercise twice daily for best results.

In a quiet, comfortable environment, preferably outdoors, stand with your feet shoulder-width apart, knees slightly bent, spine erect, tailbone tucked in, and head tilted slightly forward. Let your arms hang by your sides, with your shoulders relaxed.

Begin to breathe in a rhythmic, slow, and relaxed fashion. Inhale deeply but softly, and imagine the breath extending all the way down to the lower abdomen, about two finger-widths below the navel. Exhale gently and softly. Stay in this position for 7 breath cycles, relaxing and calming your mind.

To begin the exercise, on an inhale, bend down from your waist, letting your hands hang between your legs. Exhale and begin gently swaying your arms back and forth like a pendulum. Your arms should be totally

ASTHMA

relaxed and making a rhythmic and gentle motion. Sway your hands back and forth 3 times.

Inhale, raise your torso back to the standing position, and raise your arms to your chest, bringing energy to the chest area. Bend your knees more deeply, putting yourself into a squatting position.

Exhale, and spread your arms with your palms facing out to both sides, pushing out to the left and right. As you exhale, push your hands out 3 times. Repeat the exercise 7 times, then return to the starting standing posture. Place your hands on your lower abdomen, palms down, one hand overlapping the other. Rub your lower abdomen 7 times in small, clockwise circles just below the navel.

--------------------- ❋ ACUPRESSURE ❋ ---------------------

• Find the acupoint Cubit Marsh (LU-5): Bend your right arm at the elbow and locate the point in the elbow crease, on the outer side of the large tendon in the middle of the crease. Apply moderate pressure with your left thumb until you feel soreness. Hold for 2 minutes. Repeat on the left arm.

....

• Locate the Asthma Relief (Dingchuan) acupoints on the upper back— there are two points located one finger-width to either side of the large bony structure at the base of the neck (seventh cervical vertebra). Apply steady pressure with your index fingers until you feel soreness. Hold for 3 minutes.

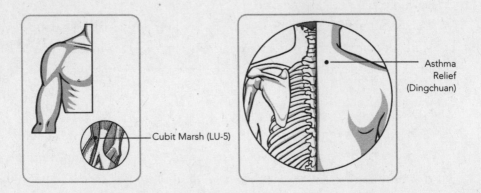

Cubit Marsh (LU-5)

Asthma Relief (Dingchuan)

• Excessive physical activity, and get plenty of rest.

• Alcohol, smoking, and caffeine; these stimulants can worsen the condition.

• Exposure to cold weather, as it can trigger an asthma attack. Bundle up and stay warm.

• Stress, anxiety, and emotional turmoil, as they can trigger asthma, especially in children.

• Certain drugs; allergic reactions can cause asthma. These include aspirin, NSAIDs (nonsteroidal anti-inflammatory drugs), and beta-blockers.

BAD BREATH

EVERYONE SUFFERS FROM BAD BREATH OCCASIONALLY. Perhaps you ate too much garlic or spicy food for lunch, or maybe you were unable to brush your teeth the night before. Transient bad breath can also occur as a result of hunger, dieting, alcohol use, or simply a dry mouth. It is easily remedied with good oral hygiene. But about 25 percent of the U.S. population suffers from more severe, chronic bad breath known as halitosis, a serious condition that can affect one's personal and professional life. Chronic bad breath is thought be caused by various bacteria in the oral cavity and gums. Gingivitis and other dental disorders are also associated with chronic bad breath. Severe cases require medical intervention with antibiotics. Prevention is the best method for avoiding halitosis. Brushing, flossing, and using oral rinses on a regular basis can dramatically reduce the risks and symptoms.

BAD BREATH

The gums and the mouth are an extension of the digestive system. According to Chinese medicine, they represent the condition of the stomach and the entire digestive system. Both gum disease and bad breath are caused by excessive heat—infection or inflammation—in the spleen-pancreas-stomach network. The heat is often combined with an accumulation of foods, dampness, and mucus. Emotions also play a role in the development of gum disease, as emotional stress can lower immune function, leading to bacterial or fungal growth in the oral and digestive tracts. Not surprisingly, Chinese medicine uses odor as one of its diagnostic techniques.

I noticed that the breath of one of my patients smelled like bread baking. This corroborated with his excessive thirst and appetite, leading me to suspect high blood sugar. I sent him to an endocrinologist, and tests came back confirming the diagnosis of diabetes. My therapy for bad breath focuses on clearing the pathogenic heat, expelling the mucus and dampness, and removing any food accumulation by educating the patient about proper oral hygiene.

✳ DIET ✳

• To prevent bad breath and gum diseases that cause bad breath, eat a varied diet consisting of fresh fruits, leafy vegetables, organic lean meat, and whole grains. Eat smaller meals, chew well, and don't skip meals. Eat to just 80 percent of your capacity to avoid overeating. Drink plenty of water. Obvious odiferous foods like garlic and onions should be consumed sparingly or along with parsley or anise to reduce odor.

....

• Avoid sugars, refined processed foods, and highly acidic foods. Hot, spicy, deep-fried, and greasy foods can injure stomach fluids and produce heat. Alcohol and coffee are also heat producing. Carbonated drinks and sour acidic foods should be avoided, as they can cause oral pH imbalance and damage the teeth.

✳ HOME REMEDIES ✳

• Make sure to brush your teeth on a regular basis to prevent gum disease. Always brush after meals and before and after sleep.

....

• Gargle with a mixture of 1 part hydrogen peroxide to 3 parts lukewarm water for 2 minutes twice a day.

....

• Drink green tea as often as possible, as it is antibacterial and cleanses the oral cavity.

....

• Make your own mouthwash by mixing 5 drops each of sage and peppermint essential oils with 8 ounces lukewarm water.

✳ DAILY SUPPLEMENTS ✳

• Using folic acid in a mouthwash and taken as a supplement can prevent and heal gum disease. As mouthwash use a 0.1% solution, and as capsules take 10 milligrams daily. It is available in liquid form sold in health food stores, certain drugstores, and some dental offices.

....

• Chlorophyll (100 milligrams) combats bad breath by helping clear toxins from the body.

....

• The probiotic supplement acidophilus (3 to 5 billion organisms) helps restore the natural flora along the mucous membranes of the lower digestive track.

✳ HERBAL THERAPY ✳

• Herbs can be found in health food or vitamin stores, online, and at the offices of Chinese medicine practitioners. Herbs should be used according to individual needs; consult with a licensed practitioner for a customized formulation. To learn more about the herbs listed here, go to www.ask drmao.com.

....

BAD BREATH

• Massage essential oils of caraway, sage, peppermint, or myrrh into the gums to support healthy gums.

....

• Chew on anise, cloves, fennel, or parsley to combat bad breath.

....

• Traditional Chinese herbs for treating bad breath include gardenia, siler, patchouli, and licorice.

———————————— ❊ EXERCISE ❊ ————————————

Physical activity not only helps maintain good digestion, but it can also reduce stress, anxiety, and strong emotions, which can cause stomach heat. A daily fitness program of 30-minute daily walks and a regular practice of qi gong or tai chi is very beneficial for a healthy digestive system, starting with the gums.

The following is part of the Eight Treasures Qi Gong practice called Drawing the Bow. It is beneficial in that it drains stomach heat, improves circulation, and clears the breath.

In a quiet, comfortable environment, preferably outdoors, stand with your feet shoulder-width apart, knees slightly bent, spine erect, tailbone tucked in, and head tilted slightly forward. Place your arms palms down on your lower abdomen just below the navel, one hand overlapping the other.

Begin with rhythmic, slow, and relaxed breathing. Inhale deeply but softly, and imagine the breath extending all the way down to the lower abdomen, about two finger-widths below the navel. Exhale gently and softly. Stay in this position for 7 breath cycles, relaxing and calming your mind.

Now begin the exercise—you will be collecting energy with a sweeping motion of your arms in front of you and then imitating the motion of stretching a bow to the left and right.

Inhale, and sweep your right arm in front of you from right to left and to your chest as you raise your left arm to your chest.

Exhale as your right arm completes the sweep. Extend it out to the right with your index finger extended and palm making a loose fist pointing to the right, while you make a loose fist with your left hand and draw the bow back to the left in front of your chest. Turn your head to the right, looking beyond the index finger of the right arm as though you were aiming at a distant target.

Return to the standing posture.

Now repeat on the left side: Inhale and sweep your left arm in front of you from left to right and to your chest as you raise your right arm to your chest.

Exhale as your left arm completes the sweep. Extend it out to the left with your index finger extended and make a loose fist pointing to the left, while you make a loose fist with your right hand and draw the bow back to the right in front of your chest. Turn your head to the left to look beyond the index finger of the left arm as though you were aiming at a distant target.

Repeat the exercise for a total of 3 times on each side, and then return to the starting posture. Conclude with a 1-minute quiet meditation.

--- ❋ ACUPRESSURE ❋ ---

• Find the acupoint Nectar Receptor (REN-24), in the depression at the center of the lower chin about a finger-width below the lower lip. Apply steady pressure until you feel soreness. Hold for 1 minute. This stimulates saliva and enzyme release.

· ·

• Find the acupoint Inner Court (ST-44), in the web between the second and third toes of your right foot. With your left index finger and thumb, pinch the web between the two toes. Hold for 3 to 5 minutes and then repeat on the left foot.

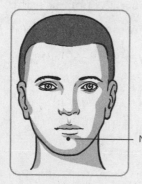
Nectar Receptor (REN-24)

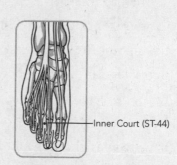
Inner Court (ST-44)

BONE LOSS

JUST AS YOU REMODEL YOUR HOME EVERY SO OFTEN, your bones undergo constant remodeling. Specialized cells in your bones are hard at work, constantly breaking down and rebuilding your bone tissue and reshaping your skeletal structure. Osteopenia, low bone density, and osteoporosis are names given to describe a condition in which the body breaks down more bone than is created. In essence, there is more demolition happening than construction. In the United States over 1.5 million fractures a year are attributed to osteoporosis. Over 10 million individuals, primarily postmenopausal women, have been diagnosed with osteoporosis. An additional 18 million people have very low bone density, placing them at higher risk of developing the condition.

Perhaps one of the most dangerous things about osteoporosis is the relative lack of obvious symptoms to serve as warning signs. Most of the time the disease makes itself known through a minor fall that results in fractures or broken bones. The one place that osteoporosis may actually be seen is the spine. As bone mass is reduced, the vertebrae collapse, causing curvature, loss of height, and humps. It is important to have regular checkups to determine whether you are suffering from bone loss, especially if you are at higher risk due to family history, history of steroid use, or if you're postmenopausal. If the condition is identified early on, there are good medical and alternative treatments available to help prevent progression of the disease.

According to Chinese medicine, bones, bone marrow, and the skeletal structure rely heavily on the kidney essence. The kidney essence is built during the prenatal period and tends to get consumed at a regular pace throughout life. Replenishment of kidney essence is a difficult and a slow process but is not impossible. It is essential, according to Chinese medical theory, to prevent its unnecessary loss so it can serve you well into your old age. Fortunately, through tai chi and qi gong exercises, specialized herbs, and a proper diet and lifestyle, you can prevent depletion of kidney essence and slow down the progression of osteoporosis. In fact, tai chi has been shown to be excellent for increasing balance and strength.

I work with orthopedists and gynecologists in designing natural ways to support healthy bones in patients who are unable or unwilling to take drug medication. I identify lifestyle and diet elements that weaken the kidney essence, use acupuncture and herbal remedies to stimulate bone growth and strengthen the kidney-bladder network, and offer specialized exercises that generate appropriate pressure on the skeletal structure to stimulate bone rebuilding without putting patients at risk of falls and fractures.

Here are some of my recommendations.

———————————————— ☀ DIET ☀ ————————————————

• A healthy, well-balanced diet rich in complex carbohydrates, whole grains, fresh vegetables, and organic proteins is important for a healthy body. Bones, however, have additional nutrition requirements, as they are made of calcium and other minerals. Foods high in calcium and vitamin D (required to enhance calcium absorption) include broccoli, chestnuts, clams, dark green leafy vegetables, and saltwater fish such as flounder, salmon, sardines, and shrimp. These foods should not be combined with grains, as grains can impair the absorption of vital nutrients. Sulfur, phosphorus, and other minerals required for healthy bones can be obtained from garlic and onions. Kale, soy products like tofu and tempeh, pineapple, grapes, and prunes are also good for the bones.

....

• Avoid carbonated soft drinks, alcohol, and smoking. Yeast and sugars—especially processed bleached sugars—should be eliminated as well. Take it easy with citrus fruits, as they can disrupt calcium absorption. Salt in small quantities can help strengthen the bones but should be used in moderation.

———————————— ✳ HOME REMEDIES ✳ ————————————

• Prepare a calcium-rich broth such as one featuring oxtail, or ox bone stew with onions, garlic, tomatoes, and ginger to nourish the bones. Place 2 pounds cut oxtail or 4 pounds ox bone in a large pot filled with water. Add 2 chopped onions, 1 head of garlic, 3 chopped tomatoes, and 10 slices ginger root, and simmer for 2 hours.

....

• Make a tea by boiling 1/3 cup soybeans and 1/3 cup dried, diced wild yams (available in Asian markets) in 5 cups of water for 30 to 40 minutes. Strain and drink 3 cups daily. This will provide plant-based phytoestrogens, which support a hormonal system that has weakened with age, especially after menopause.

....

• Sunbathe daily for 30 minutes—but before 10:00 A.M. and after 3:00 P.M. to avoid the strongest UV rays. This increases your body's production of vitamin D, which is essential for healthy bones.

———————————— ✳ DAILY SUPPLEMENTS ✳ ————————————

• Supplementing with calcium citrate (1,000 milligrams) combined with magnesium (500 milligrams) and vitamin D (600 IU) promotes bone health.

Boron (3 milligrams), a trace mineral, is also important in calcium absorption.

• Taking zinc (20 milligrams), silica (50 milligrams), and manganese (10 milligrams), can also be helpful for increasing bone density.

• Glucosamine sulfate (1,000 milligrams) and chondroitin sulfate (400 milligrams) taken together can help strengthen bones and joints.

_____ ✳ HERBAL THERAPY ✳ _____

• Herbs can be found in health food or vitamin stores, online, and at the offices of Chinese medicine practitioners. Herbs should be used according to individual needs; consult with a licensed practitioner for a customized formulation. To learn more about the herbs listed here, go to www.ask drmao.com.

• Black cohosh, barley grass, alfalfa, nettle, and rose hips have traditionally been used to help support healthy bones.

• Kelp, horsetail, wild yam, and red clover are also used by herbalists to nourish the bones.

• Dura-Bone, a Chinese herbal formula I make for my patients, includes shark cartilage, oyster shells, Siberian ginseng, bone mender root, astragalus, eucommia bark, Fo-Ti, dipsacus root, mulberry, Job's tears, and other Chinese herbs.

_____ ✳ EXERCISE ✳ _____

Research has shown conclusively that exercise early in life builds bone mass and strengthens the skeletal structure, thus preventing osteoporosis. Even later in life, regular exercise can slow the progress of many degenerative bone disorders. I recommend a combination of weight-bearing exercises: a 30-minute daily walk, light weight training to strengthen muscles

BONE LOSS

and build endurance, and flexibility exercises such as tai chi or qi gong. All my patients receive instruction on my favorite qi gong practice, Eight Treasures Qi Gong, which supports the hormonal system, helps restore the vital kidney essence, and enhances balance, flexibility, and coordination. The section of the practice known as Bringing the Stream Back to the Sea is especially helpful. Practice twice a day and you'll see the results for yourself.

In a quiet, comfortable environment, preferably outdoors, stand with your feet shoulder-width apart, knees slightly bent, spine erect, tailbone tucked in, and head tilted slightly forward. Place your arms palms down on your lower abdomen just below the navel, one hand overlapping the other.

Begin with rhythmic, slow, and relaxed breathing. Inhale deeply but softly, and imagine the breath extending all the way down to the lower abdomen, about two finger-widths below the navel. Exhale gently and softly. Stay in this position for 7 breath cycles, relaxing and calming your mind.

Now begin the exercise, a gentle, rhythmic back and forth rocking of the body using the soles of your feet as the rocking surface.

Inhale, and raise your heels to elevate your body, moving your abdomen slightly forward to assist in the movement.

Exhale and rock backward on your heels in a gentle, back-and-forth fashion, raising the balls of your feet. The movement should send a mild shock up the legs and upper spine. Be sure to be gentle, as this movement stimulates the spinal column.

Repeat the movement 24 times, inhaling while raising the heels, exhaling while rocking down and back on the heels.

Conclude the exercise with a standing meditation for 1 to 3 minutes.

❋ ACUPRESSURE ❋

• Find the acupoint Forceful Torrent (KID-3), in the depression midway between the inner anklebone and Achilles tendon on the right foot. Apply pressure with your right thumb until you feel soreness. Hold for 3 minutes.

Repeat on the left foot. This supports healthy kidney function, which is important in maintaining good calcium levels.

• Find the acupoint Kunlun Mountain (UB-60), between the outer anklebone and the Achilles tendon. Apply pressure with your right thumb until you feel soreness. Hold for 3 minutes. Repeat on the left foot.

• Engaging the combination of these points is good for the spine, strengthening the kidneys, and fortifying the kidney essence.

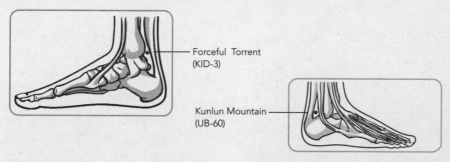

Forceful Torrent
(KID-3)

Kunlun Mountain
(UB-60)

AVOID

• Smoking and excessive use of alcohol, which can deplete the body of vital nutrients needed for bone health. Nicotine especially impairs bone formation.

• Excess coffee consumption, as it increases urinary passage of calcium from the body.

• Overconsumption of vitamin A, which can speed up bone loss.

• Overuse of steroids, thyroid medications, blood thinners, diuretics, and aluminum-containing substances. This can deplete bone mass and speed up osteoporosis. Consult your physician.

• Excessive stress, worry, tension, and sexual activity, which deplete the vital essence.

BONE LOSS

BRONCHITIS

THE AIRWAY PASSAGES IN THE LUNGS, called bronchi, are susceptible to viral and bacterial infections. Following a common cold or flu, the pathogen often settles in the bronchi, causing an acute infection called bronchitis. Severe cough, mild fever, and chest tightness and pain accompanied by fatigue and exhaustion are common symptoms. Over 90 percent of acute bronchitis is caused by viral infections that do not respond to antibiotics. Chronic bronchitis, on the other hand, is often associated with smokers, people with asthma, immune-compromised individuals, and the elderly. About 1 in 20 Americans suffer from bronchitis as a result of common colds and flu, and over 12 million develop chronic bronchitis over their lifetime.

In Chinese medicine, respiratory infections are classified as heat in the lungs due to exterior pathogens. Weakened immunity as a result of lung–large intestine network deficiency is considered in chronic cases. Bronchitis is often remedied first with cupping, a practice using suction cups on the upper back, and acupuncture to relax the bronchial constriction and relieve the cough. These treatments are followed by fast-acting herbal therapy to remove the pathogen, clear the lungs, and further subdue the cough.

For chronic bronchitis, it is also essential to support the healthy functioning of the lung, stomach, and kidney networks, and to provide dietary and lifestyle advice. Stopping smoking is a must. Many cases of chronic bronchitis are caused by stomach imbalance. For example, a woman came to me after suffering from chronic bronchitis for more than two years. She took various medications and used inhalers but still had a constant cough. I discovered that she also suffered from indigestion and postnasal drip. I decided to tackle the postnasal drip and the acid reflux first—in other words, I wanted to support the spleen-pancreas-stomach network to stop mucus production and to rebalance acid production. As soon as her indigestion and postnasal drip cleared up, her two-year-old bronchitis went away.

Chronic bronchitis is a serious condition that requires a collaborative effort. In these cases I work with pulmonary specialists to develop and administer comprehensive treatment plans integrating Western and Eastern medicine.

Here are my recommendations.

❊ DIET ❊

• For specific dietary advice for bronchitis following the common cold, refer to the section on colds (page 240).

• Follow a balanced diet rich in complex carbohydrates, low in fat, and with organic sources of lean protein such as egg whites, skinless chicken, ostrich, and turkey. Favor green vegetables and include green and red cabbage, kale, asparagus, bell peppers, Brussels sprouts, celery, daikon radish, garlic, green beans, carrots, papaya, lotus root, seaweed, button mushrooms, reishi mushrooms, mustard greens, onions, leeks, parsnips, seaweed, turnips, water chestnuts, watercress, apples, bananas, apricots, figs, grapefruits, mulberries, oranges, Asian pears (also known as pear apples), persimmons, almonds, ginkgo nuts (available in Asian markets), chestnuts, walnuts, olives, and honey. During an infection, increase fluid intake to 80 ounces of room temperature or lukewarm beverages a day.

• Eliminate foods that promote mucus, including dairy products, but especially ice cream, cold and raw foods, sweet foods containing simple processed sugars or processed flour, and soft drinks.

• Juice 3 large daikon radishes, strain, and add 1 teaspoon fresh ginger juice and 1 tablespoon honey. Drink it lukewarm, 1 cup 3 times daily until the condition improves.

• Add 1/2 cup crushed water chestnuts and 1/2 cup honeysuckle (available in health food stores) to 20 ounces of water and boil for 20 minutes. Strain, and drink 1 cup of this tea twice daily until the condition improves.

• Core 1 Asian pear, spoon 1 tablespoon honey in the center, and steam or bake for 10 to 15 minutes. Eating 3 daily will nourish the lungs and soothe a cough.

• To open the passageways and relieve joint pain, boil a stockpot of water and turn off the heat. Add 10 drops of my Tonic Oil (available at www.askdr mao.com), which consists of oils of camphor, peppermint, eucalyptus, fennel, and wintergreen. Inhale the fumes deeply for 10 minutes with a towel covering your head and the pot.

• Make a honey and onion syrup: Finely chop 1 onion and mix with 2 tablespoons of honey. Store in sealed container for 8 hours. Take 1 tablespoon straight or dissolve it in 1 cup hot water and drink 4 to 5 times a day until the condition improves.

━━━━━━━━━━━ ❋ DAILY SUPPLEMENTS ❋ ━━━━━━━━━━━

• Vitamins A (200 IU), C (1,000 milligrams), E (800 IU), and bromelain (450 milligrams), garlic (900 milligrams), and zinc (50 milligrams) are beneficial for treating bronchitis.

• Methylsulfanylmethane or MSM (1,000 milligrams) and pycnogenol (450 milligrams), a bioflavonoid found in grape seeds, can protect the lungs and prevent infections.

• Quercetin (500 milligrams) is useful for its antihistamine properties in allergic bronchitis.

────────────── ✳ HERBAL THERAPY ✳ ──────────────

• Herbs can be found in health food or vitamin stores, online, and at the offices of Chinese medicine practitioners. Herbs should be used according to individual needs; consult with a licensed practitioner for a customized formulation. To learn more, go to www.askdrmao.com.

. . . .

• Linden, marshmallow, and peppermint are traditionally used to suppress cough.

. . . .

• Lily bulb, apricot kernel, stemona root, fritillaria, mulberry, Chinese basil, mustard seed, daikon seed, ginger, and schizandra berry are among the many herbs used in Chinese medicine to calm cough and ventilate the lungs.

. . . .

• For chronic bronchitis accompanied by kidney weakness, tonic herbs such as ginkgo seed, goji berry, cornus berry, astragalus, and ginseng are recommended.

────────────── ✳ EXERCISE ✳ ──────────────

Don't exercise strenuously while suffering from acute bronchitis, as exercising can worsen the condition. Calm and restful walks in fresh air can help. During remission, moderate physical exercise can be integrated. I recommend daily qi gong exercises to strengthen the body, open and strengthen the lungs, and redirect the flow of qi downward. The Eight Treasures Qi Gong exercises can be of great benefit to the mind and body, when performed daily for 30 minutes. In particular, the fifth movement of the practice, called Water and Fire Meet, is targeted to bring the cooling energy of the kidneys to the chest, redirect the qi downward, and calm a cough. Perform this exercise twice daily. The time corresponding to the lung energy is around 5 A.M., so between 5 and 7 A.M. is the best time to practice tai chi or qi gong exercises targeted to the lungs.

In a quiet, comfortable environment, preferably outdoors, stand with your feet shoulder-width apart, knees slightly bent, spine erect, tailbone tucked in, and head tilted slightly forward. Place your arms palms down on your lower abdomen just below the navel, one hand overlapping the other.

Begin with rhythmic, slow, and relaxed breathing. Inhale deeply but softly, and imagine the breath extending all the way down to your lower abdomen, about two finger-widths below the navel. Exhale gently and softly. Stay in this position for 7 breath cycles, relaxing and calming your mind.

Then begin the exercise: Exhale, bending down from your waist. Begin a gentle massage of your inner legs, starting at the inner ankles by rubbing rhythmically in a circular motion.

Inhale as you continue the massage, slowly coming up the inner legs to your inner thighs. Raise your arms slowly to your chest with the backs of your palms touching each other and your elbows bent.

When you reach your chest, make small circles by moving your hands from the middle to the outside of the chest with palms facing down, expanding your chest. Then move from the outer to the middle of your chest with your palms facing up.

Inhale, and in alternating fashion make circles with the bent elbows, moving from front to back and bending at the hips to exaggerate the motion slightly. Alternate between your left and right arms 3 times.

Repeat the circles now in the reverse direction from the back to the front, inhaling and exhaling with each circle. Repeat with each arm 3 times.

Bring the arms back to the center of the chest, with the backs of the palms facing each other, elbows bent. Inhale and open the chest with both arms stretching back and to the sides, again with elbows bent and palms relaxed. Exhale and stretch both arms out to the sides, palms facing out, pushing out to the left and right. As you exhale, push your hands out 3 times.

To complete the exercise, return to the initial standing posture. Place your hands on the lower abdomen, palms down, one hand overlapping the other. Rub your lower abdomen 7 times in small clockwise circles just below the navel.

• Find the acupoint Cubit Marsh (LU-5) by bending your right arm at the elbow—the point is located in the elbow crease, on the outer side of the large tendon in the middle of the crease. Apply moderate pressure with your left thumb until you feel soreness. Hold for 2 minutes. Repeat on the left arm.

• Locate the acupoint Upward Thrust (REN-22) on the chest—it's level with the clavicle and shoulders, in the depression at the center of the sternum just below the 'V' of the neck. Apply steady pressure with your index fingers until you feel soreness. Hold for 3 minutes.

• Both of these points are traditionally used to soothe breathing, redirect lung energy downward, and stop cough.

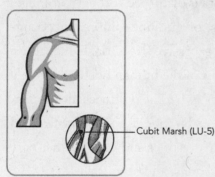

Cubit Marsh (LU-5)

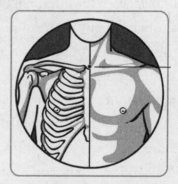

Upward Thrust (REN-22)

── AVOID ──

• Exposure to airborne irritants, which can aggravate the condition.

• Alcohol, smoking, and caffeine, stimulants that can worsen the condition.

• Exposure to cold weather, which can trigger bronchial constriction and worsen cough.

• Stress, anxiety, and emotional turmoil, which can aggravate the symptoms.

BRONCHITIS

CANDIDA (DYSBIOSIS OR YEAST OVERGROWTH)

OVER 500 SYMBIOTIC SPECIES OF BACTERIA and yeast live in our gastrointestinal tract. These intestinal flora play a key role in digestion and the absorption of essential nutrients. They're also responsible for producing essential fatty acids from ingested foods, producing valuable nutrients (including B vitamins and vitamin K), facilitating the metabolism of drugs, protecting us from infection by pathogenic bacteria, maintaining a healthy intestinal acid-base balance, and enhancing immune functions. One of the most common intestinal flora is the yeast *Candida albicans.*

If the balance of the intestinal flora is disturbed through prolonged use of antibiotics, birth control pills, or immune-suppressant drugs, hormonal imbalance, improper diet, excessive stress, or alcohol abuse, candida can flourish, to the detriment of the human host. At first the outgrowth is limited to the intestines, where it produces alcohol and other toxic by-products, putting stress on the body. If left untreated, the condition can expand beyond the intestines and invade other parts of the body, including the abdomen, lungs, and other cavities.

The resulting infection overburdens the immune system, causing symptoms such as fatigue, weakness, muscle and joint pains, and gastrointestinal disturbances, including diarrhea, constipation, nausea, and bloating after eating. Severe infections can also cause depression, memory problems, infertility, and allergies. Recent research suggests that gluten allergies may be linked to chronic candida infestation. Other common manifestations linked to candida overgrowth include oral thrush, skin infections, and vaginal yeast infections.

Chinese medicine classifies candida as an accumulation of excessive dampness and heat in the body. Because the functions of the spleen-pancreas-stomach network are weakened, normal digestion is impaired, causing buildup of dampness, which is heavy in property and tends to occupy the lower parts of the body. Dampness is the ancient way of describing mold or fungal infestation. The sticky, congealing nature of dampness combined with emotional stress blocks the free flow of energy, producing pathogenic heat. This dampness and heat together cause the symptoms of candida infection.

I have seen many patients suffer from fatigue, muscle weakness, digestive disturbances, and even infertility as the result of a candida infestation. Often these patients have a history of abusing sugar and wheat products, of being exposed to mold, or of being emotionally and physically run-down. By identifying the causes, and by using herbal and dietary therapy and acupuncture, I have been able to help my patients return their bodies to a healthy state.

Here are some recommendations.

✳ DIET ✳

• The most important line of defense against candida is a proper diet. The diet should be low in refined carbohydrates and high in protein and essential fatty acids. All breads, including refined wheat and rye breads, dairy products, cheeses of all kinds, alcohol, sugar, pastries, pickled foods, and vinegar should be eliminated. Whole grains are fine, but limit the quantity. Cold and raw foods, in which microbes are naturally present, can cause digestive dampness and should be avoided. Most fruits and juices, as well as starchy vegetables, such as potatoes, carrots, and squash, should also be minimized. Leftovers should be frozen, not refrigerated, since mold or fungus has a great opportunity to grow overnight.

• Foods should be rotated in your diet. The easiest way to acquire a food allergy is to consume the same foods repeatedly.

• Include more dandelions, beet tops, carrot tops, barley, garlic, cayenne pepper, mung beans, citrus fruits, kohlrabi, cabbage, shiitake mushrooms, ginger, turmeric, oregano, cilantro, rosemary, dill, sage, fennel, cardamom, and anise in your diet.

❋ HOME REMEDIES ❋

• Boil a handful of fresh dandelion greens in 3 cups of water for 10 minutes. Strain, and drink 3 cups a day.

• Eat 2 to 3 fresh garlic cloves a day, with or without food.

• Make a tea by boiling 1 teaspoon oregano, 1/4 teaspoon cayenne pepper, and 1/2 teaspoon ginger in 3 cups water for 10 minutes. Strain, and drink 2 to 3 cups a day.

❋ DAILY SUPPLEMENTS ❋

• Taking probiotics such as acidophilus (3 to 10 billion cultures daily) can help control candida overgrowth.

• Mix 1 tablespoon of soluble fiber—guar gum, psyllium husks, flaxseeds, or pectin—in 1 cup of water. Drink 2 times a day on an empty stomach. This is essential for healthy bowels.

• Enteric-coated garlic pills (900 milligrams) can inhibit growth of candida.

• Caprylic acid (300 milligrams) is used as a mild antifungal.

❋ HERBAL THERAPY ❋

• Herbs can be found in health food or vitamin stores, online, and at the offices of Chinese medicine practitioners. Herbs should be used according to individual needs; consult with a licensed practitioner for a customized formulation. To learn more about the herbs listed here, go to www.askdrmao.com.

• Taheebo bark tea taken 3 times a day can have an inhibitory effect on yeast overgrowth.

• Taking tea tree, peppermint, oregano, and lavender oils in enteric-coated capsules can be helpful for controlling yeast overgrowth.

• Chinese herbs with specific and general antifungal abilities include pagoda tree fruit, chaulmoogra seeds, erythrina bark, aloe vera, and genkwa flower.

• A traditional herbal formula for clearing up damp heat consists of the herbs gentian root, skullcap, gardenia, akebia, plantain, alisma, bupleurum, rehmannia, dong quai, and licorice. This formula is often combined with or followed by formulations that support the spleen, stomach, and digestive functions and that contain herbs such as astragalus, codonopsis, atractylodes, tangerine, cardamom, and dioscorea.

❋ EXERCISE ❋

In addition to a regular physical exercise regimen, I recommend qi gong exercises to strengthen the stomach, spleen, and digestive system and promote the flow of energy in the abdomen. Perform the following exercise twice a day on an empty stomach.

Lie down on your back comfortably, with your hands at your sides. Focus on your navel. Visualize a golden disk the size of a Frisbee spinning around your entire abdomen with its center at your navel.

With every inhalation the disk spins half of a full circle. With every exhalation the disk completes the other half of the circle.

Breathe deeply so that the disk spins slowly, corresponding to your respiration, for a total of 21 times in the clockwise direction.

Reverse the direction of the disk's rotation and repeat the breathing-spinning sequence.

• Locate the acupoint Foot Three Miles (ST-36), four finger-widths below and to the outside of the right kneecap. Apply moderate pressure with your right thumb. Hold for 5 minutes. Repeat on the left leg.

• Locate the acupoint Winding Gulch (LI-11), in the depression at the outer part of the left elbow crease, between the elbow tendon and the bone. The point is best located when the arm is bent at 90 degrees with the palm facing the abdomen. Apply steady pressure with your right thumb until you feel soreness. Hold for 3 minutes. Repeat on the right arm.

• Both of these points have traditionally been used to strengthen digestive function and enhance immunity.

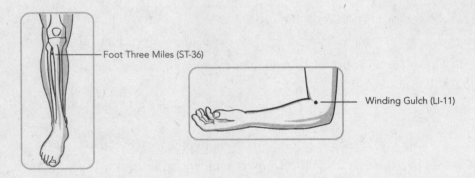

Foot Three Miles (ST-36)

Winding Gulch (LI-11)

—————————— AVOID ——————————

• Excessive activity, straining the body, and overeating. Get plenty of sleep.

• Alcohol, smoking, and caffeine, as they weaken the qi.

• Eating foods you're allergic to, which can aggravate candida. Rotate foods and eliminate gluten.

- Stress, anxiety, and emotional turmoil, which cause the qi to stagnate and complicate the condition.

- Excessive use of antibiotics and hormones, which can cause candida.

 ## CARPAL TUNNEL SYNDROME

YOUR HAND IS ONE OF THE MOST COMPLEX STRUCTURES in your body. Each hand is made up of twenty-seven bones, numerous muscles and tendons, and thousands of tiny blood vessels and nerve endings. Eight bones called the carpals form the base of the hand. The carpals attach the hand to the arm and form a tunnel filled with the many tendons required for fine, coordinated finger movements. A major nerve that controls the hand—particularly the thumb, index finger, and middle finger—also passes through this tunnel. Repetitive, forceful movements of the hand can cause the carpal tendons to get inflamed, pinching the nerve. Hence the name carpal tunnel syndrome (CTS).

CTS can be triggered by repetitive use of a computer keyboard and mouse, using cell phones with tiny keypads, or BlackBerrys, or playing video games. Even excessive knitting can cause numbness, tingling, weakness of the hands and fingers, loss of grip strength, and pain that originates in the wrist and radiates to the shoulders. The muscles of the affected fingers—especially the base of the thumb—are often weakened as well. Repetitive activities with hands using fine tools, and extended use of computer keyboards, put people at risk for CTS. Pregnancy, menopause, and inflammatory diseases like Lyme disease and rubella can also increase the risk of developing CTS. Women are more likely to develop CTS than men are, and age of onset is typically from forty to sixty years old.

CARPAL TUNNEL SYNDROME

In Chinese medicine, wrist and hand pain, numbness, and tingling are attributed to stagnation of energy and blood flow. These symptoms can be compounded by the accumulation of dampness and phlegm. The inflammation of the carpal tendons creates swelling, diminishing the nerve impulses to and from the hand. Since our practice at Tao of Wellness serves many pregnant and postpartum women, localized therapies that reduce inflammation and release stagnation have shown the best results. These include acupuncture and electrostimulation, topical herbal patches and liniments combined with herbal and nutritional therapies, and specialized hand exercises. Some simple lifestyle changes and exercises can relieve the symptoms of CTS, including regularly stretching and relaxing your arms and fingers, modifying your work environment to reduce stress on your hands, and alternating repetitive tasks. Below are some other recommendations.

❋ DIET ❋

• Because CTS is an arthritic condition, I suggest a healthy, well-balanced diet rich in complex carbohydrates, whole grains, and fresh vegetables. Scallions, grapes (with seeds), mulberries, black beans, and green leafy vegetables, as well as dampness-reducing foods such as barley, mung beans, mustard greens, red beans, millet, and cornsilk tea, are beneficial.

• Avoid cold foods, raw fruits and vegetables, dairy products, and greasy, fried, and salty foods. Meat, shellfish, sugars, and alcohol, smoking, and other stimulants can aggravate the condition.

❋ HOME REMEDIES ❋

• Ample rest for your hands is the most important remedy for CTS.

• Give your hands a day off every week. Treat them to a warm soothing bubble bath with lavender essential oil and massage them with rosemary and St.-John's-wort oils.

• Favor fruits such as pineapple, papaya, cherries, and grapes, which possess enzymes and antioxidants that are nature's anti-inflammatory remedies.

• Boil 1/4 cup chopped scallions or Chinese parsley in 2 cups of water for 10 minutes. Strain, and drink this tea 3 times a day.

• For damp arthritis, boil 1/3 cup each of soaked mung beans, pearl barley, and red adzuki beans in 4 cups of water for 1 hour. Eat daily for 1 month. Cornsilk tea is also beneficial for damp-type arthritis. Boil a handful of cornsilk for 20 minutes in 4 cups of water. Strain, and drink 3 cups a day.

❋ DAILY SUPPLEMENTS ❋

• Taking vitamin B complex and additional B_6 supplements can help with nerve pain and inflammation.

• Supplementing with essential fatty acids like those in fish oil or in flaxseed oil (1,000 milligrams EPA; 800 milligrams DHA), the enzyme bromelain (450 milligrams), and alpha lipoic acid (50 milligrams) daily can help reduce swelling and support circulation.

• Borage and evening primrose oil are both rich in gamma-linolenic acid (GLA; 240 milligrams), which the body converts to its own anti-inflammatory agent.

❋ HERBAL THERAPY ❋

• Herbs can be found in health food or vitamin stores, online, and at the offices of Chinese medicine practitioners. Herbs should be used according to individual needs; consult with a licensed practitioner for a customized formulation. To learn more about the herbs listed here, go to www.askdrmao.com.

• Turmeric, St.-John's-wort, wild yam, and cramp bark are useful for alleviating pain and relieving inflammation.

....

• I recommend Arthritis/Joint Elixir, our Chinese herbal formula that supports healthy functioning of joints, tendons, and ligaments. The formulation includes angelica du huo, notopterygium, siler, white peony, Chinese lovage, peach kernel, safflower, eucommia, mulberry stem, astragalus, dong quai, and cinnamon.

—————————————— ✳ EXERCISE ✳ ——————————————

At work do some simple stretching exercises for 5 minute every hour. And when you sleep, wear a wrist brace to avoid bending or twisting your wrist.

The benefits of regular physical exercise for a healthy body and strong joints are well documented. I recommend adding a regular practice of tai chi or qi gong to your fitness program to strengthen your muscles, tendons, and bones, and to build endurance and flexibility. One such practice that I often recommend is the Eight Treasures Qi Gong, which enhances physical strength and endurance and increases joint flexibility and coordination without putting extra stress on the body. The warm-up sequence to the practice includes exercises targeting the hands, which I am including here. Performing the practice for 5 minutes every hour during the workday can provide healing and preventive benefits for CTS.

In a quiet, comfortable environment, preferably outdoors, stand with your feet shoulder-width apart, knees slightly bent, spine erect, tailbone tucked in, and head tilted slightly forward. Place your arms palms down on your lower abdomen just below the navel, one hand overlapping the other.

Begin with rhythmic, slow, and relaxed breathing. Inhale deeply but softly, and imagine the breath extending all the way down to the lower abdomen, about two finger-widths below the navel. Exhale gently and softly. Stay in this position for 7 breath cycles, relaxing and calming your mind.

Now begin the exercise, a gentle workout for your hands and wrists that stimulates circulation and relaxes the muscles and tendons.

Inhale, and raise your arms to chest level. Turn the palms to face each other and interlock the fingers of both hands.

Exhale, and begin gently rotating your hands in unison at the wrist, beginning with small circles, and gradually increasing the radius of the circles. Alternate a forward and backward motion for 16 rotations in each direction.

Return to the standing position and let your hands hang at your sides.

Inhale, and shake your hands loosely at your sides. Shake up and down as if you were trying to shake off dirt from your hands.

With each breath, focus your attention on relaxing your wrists, palms, and each finger until you feel your hands just dangling from your arms.

Continue shaking for 1 to 3 minutes. To enhance the shaking process, you can bounce gently on your feet.

Conclude the exercise with a gentle massage of the wrists and hands by imitating the motion of washing your hands.

✳ ACUPRESSURE ✳

• Find the acupoint Great Hill (P-7), at the center of the right wrist crease between the two tendons. Apply pressure with your left thumb until you feel soreness. Hold for 2 minutes. Repeat on your left hand.

. . . .

• Find the acupoint Outer Gate (SJ-5), two thumb-widths above the outer wrist crease of the right hand, between the two tendons. Apply pressure

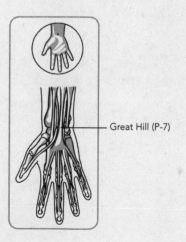

Great Hill (P-7)

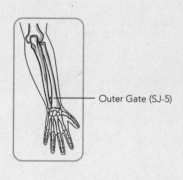

Outer Gate (SJ-5)

with your left thumb until you feel soreness. Hold for 3 minutes. Repeat on your left hand.

•Engaging the combination of these points has been used to successfully treat CTS in many clinical cases. Acupuncture has also been shown to be very effective in treating CTS, especially when combined with electrostimulation.

AVOID

•Smoking, coffee, and excess salt and alcohol intake, as they irritate inflammatory conditions and can cause CTS to flare up.

•Harsh, jolting, and strenuous activities using your wrists. Protect your wrists with braces if you must use them for repetitive tasks.

•Stress, worry, and tension, which weaken your body's ability to heal.

CHRONIC FATIGUE SYNDROME

IF YOU SUFFER FROM SEVERE EXHAUSTION and recurrent fatigue that does not improve with rest and that gets worse with the simplest activities, and if it is accompanied by muscle aches, headaches, sore throat, and recurrent colds that linger for long periods of time, you may be suffering from chronic fatigue syndrome (CFS). The medical community has classified CFS as a syndrome because it is a variable group of symptoms that are present at the same time with no discernable underlying medical condition. CFS affects more people than statistics show since there are no definitive tests for diagnosis. In recent years CFS has been on the rise—more than half a million Americans may suffer from this condition without being aware of it. There are no known biomedical causes for CFS, but some think that severe emotional or physical stress or trauma and prolonged viral or bacterial infections precede the appearance of symptoms. There are speculations that CFS is caused by an overstressed immune system that fails to protect the body properly or becomes overstimulated and attacks the body itself.

I saw my first case of CFS in 1986. A patient from the Lake Tahoe area flew to Los Angeles to see me after seeing a number of specialists, without success. After I helped her recover, many people with CFS from the same area came to see me. Initially I thought it was a geographically unique condition limited to Lake Tahoe, but soon I was seeing patients from around the country. Over the years I've worked with immunologists and holistic internists to design a comprehensive program to help CFS patients regain their quality of life. CFS can be debilitating—many patients aren't sick enough to be bedridden, but they're not well enough to live a normal active life. The most frustrating thing for many CFS patients is that since they don't appear sick, their family and friends have difficulty understanding why they're unable to live normally.

In Chinese medicine, in order to function properly, the body requires vital substances, including blood, fluids, energy produced by a healthy digestive system, and the vital essence from the kidney-bladder network which maintains healthy immune function. When these energies are exhausted, the body cannot function properly. Breakdown is the consequence. Many classical medical texts attribute conditions similar to CFS to the exhaustion of these vital substances as a result of being overworked, prolonged illness, emotional trauma, physical stress, or overindulgence. Most of my patients with CFS have experienced one or more of these. My success in treating CFS can be attributed to understanding the intricate balance of the body's vital substances and restoring deficiencies with herbal and nutritional therapies, acupuncture, and lifestyle counseling.

Here are some of my typical recommendations.

❋ DIET ❋

• Proper nutrition and a balance of the right foods can help the body heal itself. Improper nutrition and lifestyle, on the other hand, can complicate disease and prolong its course. I recommend a seasonal diet rich in substances that help regenerate blood, energy, and vital essence. Favor winter melon and squash, pumpkin, pumpkin seeds, yams, sweet potatoes, lima beans, black beans, soybeans, mung beans, adzuki beans, daikon radish, pearl barley, white fungus (an Asian mushroom), egg, cabbage, carrots, and buckwheat. Incorporate more fresh fruits, including a variety of berries, watermelon, pineapple, papaya, figs, pears, and jujube dates. Ginger, scallions, garlic, oregano, cilantro, rosemary, sage, dill, turmeric, and cayenne pepper are all energy tonics that support healthy immune function. Organic sources of protein, such as chicken, turkey, and lamb, as well as wild-caught deep-sea fish are helpful for energy, blood, and essence building.

• Eat smaller meals at regular intervals and more frequently. Don't eat late in the evening and don't eat very heavy meals. Drink at least 60 ounces of room temperature water every day.

• Avoid dairy products (especially cheese), simple sugars, processed flour, all processed and artificially flavored foods, and fatty, oily foods, which create dampness and injure the vital energy. Tomatoes, potatoes, eggplant, bell peppers, and shellfish should also be avoided. Avoid coffee and alcohol, as they produce heat in the body and cause confusion of the body's energy.

• Take an invigorating bath with Epsom salts and essential oils of wintergreen, eucalyptus, and menthol for 20 minutes every day.

• Always go to bed at the same time every night, before 11 P.M., and get at least 8 hours of sleep. If you can, take a 30-minute nap in the middle of the day, or at least try to get some relaxation time in by lying down in your car for a little while. Never nap for more than 30 minutes at a time, or you may wake up groggy.

• Make a garlic–egg white omelet with 2 egg whites and include 1 finely chopped garlic clove, 1/3 cup diced sauteed yam, and 1/2 cup chopped parsley

————————— ✳ DAILY SUPPLEMENTS ✳ —————————

• Taking beta carotene (800 milligrams), vitamins C (1,000 milligrams), E (800 IU), and B complex, and omega-3 fatty acids (1,000 milligrams EPA; 800 milligrams DHA) can help alleviate the symptoms of CFS. Many of these nutrients are depleted in CFS patients.

• The mineral supplements zinc picolinate (50 milligrams), magnesium glycinate (500 milligrams), calcium citrate (1,000 milligrams), vitamin D (400 IU), and manganese (25 milligrams) support healthy immune function.

• The amino acids L-carnitine (500 milligrams), L-lysine (1,000 milligrams), and L-glutathione (100 milligrams), and alpha lipoic acid (50 milligrams), and the antioxidant coenzyme Q-10 (50 milligrams), can help the body to recover from CFS.

————————— ✳ HERBAL THERAPY ✳ —————————

• Herbs can be found in health food or vitamin stores, online, and at the offices of Chinese medicine practitioners. Herbs should be used according

CHRONIC FATIGUE SYNDROME

to individual needs; consult with a licensed practitioner for a customized formulation. To learn more about the herbs listed here, go to www.ask drmao.com.

. . . .

• Ginseng, licorice, astragalus, green tea, gotu kola, codonopsis, schizandra, Siberian ginseng, and cordyceps have adaptogenic capabilities and are used to relieve the symptoms of CFS.

. . . .

• I recommend Abundant Energy and High Performance, our Chinese herbal formulas for supporting healthy digestive function. The formulas contain ginseng, codonopsis, polygonatum, glehnia root, longan, Japanese apricot, astragalus, schizandra, Siberian ginseng, and other Chinese herbs.

. . . .

• Another formula we often use is Perpetual Shield Immune Booster, which helps support healthy functioning of the immune system. It includes Fo-Ti root, ligustrum, Cherokee rose, white mulberry, sesame, eclipta, achyranthes, honeysuckle, siler, goji berry, and other Chinese herbs.

✳ EXERCISE ✳

I recommend light to moderate exercise, since people with CFS are prone to setbacks from overexertion. Start by exercising 10 minutes a day, and increase by 5 minutes each week until you reach 45 minutes. Be patient and amp up gradually. Excessive exercise can further injure the energy. Walking is a good start—30 minutes of gentle walking every other day can invigorate the body, raise basal metabolism, and help with energy. I often prescribe tai chi or a self-healing qi gong exercise to strengthen the vital qi of the spleen and stomach. It's called Spleen-Stomach Strengthening Qi Gong. This exercise should be done daily for 15 minutes, preferably in the morning and not too vigorously.

Lie down comfortably on your back, with your hands at your sides. Focus on your navel. Visualize a golden disk the size of a Frisbee spinning around your entire abdomen with its center at your navel.

With every inhalation the disk spins half of a circle. With every exhalation the disk completes the other half of the circle.

Breathe deeply so that the disk spins slowly, corresponding to your respiration for a total of 21 times in the clockwise direction.

Reverse the direction of the disk's rotation and repeat the breathing-spinning synchronization.

❊ ACUPRESSURE ❊

• Locate the acupoint Foot Three Miles (ST-36), four finger-widths below and to the outside of the right kneecap. Apply moderate pressure with your right thumb. Hold for 5 minutes. Repeat on the left leg.

....

• Locate the acupoint Hundred Meeting (DU-20), on top of your head, midway between your ears. Apply steady pressure with your index finger until you feel soreness. Hold for 3 minutes.

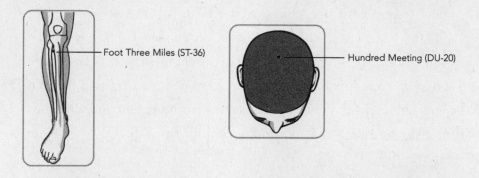

Foot Three Miles (ST-36)

Hundred Meeting (DU-20)

AVOID

• Excessive physical and mental activity, all kinds of stress, and overeating. Get plenty of sleep.

....

• Alcohol, smoking, and caffeine, as using them will weaken vital energy in the long run.

- Developing food allergies, and practice food rotation—don't repeat any one food within four days of eating it. For CFS, eliminate nightshade vegetables including tomatoes, potatoes, bell peppers, and eggplant.

- Anxiety and emotional turmoil, which burn out the vital energy.

COLD AND FLU

ONE IN THREE AMERICANS SUFFERS a seasonal cold at least once a year. The incidence rate is higher in schoolchildren, the elderly, and immune-compromised individuals. Though considered common, a cold can have severe health repercussions. Colds occur more during the fall and winter seasons, and the influenza virus likes to make its annual visit sometime in the fall. The early symptoms of a common cold include general malaise, chills, stiff neck, stuffy or runny nose, sneezing, and headaches. As the condition progresses, fever, sore throat, cough, stomach disturbances, and diarrhea may occur. The flu, as a result of the mutating influenza virus, is a more severe form of the common cold. It displays most of the same symptoms, though with more intensity and with the addition of rapidly rising fever, body aches, and vomiting.

Chinese medicine classifies the common cold as a wind pathogen that invades from the exterior. Wind cold is differentiated from wind heat, based on the finer differences between a cold and the flu. Wind cold usually occurs during seasonal changes and as a result of exposure to drafts, or even excessive exposure to air-conditioning. At this early stage, Chinese medicine suggests that perspiration is helpful in removing the pathogen from the skin. Common warming foods are used for this. Wind heat, in contrast, is characterized by high fever, sweating, sore throat, cough, headaches, and a yellow nasal discharge. It requires herbal prescriptions to clear the pathogen and relieve the symptoms. Acupuncture is widely used to treat the common cold, and there are many time-tested herbal formulations for upper respiratory infections. During the SARS epidemic in Asia, many hospitals and doctors' offices were offering these formulas as preventives. During the cold and flu seasons, I see many patients in my office. In addition to administering treatments, I educate them on simple ways to avoid catching a cold or the flu.

Here are some recommendations.

✳ DIET ✳

• For wind cold, warming and dispersing foods are encouraged to promote perspiration and expel the pathogen. These include ginger, garlic, mustard greens and seeds, grapefruit peel, cilantro, parsnips, scallions, basil, and cinnamon. Eat as little as possible so as not to burden the immune system, and drink plenty of warm fluids such as soups, porridges, and tea.

• For wind heat, cooling, soothing, and heat-clearing foods are best. Favor fresh fruits and vegetables like cabbage, burdock root, cilantro, dandelion, mint, chrysanthemum flowers, apples, pears, and bitter melon. Drink plenty of room temperature water or tea.

• For both wind cold and wind heat, avoid overeating. Avoid heavy, rich, greasy foods and meats and shellfish. Also stay away from astringent substances, such as vinegar, which close the pores and "trap the thief in the house."

✳ HOME REMEDIES ✳

• For wind cold, make a tea by boiling 1 chopped garlic clove, 3 slices of ginger, 1 chopped scallion, some basil, and a pinch of cinnamon in 3 cups of water for 5 minutes. Strain. Drink the tea hot and get into bed. Cover up and prepare to sweat. Sweating opens the pores, releasing trapped pathogens from the skin. Drink at least 3 cups of this tea every day until symptoms subside.

• Fill an 8-ounce squeeze bottle with 1 teaspoon sea salt. For wind cold, irrigate your sinuses with warm salt water twice daily to clean your nasal passageways. Gargle with warm salt water to relieve sore throat and take hot baths with Epsom salts to sweat.

• For wind cold, make a tea by boiling 1 whole lemon, 1 teaspoon cayenne pepper, and 1 tablespoon honey in 3 1/2 cups of water for 10 minutes. Strain, and drink 3 cups a day.

• For wind heat, juice a head of cabbage, 1 cup dandelion greens, 2 cucumbers, and 2 oranges. Drink 3 glasses daily.

• Boil a pot of water and turn off the heat. Add 10 drops of Tonic Oil (available at www.askdrmao.com), which consists of oils of camphor, peppermint, eucalyptus, fennel, and wintergreen, traditionally used for opening passageways and relieving joint pain. Inhale the fumes deeply for 10 minutes, covering your head and the pot with a towel.

• Make a tea with 1/2 cup fresh mint leaves and 1/2 cup dried chrysanthemum flowers by boiling in 4 cups of water for 20 minutes. Strain, and drink 3 cups daily. Drink throughout the day.

❋ DAILY SUPPLEMENTS ❋

• Up to 50 milligrams of zinc taken daily can help reduce the symptoms of a common cold.

• Up to 3,000 milligrams of vitamin C taken daily has been shown to reduce the duration of a cold.

• Vitamins E (800 IU), A (200 IU), and the B complex are antioxidants that help support healthy immune function.

• Thymus extract (200 milligrams) can help stimulate the immune system.

──────────── ✳ HERBAL THERAPY ✳ ────────────

• Herbs can be found in health food or vitamin stores, online, and at the offices of Chinese medicine practitioners. Herbs should be used according to individual needs; consult with a licensed practitioner for a customized formulation. To learn more about the herbs listed here, go to www.askdrmao.com.

• Ginger, kudzu, osha, yarrow, garlic, and astragalus can help fight off a cold at the onset. Take at the first signs of a cold.

• Andrographis has been shown to reduce the symptoms of a cold and shorten its duration.

• Make a tea by boiling 2 tablespoons of dried elderberry in 1 1/4 cups of water for 10 minutes. Strain, and drink 3 cups a day until the symptoms subside.

• I recommend our Cold/Flu Elixir, a Chinese herbal formula that supports a healthy immune system and can temporarily relieve cold symptoms. It contains honeysuckle, forsythia, schizonepetae, siler, kudzu, isatis, arctium, peppermint, figwort, apricot kernel, licorice, and other Chinese herbs.

──────────── ✳ EXERCISE ✳ ────────────

When you have a common cold, excessive exercise will deplete the body of vital qi, which is needed to fight the pathogen. I recommend rest and calm. A qi gong exercise called the Dragon Dance helps with circulation and promotes opening of the pores. It should be done indoors and not too vigorously.

COLD AND FLU

This exercise resembles a belly dance—it is a wriggling rhythmic dance of the torso that burns energy and promotes fat burning in the abdomen.

In a comfortable, quiet place stand with your feet together and ankles touching, or as close together as you can get them. Place your hands over your head, with palms together and fingers pointing up. Be sure to keep your palms together during the entire exercise.

Inhaling, push your waist out to the right side while keeping your head and upper torso straight. Simultaneously move your right elbow to the right, so that it rests at shoulder height.

Exhaling, push your waist out to the left side while keeping your head and upper torso straight. Simultaneously move your left elbow fully to the left at shoulder height.

Repeat this movement several times. Every time you move your waist to the right, bend your knees a little more, lowering your entire body as you squat. Be sure to keep your upper torso and head straight.

With each movement to the right, move your hands lower, keeping your palms together and fingers pointing up. When your arms reach your chest, turn your fingers toward the ground and continue the movement.

When your arms reach your knees, you should be squatting. Continue the movements, now rising with each right movement until you reach the standing position. When your arms reach your chest, switch the direction of your fingers so that they're pointing up again.

Throughout this exercise your hands should make an S-shaped movement and your body should perform a rhythmic belly dance. Remember to inhale on the rightward movement and exhale to the left.

Do this exercise during the day on an empty stomach. Begin slowly and increase speed and vigor, warming up the whole body, but not to the point of perspiration

---

✳ ACUPRESSURE ✳

• Locate the acupoint Valley of Harmony (LI-4), in the web between your thumb and index finger on your right hand. Apply steady pressure with your left thumb until you feel soreness. Hold for 2 minutes. Repeat on the left hand. This is traditionally used to support immune functions and detoxification.

• Locate the acupoint Wind Pond (GB-20), in the natural indentation at the base of your skull on either side of your neck. Press and lift up toward the base of your skull with your thumbs and lean your head back. Use the weight of your head against your thumbs for a steady pressure. Hold for about 5 minutes, breathing deeply and slowly.

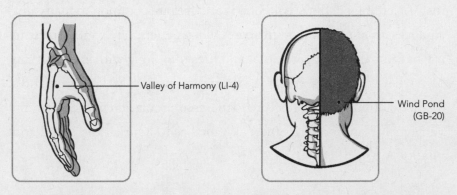

Valley of Harmony (LI-4)

Wind Pond (GB-20)

AVOID

• Excessive activity, straining, and overeating. Get plenty of sleep.

• Alcohol, smoking, and caffeine, which adversely affect energy and immunity.

COLD HANDS AND FEET

LIMBS GET COLD WHEN BLOOD VESSELS constrict or become obstructed. The hands or feet may change in color from pink to purple, blue, or white. Causes include exposure to extreme cold, poor circulation due to heart disease, frostbite, stress, side effects of medications, and prolonged work with vibrating equipment such as jackhammers. Raynaud's syndrome is a disorder that constricts the flow of blood to the fingers and toes, and shows up as cold hands and feet. Some people who suffer from low thyroid function experience cold hands and feet, as the thyroid controls and maintains body temperature. Cold extremities are more common in women than in men.

Chinese medicine considers coldness in the body to be a lack of or diminished flow of the body's yang, or fire energy, or as the result of insufficient blood. Since cold hands and feet are common to many imbalances, this symptom often abates when patients are well. I stress to my patients that changes to diet and lifestyle, along with exercise, can help relieve the symptoms. If the symptoms persist, as with Raynaud's disease, I often use acupuncture to increase circulation of the warming yang energy and prescribe herbal remedies to nourish the blood and vitality.

Here are some of my favorite recommendations.

❊ DIET ❊

• Eat plenty of omega-3–rich foods, such as mackerel, herring, salmon, and anchovies. Emphasize blood-building meats such as lamb, beef, and wild game as well as iron-rich foods like spinach, broccoli, prunes, figs, raisins, oats, spelt, quinoa, sunflower and sesame seeds, walnuts, chestnuts, yams, squash, kale, onions, leeks, chives, garlic, scallions, parsley, parsnips, and jujube date. Liberally use spices such as cinnamon, turmeric, ginger, black pepper, fennel, anise, cardamom, and cayenne pepper. Drink only warm or hot water.

. . . .

• Avoid raw foods and icy-cold foods and beverages as well as alcohol and coffee. Avoid foods containing preservatives and additives as well. Although alcohol may temporarily be warming, it actually lowers body temperature.

• Make a tea by steeping 1 teaspoon ground cinnamon and 1 teaspoon ground cloves in 3 cups of hot water. Drink 1 cup of this tea in the evening to warm your insides, and to encourage a good night's sleep.

• Wear socks and gloves to bed to maintain warmth in the extremities.

• Take a hot spice bath by boiling the following spices in a large pot for 15 minutes: 1 tablespoon each of crushed black pepper, cayenne pepper, ginger, cinnamon, rosemary, oregano, sage, and cumin. Pour the mixture into the bathtub through a strainer and fill the tub with hot water. You'll feel warmed by the spices and you'll also smell good. Taking the bath before bedtime is preferable, but anytime will do.

———————— ❋ DAILY SUPPLEMENTS ❋ ————————

• Taking a daily dose of vitamin B_3 (100 milligrams), or niacin, can be helpful in treating Raynaud's phenomenon.

• Taking omega-3 fish oils (1,000 milligrams EPA; 800 milligrams DHA) on a daily basis may also help treat cold hands and feet.

• Evening primrose oil or borage oil provides a good source of GLA (gamma-linolenic acid; 400 milligrams), an essential fatty acid that has been shown to reduce symptoms of Raynaud's syndrome.

———————— ❋ HERBAL THERAPY ❋ ————————

• Herbs can be found in health food or vitamin stores, online, and at the offices of Chinese medicine practitioners. Herbs should be used according to individual needs; consult with a licensed practitioner for a customized formulation. To learn more about the herbs listed here, go to www.askdrmao.com.

• Using ginkgo, turmeric, cinnamon, and ginger can improve circulation in the fingers and toes.

COLD HANDS AND FEET

•I recommend our Chinese herbal formulation Dragon Male, which supports healthy circulation and warms the yang energy of the body. It contains naturally shed deer antler velvet, ginseng root, morinda root, cistanches, psoralea fruit, fennel, clove flower bud, frankincense, myrrh, horny goat weed, and other Chinese herbs.

--- ❊ EXERCISE ❊ ---

Regular physical activity is essential for smooth flow of energy in the body and for preventing blockages and promoting healthy circulation. I also recommend energy exercises like the qi gong warm-up exercise I outline below. By tapping the trunk, arms, and legs, you activate the flow of energy and blood in your body. Practice the warm-up for 15 minutes—or more often—every day.

Stand with your feet shoulder-width apart, spine erect, and head tilted slightly forward.

Make your right hand into a loose fist and begin tapping your lower abdomen with mild to moderate strength in a rhythmic fashion. Proceed to the middle and upper abdomen, then the chest.

Start tapping under the armpit of the left arm, then the inner part of the arm and down to the palm. Then tap the outer part of the arm back up to the shoulder. Tap the shoulder muscle 7 times.

Repeat the same movement with the left hand.

Begin tapping the lower back on both sides with both hands in loose fists. Move the tapping down the back of the legs to the outsides of the ankles.

Start tapping on the insides of the ankles, working your way up the insides of the calves and thighs.

Finally, return to a standing position, again tapping your lower abdomen. End by placing your palms on your lower abdomen, left hand on top of the right. Make clockwise circles, rubbing the lower abdomen 36 times.

• Locate the acupoint Valley of Harmony (LI-4), in the web between your thumb and index finger on your right hand. Apply steady pressure with your left thumb until you feel soreness. Hold for 2 minutes. Repeat on the left hand. This is used to unblock energy and blood stasis.

• Locate the acupoint Great Surge (LIV-3), in the natural indentation on the top of your right foot between the big and second toes. Apply moderate pressure with your right thumb for 5 minutes. Repeat on the left foot. This point is traditionally used to release all types of blockages.

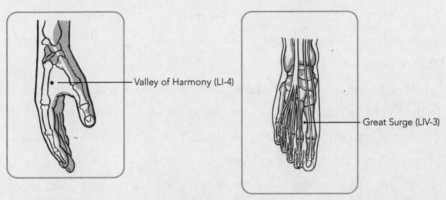

Valley of Harmony (LI-4)

Great Surge (LIV-3)

AVOID

• Smoking, as it impairs circulation.

• Caffeine, as it constricts blood vessels and can cause cold hands and feet.

• Alcohol, as its warming effects are only temporary.

 # CONSTIPATION

THE HUMAN BOWEL SYSTEM IS LIKE THE SEWER SYSTEM—if the sewers get clogged, the waste backs up and spills into the house. If your

CONSTIPATION

bowels are not moving, all the toxins and waste products of daily living remain and recirculate in your body, leading to disease. With constipation there is trouble emptying the bowels daily, and stools may be dry and hard, making them difficult to pass and forcing you to strain. In some cases, you may experience incomplete passing of the stool and feel the urge to have a bowel movement after you've just had one. Many people suffer from constipation in Western cultures, where sedentary lifestyle, unhealthy diet, and stress are prevalent. Constipation is caused by a fiber-deprived diet, hormonal changes, side effects from pain medications, illnesses, and, in some cases, misshapen intestines. Regular bowel movements are essential for a long, healthy, and productive life.

In Chinese medicine, the bowels are recognized as being connected to the liver and spleen digestive systems. Besides improper diet, many cases of constipation are due to prolonged stress and emotional imbalance, causing the liver energy to stagnate and preventing natural peristaltic bowel movements. Other cases of constipation involve prolonged blood and fluid deficiency, drying up the stools and making them hard to pass.

I've seen many patients suffering with constipation, and I often work with them in consultation with a gastroenterologist. Usually constipation is one of many symptoms of a medical condition such as irritable bowel syndrome (IBS), gallstones, colitis, Crohn's disease, bacterial overgrowth in the small bowel, or endometriosis. My treatment for constipation focuses on discovering the primary condition and then freeing the liver energy, stimulating the natural movements of the bowels. I also address the underlying cause, be it emotional, dietary, or deficiencies of blood and fluids. I find the best success comes when the patient participates by changing his or her lifestyle. Below are some of my favorite home remedies that have been used successfully in my practice. If you experience sudden constipation lasting more than a week, you should consult your physician, as this may be a sign of a more serious condition requiring immediate attention.

※ DIET ※

• It is important to keep the bowels in healthy peristalsis with a diet rich in high-fiber foods. Favor whole grains with fiber-rich bran, legumes, fruits, and vegetables. Bananas, apples, prunes, figs, walnuts, spinach, peaches, pears, pine nuts, sesame seeds, mulberries, grapefruit, yams, avocados, adzuki beans, apricot kernels, yogurt, sprouted greens, beets, cabbage, bok choy, cauliflower, and broccoli all help keep the intestines hydrated. Fish, nuts, and seeds are rich in omega-3 fatty acids and help lubricate the intestines. Drink at least six to eight glasses of room temperature water a day.

• Do not overeat, and eliminate red meat, animal fats, fried and greasy foods, refined sugars, and simple carbohydrates, which create dampness, clogging up the digestive system.

※ HOME REMEDIES ※

• To stimulate the natural peristalsis of the bowels upon waking each morning, on an empty stomach drink a 12-ounce glass of lukewarm water mixed with 1 tablespoon honey. Walk 200 paces afterward and try to use the bathroom.

• Cook 1 cup peeled and chopped beets with 1 cup of chopped cabbage in a soup. Eat with dinner every other night for two weeks. This helps lubricate the bowels.

• Drink a glass of aloe vera juice on an empty stomach every morning for two weeks to help lubricate the bowels.

• Stew 3 to 5 prunes lightly in water for 5 minutes. Eat the prunes and drink the juice before bedtime as needed.

CONSTIPATION

--- ❋ DAILY SUPPLEMENTS ❋ ---

• Taking 5 to 10 grams psyllium (in pill or powder form) three times a day with a glass of lukewarm water can help keep you regular.

• Taking 300 to 500 milligrams of aloe vera in capsule form once a day helps stimulate the intestinal tract and move the bowels.

• Taking 2 to 4 grams of flaxseed in either liquid, ground-up powder, or pill form twice each day can deliver the necessary amount of omega-3 fatty acids to soften stool and lubricate the bowels.

--- ❋ HERBAL THERAPY ❋ ---

• Herbs can be found in health food or vitamin stores, online, and at the offices of Chinese medicine practitioners. Herbs should be used according to individual needs; consult with a licensed practitioner for a customized formulation. To learn more about the herbs listed here, go to www.ask drmao.com.

• Taking fenugreek 3 times a day can help soften the stools, and also helps regulate blood sugar.

• Senna leaf can be taken as a powerful laxative but should be used with caution. Limit its use to less than 10 days; otherwise it can become addictive.

• Chinese herbs such as peach kernel, plum kernel, apricot kernel, biota seed, pine nut, and tangerine peel have lubricating and stool-softening properties. These can be used long term without side effects.

• For supporting healthy bowel function I often recommend our Chinese Internal Cleanse Tea. It contains cassia seed, dandelion, hawthorn, chrysanthemum, mulberry leaf, and other herbs. I drink it regularly myself to support the cleansing function of my body.

One of the biggest causes of constipation is leading a sedentary life. Continual inactivity dramatically reduces stimulation to the digestive tract. Just like those of a hibernating bear, our bowels shut down. A simple activity like a 30-minute brisk walk each day helps stimulate the leg and thigh muscles, where the stomach and liver energetic meridians traverse.

Here is a simple 15-minute abdominal massage used to promote bowel movement function. Do this massage daily.

Lie on your back and bend your knees slightly to a comfortable position.

Begin a circular massage of the abdomen, with both palms moving together: Starting from the lower right side and with moderate pressure, rub your abdomen in small clockwise circles with your palms. Keep making small circles with the hands as you slowly traverse the abdomen around the navel.

When you reach the lower left abdomen lift your arms and begin again from the lower right abdomen. Continue for 10 to 15 minutes.

* ACUPRESSURE *

• Find the acupoint Valley of Harmony (LI-4), at the web between your right thumb and index finger. Apply steady pressure with your left thumb until you feel soreness. Hold for 2 minutes. Repeat on the left hand.

• Find the acupoint Upper Great Opening (ST-37) by measuring 2 hand-widths or 8 fingers below the outer indentation of your right knee next to

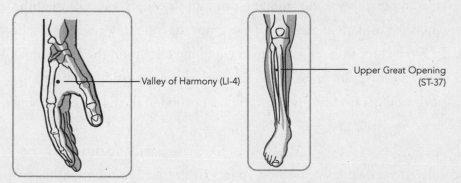

Valley of Harmony (LI-4)

Upper Great Opening (ST-37)

CONSTIPATION

your shinbone. Apply steady pressure with your left thumb until you feel soreness. Hold for 2 minutes. Repeat on the left leg.

AVOID

• A sedentary lifestyle, inactivity, and prolonged sitting, which suppress natural intestinal peristalsis.

....

• Smoking, alcohol, and coffee, which tend to be dehydrating, making constipation worse.

....

• Resisting the urge to move your bowels when necessary, which can contribute to abnormal bowel habits and constipation.

....

• Some antacids, especially those containing aluminum, calcium, and iron supplements, as they can cause constipation.

COUGH

COUGHING IS YOUR BODY'S NATURAL RESPONSE to foreign substances in the airways or the throat. It is triggered by the nervous system, which produces a spasm of the muscles in the chest, pushing the air out of the lungs at an incredible speed (measured at 300 miles per hour). Anything from a common cold to respiratory infections, chronic obstructive disorders, and smoking can cause a cough. Most of the time when the underlying condition is removed, coughing resolves itself. In some chronic cases, prolonged coughing can strain the chest muscles, causing pain, injuring the rib cage, or even causing spontaneous pneumothorax, a condition in which a portion of the tissue separating the lungs collapses.

In Chinese medicine, a cough, like nausea and vomiting, is considered a rebellious upsurge of energy. It's often a result of pathogens in the lungs, and sometimes it can be due to emotional turmoil aggravating the liver-gallbladder network, whose energy surges upward and injures the lungs. Most of the cough cases I treat are the result of common colds, allergies, or respiratory infections. As I mentioned in the bronchitis section, many are also due to acid reflux. I see the best results when I use acupuncture and cupping therapies to quickly relieve the cough, followed by fast-acting herbal therapy to soothe the bronchial tubes, redirect the energy downward, open the lungs to promote respiration, and remove the underlying condition.

Mucus or phlegm is often a culprit in a chronic cough. In Chinese medicine, the saying "The spleen creates dampness and mucus and the lungs are the storehouse" explains how diet and digestive weakness cause a buildup of dampness and phlegm that accumulates in the lungs, leading to a rebellion of the lung energy. In many cases, reducing and clearing out the mucus will ease the cough. I have worked with many pulmonary specialists over the years, and I tell my patients that if a cough persists beyond a month without improvement, they should immediately see a lung specialist for further examination.

Follow the simple recommendations below to help with your cough.

❋ DIET ❋

• For dietary advice for a cough associated with a common cold, refer to the section on common colds (page 240).

....

• I recommend a diet rich in complex carbohydrates, low in fat, and moderate in protein. Eat green vegetables, cabbage (both green and red), celery, daikon radish, garlic, green beans, button mushrooms, mustard greens, onions, leeks, parsnips, seaweed, turnips, water chestnuts, watercress, apples, bananas, apricots, figs, grapefruits, mulberries, oranges, pear apples, persimmons, almonds, chestnuts, walnuts, olives, and honey.

• Eliminate foods that promote mucus, including all dairy products (especially ice cream), cold and raw foods, sweet foods containing simple processed sugars, processed flour, and soft drinks.

———————— ❊ HOME REMEDIES ❊ ————————

• For a dry cough, finely chop 2 cups each of green and red cabbage, add 1 sliced pear apple (Asian pear), and boil in 6 cups of water for 30 minutes. Strain, and drink this broth 3 times a day.

• For a dry cough with thick yellow phlegm that is difficult to expectorate, juice 1 daikon radish and 1/2 cup water chestnuts. Warm the juice and drink with 1 teaspoon honey. Drink 3 cups a day until the mucus returns to a clear color and the cough subsides.

• For a chronic cough with excess mucus, boil 20 grapefruit seeds, 1 teaspoon mustard seeds, and 1 teaspoon parsnip seeds in 1 1/2 cups water for 10 minutes. Strain. Add 1 teaspoon honey and drink 3 times a day. Take until the cough subsides.

• For a cough with excess mucus, boil 2 oranges, including the peels, in 4 cups of water for 30 minutes. Drink 3 cups daily and eat the oranges.

• For all kinds of coughs, boil a pot of water and turn off the stove. Add 10 drops of Tonic Oil (available at www.askdrmao.com), which consists of oils of camphor, peppermint, eucalyptus, fennel, and wintergreen. Inhale the fumes deeply for 10 minutes, covering your head and the pot with a towel. This is traditionally used for opening passageways and relieving joint pain.

———————— ❊ DAILY SUPPLEMENTS ❊ ————————

• Supplementing with vitamins C (1,000 milligrams), E (800 IU), and B complex, bromelain (450 milligrams), garlic (900 milligrams), zinc (50 milligrams), and iron (25 milligrams) can help treat cough.

• Taking MSM (1,000 milligrams) and pycnogenol (200 milligrams), a bioflavonoid found in grape seeds, can help protect the lungs and prevent infections.

• Taking quercetin (250 milligrams) is useful for its antihistamine properties in allergic bronchitis.

———————————— ✳ HERBAL THERAPY ✳ ————————————

• Herbs can be found in health food or vitamin stores, online, and at the offices of Chinese medicine practitioners. Herbs should be used according to individual needs; consult with a licensed practitioner for a customized formulation. To learn more about the herbs listed here, go to www.ask drmao.com.

• Linden, marshmallow, and peppermint are traditionally used to suppress cough.

• Lily bulb, apricot kernel, stemona root, fritillaria, mulberry, Chinese basil, mustard seed, daikon seed, ginger, and schizandra berry are among the many herbs used in Chinese medicine to calm coughs and ventilate the lungs.

• For chronic bronchitis accompanied by kidney weakness, I recommend tonic herbs such as ginkgo seed, goji berry, cornus berry, astragalus, and ginseng.

———————————— ✳ EXERCISE ✳ ————————————

Don't exercise strenuously during acute stages of coughing bouts, as exercise can worsen the condition. Calm and restful walks in fresh air can help. During remission, moderate physical exercise is appropriate. I recommend daily qi gong exercises to strengthen the body, open the lungs, and redirect the flow of qi downward. Eight Treasures Qi Gong is a wonderful set of qi gong movements that, when performed daily for 30 minutes, can be of great benefit to the mind and body. The fifth movement of the practice, called Water and Fire Meet, is targeted to bring the cooling and calming energy of the kidneys to the chest, to redirect the qi downward, and to calm a cough. Perform this exercise twice daily, preferably at 5:00 A.M. and 7:00 P.M.

In a quiet, comfortable environment, preferably outdoors, stand with your feet shoulder-width apart, knees slightly bent, spine erect, tailbone tucked in, and head tilted slightly forward. Place your arms palms down on your lower abdomen just below the navel, one hand overlapping the other.

Begin with rhythmic, slow, and relaxed breathing. Inhale deeply but softly, and imagine the breath extending all the way down to the lower abdomen, about two finger-widths below the navel. Exhale gently and softly. Stay in this position for 7 breath cycles, relaxing and calming your mind.

Now begin the exercise. Exhale, and bend down from your waist. Begin a gentle massage of the inner legs, starting at the inner ankles by rubbing rhythmically in a circular motion.

Inhale as you continue the massage, slowly coming up the inner calves to the inner thighs. Raise your arms slowly to your chest with the backs of your palms touching each other and your elbows bent.

When you reach the chest, make a small circular motion with your hands, moving from the middle to the outer chest with palms facing down, expanding the chest. Then move your hands from the outer to the middle of the chest, with palms facing up.

Inhale, and in an alternating fashion make circles with the bent elbows, moving from front to back and bending at the hips to exaggerate the motion slightly. Alternate between the left and right arms 3 times.

Repeat the circles now in the reverse direction from the back to the front, inhaling and exhaling with each circle. Repeat with each arm 3 times.

Bring the arms back to the center of the chest, with the back of the palms facing each other, elbows bent. Inhale and open the chest with both arms stretching back and to the sides, again with elbows bent and palms relaxed. Exhale and stretch both arms out to the sides, palms facing out as if you were pushing to the left and right sides. As you exhale, push your hands out 3 times.

To complete the exercise, return to the initial standing posture. Place your hands on your lower abdomen, palms down, one hand overlapping the other. Rub your lower abdomen 7 times in small clockwise circles just below the navel.

❊ ACUPRESSURE ❊

- Locate the acupoint Cubit Marsh (LU-5) by bending your right arm at the elbow and finding the point in the elbow crease, on the outer side of the large tendon in the middle of the crease. Apply moderate pressure with your left thumb until you feel soreness. Hold for 2 minutes. Repeat on the left arm.

- Locate the acupoint Upward Thrust (REN-22), on the chest, level with the clavicle and shoulders, in the depression at the center of the sternum just below the V of the neck. Apply steady pressure with your index fingers until you feel soreness. Hold for 3 minutes.

- These points are used to soothe breathing, redirect lung energy downward, and stop cough.

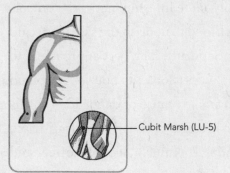

Cubit Marsh (LU-5)

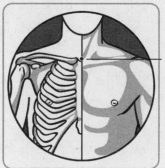

Upward Thrust (REN-22)

AVOID

- Exposure to airborne irritants, which can aggravate a cough.

- Alcohol, smoking, and caffeine, stimulants that can worsen the condition.

COUGH

> • Exposure to cold weather, which can trigger bronchial constriction and worsen a cough.
>
> • Stress, anxiety, and emotional turmoil, which can aggravate a cough.

DANDRUFF

ALMOST EVERYONE HAS SOME DEGREE OF DANDRUFF—that's normal. Your skin and scalp undergo regular regeneration and renewal; dead skin is shed to allow new skin to grow. This is especially evident in the scalp, where the dead skin gets tangled in the hair and forms a dry, flaky, crusty residue. This flaking can be worse in people with dry skin or in those with deficiencies of certain nutritional components. Hormonal imbalances, stress, and diet also play a role. Dandruff is worse during fall and winter, when the air tends to be dry.

In Chinese medicine, skin moisture relies on blood and the healthy function of the lungs, since the lung–large intestine network controls the skin. When there is insufficient blood to nourish the skin, the scalp becomes dry and flaky, producing dandruff. The best approach is to identify and resolve the underlying causes in order to nourish the blood and moisten the skin. Excess heat can also cause of dandruff—in this case the excess heat is most likely the result of a rich diet of deep-fried, greasy, spicy, and protein-rich foods. Too much alcohol, coffee, and sugar can cause the body's pH to become more acidic, directly contributing to poor scalp condition. If stress, hormonal imbalances, and nutritional deficiencies are evident, lifestyle changes can help prevent or reduce the severity of the symptoms.

I had a patient in his late twenties with dandruff so severe that he was taking antidepressants to deal with the effects of the social stigma of the condition. Though he had seen several dermatologists and had used many topical medications, his condition didn't change. I determined that he was suffering from liver energy stagnation coupled with heat from a poor diet. I put him on a cleansing and detoxification program followed by a strict vegetarian diet of fresh fruits and vegetables, beans, nuts, and whole grains for three months. I also administered weekly acupuncture and herbal therapies, and I taught him my stress release meditation, which combines simple visualization with breathing practice to reduce tension and lower stress hormones. I'm glad to report that by the end of his three-month therapy his dandruff was no longer a problem, and I hear he is dating again.

❊ DIET ❊

• A diet to relieve dandruff must focus on nourishing blood and should be moistening without being greasy. Eat a healthy organic diet with lots of fresh green leafy vegetables, fresh fruits, nuts, seeds, and whole grains. Animal products should be from organic sources with a low fat content. Drink plenty of room-temperature water to help irrigate the skin.

• Eliminate processed foods, artificial additives, bleached sugar, dairy products, soft drinks, and spicy, hot, fried, and oily foods.

❊ HOME REMEDIES ❊

• Massage aloe vera gel directly from the leaf into the scalp once a day, preferably before bedtime, for a month. Leave it on overnight and rinse it off with your morning shower.

• In the shower, wet your hands and scrub baking soda vigorously into your scalp. After rinsing off, massage Tonic Oil (available at www.askdrmao.com), which contains oils of wintergreen, eucalyptus, and menthol, into your scalp. Leave it on for 10 minutes before shampooing.

DANDRUFF

• Prepare a mild green tea, let it cool, and pour it onto your scalp. Leave it on for 10 minutes, then shampoo with olive oil or avocado oil shampoo, available at health food stores.

❋ DAILY SUPPLEMENTS ❋

• Supplementing with essential fatty acids (1,000 milligrams EPA; 800 milligrams DHA) from flaxseeds or evening primrose oil (450 milligrams GLA) is important for a healthy scalp.

....

• Taking vitamins A (200 IU), B complex, and E (800 IU) supports healthy skin and hair.

....

• Selenium (100 micrograms) is an excellent antioxidant to treat a dry, scaly scalp.

....

• Kelp (500 milligrams) supplements provide essential minerals and iodine for skin health.

❋ HERBAL THERAPY ❋

• Herbs can be found in health food or vitamin stores, online, and at the offices of Chinese medicine practitioners. Herbs should be used according to individual needs; consult with a licensed practitioner for a customized formulation. To learn more about the herbs listed here, go to www.ask drmao.com.

....

• Ginkgo biloba improves circulation to the scalp, green tea reduces sebum oil deposits, and saw palmetto helps reduce hair loss.

....

• Our Exquisite Skin Chinese herbal formula helps support healthy skin function. It contains siler, caltrop, schizonepetae, astragalus, peony, dong quai, Fo-Ti, rhubarb, and licorice.

❋ EXERCISE ❋

Regular physical exercise is important for maintaining proper circulation to the scalp. Stress-reduction exercises and meditation can also help regulate your energy and strengthen your essence. I recommend the following General Cleansing Exercise to all my patients.

Sit comfortably or lie down on your back. Slow your respiration to deep abdominal breathing. Say the word "calm" in your mind with every exhalation. You'll be visualizing the relaxation of a body part and releasing tension with every exhalation. Trace the following three pathways outlined below.

Start at the top of your head. Inhale, then exhale and visualize your scalp muscles relaxing. Say "calm" in your mind. Repeat this word for each body part as you move down through your face, throat, chest, abdomen, thighs, knees, calves, ankles, and feet. When you've relaxed your feet, visualize all the tension in your body leaving through your toes in the form of dark smoke.

Next, start at the temple region of your head. This path focuses on the sides and upper extremities. Inhale, then exhale and visualize your temple muscles relaxing. Say the word "calm" in your mind. Repeat this word for each body part as you move down through your jaws, the sides of your neck, shoulders, upper arms, elbows, forearms, wrists, and hands. Once you've relaxed your hands, visualize all the tension leaving your body through your fingertips in the form of dark smoke.

The final pathway begins on the back of your head. This path relaxes the back of your body. Repeat the breathing-visualization-word routine, as you go from the back of your neck to your upper back, middle back, lower back, back of thighs, calves, and heels. Then focus on the acupoint Bubbling Spring (KID-1), on the soles of your feet, for 1 minute.

Practice this exercise for at least 15 minutes twice a day.

❋ ACUPRESSURE ❋

• Find the acupoint Three Yin Crossing (SP-6), which is traditionally used to support yin and balance hormones. Four finger-widths above the inner ankle of the right foot. Apply steady pressure with your right thumb until you feel soreness. Hold for 2 minutes. Repeat on the left foot.

• Locate the acupoint Valley of Harmony (LI-4), in the web between your thumb and index finger on your right hand. It is traditionally used to open blockages and detoxify. Apply steady pressure with your left thumb until you feel soreness. Hold for 2 minutes. Repeat on the left hand.

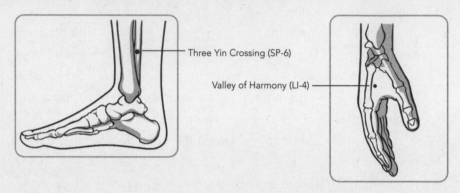

Three Yin Crossing (SP-6)

Valley of Harmony (LI-4)

— AVOID —

• Eating chemicals, additives, and preservatives, as they can interfere with the nourishment and lubrication of the skin.

• Stress and overwork, as they can deplete the vital essence, leading to dry skin.

 DIABETES

SUGAR—GLUCOSE, SPECIFICALLY—is the primary source of energy for every cell in the body, whether in the brain, the heart, or the muscles that help you walk. As food is digested, the sugars are changed into glucose. The glucose then travels throughout the body via the blood, and is absorbed by cells for energy. A tiny molecule called insulin, which is produced by the pancreas, makes this absorption possible. Under normal circumstances your blood sugar is usually balanced, with minor peaks after a meal. But consuming an excess of cookies, soft drinks, and processed foods that contain simple sugars, combined with inactivity and a sedentary life, can cause blood glucose levels to rise rapidly. In response, the pancreas produces excess insulin, which rapidly shuffles the blood sugar into cells, dropping levels to far below normal and resulting in cravings for more sugar. Over time this yo-yo effect can make the cells less sensitive to insulin and more sugar stays in the blood, resulting in diabetes. This phenomenon is called insulin resistance.

In ancient times diabetes was diagnosed by tasting a person's urine for sugar content. Excess sugar in the blood eventually drains out of the kidneys, causing frequent urination, and with loss of the fluids comes thirst. Frequent urination and excessive thirst are the hallmark characteristics of diabetes. Affecting more than 20 million people in the United States, diabetes is a complex syndrome involving many of the body's systems and has the potential to damage the heart, kidneys, nervous system, and hormonal system. If left unmanaged, diabetes can cause many complications, including heart disease, kidney failure, peripheral neuropathy, decreased wound healing, skin ulceration, and infections.

Type 2—or adult-onset diabetes—is the most common of the two main types of diabetes. Though there is no cure for diabetes, there are ways to control blood sugar. With proper diet and an approach that integrates Western and Eastern medicine, type 2 diabetes can be controlled. I work with endocrinologists to reverse or control diabetes— our patients are put on a strict diet that includes quality protein from fish, fowl, nuts, seeds, beans, and legumes. Fresh vegetables and whole grains are also part of the diet. Patients eat small but frequent meals, do at least one hour of cardiovascular exercise a day, and keep their stress levels low with meditation. I also administer weekly acupuncture treatments and Chinese herbal therapy. Initially my diabetes patients are on medication prescribed by their endocrinologist, but as their glucose levels normalize, the medications are reduced until they're no longer necessary. This type of treatment can only be accomplished through a close collaboration between Eastern and Western medicine.

Chinese medicine has recorded many observations of diabetes throughout the millennia and classifies it as "wasting and thirsting disorder." It has differentiated the condition into upper, middle, and lower regions of the body, depending on where the most symptoms occur. For example, excess thirst is the upper body, attributed to deficiency of the lung–large intestine network. Excess hunger is attributed to the middle and linked with the spleen-pancreas-stomach network. Excess urination is linked to the lower body organs, namely the kidneys. Depending on the symptoms, treatments focus on harmonizing these organs, strengthening weaknesses, and adjusting the body's ability to absorb and metabolize sugar. The best approach to diabetes is, of course, prevention. With simple changes to your diet and lifestyle, along with regular checkups, you can keep this debilitating condition from entering your life.

Please note: Never go off medications or insulin without the consent of your physician.

✳ DIET ✳

• The key to maintaining normal sugar levels in the body is to eat a balanced diet of complex carbohydrates, organic sources of protein, and healthful fats. Eat at regular intervals and eat more often in smaller amounts. Skipping meals is a sure way of causing blood glucose to bounce up and down. Favor black beans, soybeans, tofu, garbanzo beans, mung beans, yams, peas, artichokes, pumpkin, celery, spinach, daikon radish, cabbage, water chestnuts, millet, oats, amaranth, quinoa, bran, lentils, organic chicken and turkey, fish, egg whites, unsweetened low-fat yogurt, nuts, seeds, olive oil, flaxseed oil, virgin coconut oil, and fresh berries.

- Eliminate all simple sugars and foods high in sugar, such as soft drinks, candy, honey, and molasses. Alcohol should be eliminated. Smoking and caffeine also have an adverse effect on sugar metabolism.

- Learn to read food labels. Look out for sugar, corn syrup, and dextrose as ingredients. It's best to stay away from processed and refined products, which are devoid of healthful fiber and nutrients.

❋ HOME REMEDIES ❋

- Eat a slice of baked pumpkin topped with olive oil and rosemary every day.

- Boil 1/2 head chopped cabbage, 1 diced yam, and 1/3 cup lentils in 8 cups of water for 30 to 45 minutes. Season lightly with herbs and spices and eat as a soup for dinner. Have this dish 2 to 3 times a week for a month.

- Juice 1 daikon radish, 3 stalks of celery, 1 cucumber, and 1 bunch of spinach. Drink 2 glasses a day.

- Drink a tea made with 1/2 cup chrysanthemum flowers boiled for 15 minutes in 5 cups of water. Strain, and drink 3 to 4 cups a day.

❋ DAILY SUPPLEMENTS ❋

- Alpha lipoic acid (50 milligrams) is a powerful antioxidant used to prevent damage to the cells. It is being studied for its ability to absorb glucose in muscle tissue to relieve diabetic neuropathy and reduce sensitivity to insulin.

- Chromium (200 micrograms) can reduce sugar levels during fasting periods if taken for a period of at least two months.

- Vitamins E (800 IU) and B complex, coenzyme Q-10 (50 milligrams), and L-carnitine (500 milligrams) have been shown in some studies to support healthy blood glucose levels.

• Brewer's yeast (500 milligrams) contains a natural glucose-tolerance factor that is necessary for producing and using insulin.

———————— ❊ HERBAL THERAPY ❊ ————————

• Herbs can be found in health food or vitamin stores, online, and at the offices of Chinese medicine practitioners. Herbs should be used according to individual needs; consult with a licensed practitioner for a customized formulation. To learn more about the herbs listed here, go to www.askdrmao.com.

• Fenugreek, garlic, bilberry, ginseng, and gymnema are beneficial for treating diabetes.

• Traditional herbs that have been used for wasting and thirsting disorders include rehmannia, Asian cornelian cherry, Chinese yam, poria, mouton, ganoderma, astragalus, ginseng, and water plantain.

———————— ❊ EXERCISE ❊ ————————

Keeping fit and maintaining proper weight is the best thing you can do to prevent diabetes. Exercise also plays a direct role in how your body stores and uses the energy you consume. A daily 30-minute cardiovascular activity that stimulates circulation, conditions the heart, and builds muscle will encourage your body to properly metabolize sugar, helping to prevent diabetes. Studies show that tai chi and qi gong exercises have a beneficial effect on the hormonal system. With daily practice of qi gong exercises such as the Eight Treasures you can strengthen your hormonal system, help balance your blood sugar levels, and avoid the serious complications of diabetes. Below I describe a simple walking exercise called Merry-Go-Around that I recommend to many of my patients to help manage diabetes.

In a quiet outdoor setting find a tree with at least five feet of clear space around the trunk in all directions. If you were to draw a circle around the tree, its diameter would be around 10 to 12 feet, though larger or smaller circles are also fine.

Walk around the tree with a relaxed but steady gait, with your hands raised to your trunk. With each completed circle change the position of your arms by slightly raising or lowering your hands in front or on the sides of your trunk.

For the first half of the exercise, walk clockwise around the tree. For the second half, walk counterclockwise.

Do this exercise twice a day for 15 minutes.

❋ ACUPRESSURE ❋

• Find the acupoint Foot Three Miles (ST-36), four finger-widths below the kneecap on the right leg. Apply moderate pressure with your right thumb until you feel soreness. Hold for 2 minutes. Repeat on the left leg.

• Find the acupoint Three Yin Crossing (SP-6), four finger-widths above the inner anklebone, in the depression near the bone on the right leg. Apply steady pressure with your right thumb until you feel soreness. Hold for 3 minutes. Repeat on the left leg.

• Engaging both of these points helps regulate digestion and metabolism, strengthens the vital qi, and tones the yin of the kidneys, spleen, and liver, which are involved in endocrine function.

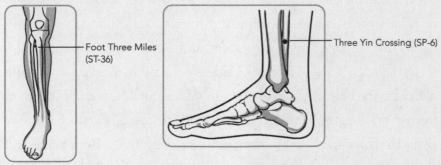

Foot Three Miles (ST-36)

Three Yin Crossing (SP-6)

AVOID

• A sedentary life, which is a major contributor to diabetes. Get out and get physically active.

DIABETES

- Sugar and sweets, alcohol, and coffee; they should be off-limits.

- Stress, anxiety, and emotional turmoil.

DIARRHEA

MOST OF US GET THE RUNS NOW AND THEN. Something we eat or drink disagrees with our system and our body rejects the offending substance by expelling it through the bowels. The diarrhea soon passes and we are back to normal. But when diarrhea is a recurring condition, the impact on daily life becomes unbearable. The two biggest causes of diarrhea are diet and a stressful lifestyle. Bacteria or parasites found in uncooked or contaminated foods can cause acute diarrhea. Most chronic diarrhea is associated with either irritable bowel syndrome (IBS) or inflammatory bowel disease (IBD), which includes colitis, ulcerative colitis, Crohn's disease, and proctitis. Dehydration is often a complication of chronic diarrhea; if unchecked, dehydration can have serious, life-threatening consequences.

In Chinese medicine, there are three possible causes of diarrhea: emotional imbalances affecting the liver system, unhealthy eating habits that damage the spleen system, and exhausting work and excess sexual activity, which deplete the kidney system. In most cases of acute diarrhea, the culprit is a pathogen from the outside, such as bacteria from contaminated food, a flu virus, or parasites. Chronic conditions always involve the liver, spleen, and kidney systems. Both acute and chronic diarrhea respond well to acupuncture and herbal therapy together with nutrition and stress management.

Often when steroids and immunosuppressant drugs fail to relieve diarrhea in IBD patients, I will get a referral from one of my gastroenterologist colleagues. The collaboration of Eastern and Western medicine has helped many patients go into remission—and stay there. Below are some remedies that my patients have found to be helpful. If you experience uncontrollable, constant diarrhea for more than forty-eight hours and experience dizziness and shortness of breath, you may be dehydrated and should go to the emergency room immediately.

❋ DIET ❋

• What goes in goes out, so proper eating habits are essential. Eat regularly, more often, and in smaller quantities. Favor blueberries, cinnamon, raspberry leaves, lotus seeds, white rice, green apples, toasted white bread, carob, amaranth, barley water (boil barley in water for 30 minutes; strain), sauerkraut, yams, sweet potatoes, taro root, daikon radish, winter melon, fresh fig leaves, peas, buckwheat, litchi, guava, apples, ginger, pearl barley, basil, and umeboshi plum or pickled green plum. Drink plenty of pure water. Avoid dehydration by drinking at least eight to ten 6-ounce glasses of water a day during the acute phase of diarrhea.

• Do not overeat. Avoid cold and raw foods, including ice cream and iced drinks. Keep raw vegetables to a minimum—cook or steam your vegetables. Keep dairy to a minimum, and eliminate spicy, stimulating, fried, and oily foods as well as preservatives, artificial colors, flavorings, and sweeteners. Avoid simple sugars and whole grains with the bran layer, as they may be too hard on the digestive system. Keep your kitchen clean as you prepare your food. Make sure to cut meat and animal products on cutting boards separate from those used for other foods, and wash the boards well. Avoid alcohol, as it impairs the intestinal wall's ability to absorb water and can contribute to diarrhea.

❋ HOME REMEDIES ❋

• Take charcoal tablets (500 milligrams) 3 times a day until the diarrhea stops.

• Eat yogurt containing live cultures—the friendly bacteria help subdue diarrhea.

• Steep black tea in a cup of boiling water for 10 minutes. Drink 3 cups a day until the diarrhea stops.

• Eat rice cakes or dry toast sprinkled with sea salt.

• Make a tea by boiling 1 teaspoon each of ground ginger, fennel, and basil in 3 1/2 cups of water for 15 minutes. Strain, and drink 3 cups a day.

• Drink 3 cups of blackberry tea daily. Blackberry is an astringent, and it is especially good for children.

❊ DAILY SUPPLEMENTS ❊

• During the active phase of diarrhea it is important to keep hydrated. Drink fluids rich in electrolytes and supplement with potassium (25 milligrams) to make up for potassium loss.

• Take bromelain (450 milligrams), found in pineapples, or another digestive enzyme such as papain (300 milligrams), 3 times a day, with each meal to aid digestion and suppress diarrhea.

• Taking quercetin (400 milligrams) 3 times a day can be useful for dysenteric diarrhea.

• Taking probiotics such as acidophilus (3 to 5 billion organisms) supports healthy flora in the bowels.

• Psyllium (2 to 4 grams) and pectin powder (1 to 2 grams) are useful as bulking agents for treating diarrhea.

❊ HERBAL THERAPY ❊

• Herbs can be found in health food or vitamin stores, online, and at the offices of Chinese medicine practitioners. Herbs should be used according to individual needs; consult with a licensed practitioner for a customized formulation. To learn more about the herbs listed here, go to www.ask drmao.com.

• For urgent, foul-smelling diarrhea accompanied by a burning sensation in the anus and abdominal pain, herbs containing berberin, such as coptidis or goldenseal, are useful, as they're naturally antibacterial.

• Traditional Chinese herbs to support healthy digestion and bowels include patchouli, atractylodis, magnolia bark, peony, ginger, tangerine, cardamom, fennel, and licorice.

• For IBS and diarrhea due to emotional stress, I often recommend our Chinese herbal formula Emotional Tranquility Tea, which supports healthy nervous system function and maintains calm and peace. It contains Chinese senega, lily bulb, poria, bamboo, zizyphus, dragon bone, and licorice.

✳ EXERCISE ✳

To help stop acute diarrhea, try this simple 15-minute abdominal massage. Note that the direction of the circles is the opposite of those in the massage for constipation.

Lie on your back and bend your knees slightly to a comfortable position.

Begin a circular massage of the abdomen, with both palms moving together: Starting from the lower left side and with moderate pressure, rub your abdomen in small counterclockwise circles with your palms.

Keep making small circles with your hands as you slowly traverse a counterclockwise path around the navel. The idea is to move opposite to the peristaltic flow of the colon.

When you reach the lower right abdomen lift your arms and begin again from the lower left side. Repeat for 10 to 15 minutes, 3 times daily.

If you have chronic diarrhea, mild exercise like tai chi or qi gong can help strengthen your energy and digestive function. I suggest the Stomach-Spleen Strengthening Qi Gong exercise to strengthen the digestive system and promote the flow of energy in the abdomen. Perform this exercise twice a day on an empty stomach.

Lie on your back, comfortably, with your hands at your sides. Focus on your navel. Visualize a golden disk the size of a Frisbee spinning around your entire abdomen with its center at your navel. With every inhalation the disk spins half of a circle. With every exhalation the disk completes the other half of the circle.

Breathe deeply so that the disk spins slowly, corresponding to your respiration, for a total of 21 times in the clockwise direction. Reverse the direction of the disk's rotation and repeat the breathing-spinning sequence.

⁕ ACUPRESSURE ⁕

• Locate the acupoint Foot Three Miles (ST-36), four finger-widths below and to the outside of the right kneecap. Apply moderate pressure with your right thumb. Hold for 5 minutes. Repeat on the left leg. This point is often tender to the touch in people with digestive disturbances.

. . . .

• Locate the acupoint Heaven's Axis (ST-25), three finger-widths to either side of the navel. Apply steady, moderate pressure with your index fingers. Hold for 5 minutes.

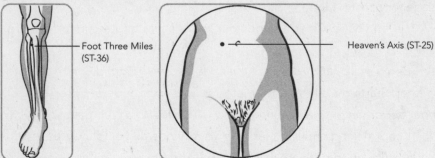

Foot Three Miles (ST-36)

Heaven's Axis (ST-25)

AVOID

• Alcohol and coffee, as they tend to irritate the intestinal lining.

. . . .

• Foods that irritate the intestinal tract, including products containing MSG, preservatives, artificial sweeteners, and chemical additives.

• Some antiviral and most antibiotic drugs, as they destroy the friendly and helpful intestinal bacteria. Some beta-blockers such as atenolol can cause diarrhea, as can heart medications such as digitalis and its derivatives. Many prescription and over-the-counter drugs can also cause diarrhea. Be sure to consult with your physician about possible side effects.

• Stress, anxiety, and emotional turmoil, as they stimulate the sympathetic nervous system, which, in turn, stimulates the bowels.

DIZZINESS

DIZZINESS IS OFTEN DESCRIBED as feeling light-headed, losing your balance, or having the sensation that your head is spinning. There are many causes for dizziness, including central nervous system dysfunction, inner ear infection, sinus problems, Ménière's disease, anemia, low or high blood pressure, low blood sugar, and fatigue. In some cases, because of a brief lack of blood flow to the brain, dizziness results from a sudden movement of the head or a sudden rise from a sitting position. This is normal, and no treatment is necessary.

In Chinese medicine, dizziness is often seen in patients with anemia, dampness accumulation, or internal wind, which blocks the clear energy from rising to the head. Once the cause is determined, I use acupuncture for symptomatic relief and herbal therapy to nourish the blood, remove dampness, channel wind, and balance inner ear pressure and blood pressure. Dizziness can also be a warning sign of a more severe problem. I once treated a young woman who suffered from intermittent dizziness. She nearly passed out a couple of times in my office. I observed that her pupils weren't adapting to changing light conditions, and I also saw purple spots on her tongue, a possible sign of a tumor. I sent her to a neurologist for a brain scan. It turned out that she

DIZZINESS

had a tumor in her brain that was causing the dizziness and fainting. I treated her through her surgery and recovery, managing her energy and symptoms successfully. When the pathology came back nonmalignant we all breathed a sigh of relief.

The following are dietary, herbal, and exercise recommendations I have given to my patients. If dizziness is accompanied by vomiting or lingers without relief, work with your physician to rule out serious neurological or vascular disease.

✳ DIET ✳

• Eating nutritious meals helps build abundant energy and blood, and it is crucial to avoid foods that create dampness and stagnation. Eat frequently and in smaller amounts. Eat foods rich in essential nutrients, including whole grains, green leafy vegetables, mint, green tea, onions, ginger, pearl barley, apples, oranges, tangerines, peach kernels, and almonds. Drink plenty of room-temperature water; dizziness can often be caused by dehydration. If you suffer from iron deficiency or blood deficiency, consume more spinach, beets, dandelion greens, and organic red meat. Vegetarians should take vitamin B_{12} supplements or shots because B_{12} deficiency often leads to anemia, a cause of dizziness.

......

• Avoid spicy foods, lettuce, and heavy starchy foods. Moderate your dairy intake. Salt, caffeine, and alcohol should also be avoided. Foods that form mucus, such as dairy, sugar, and wheat, should be avoided, as they block the clear energy from rising to the head.

✳ HOME REMEDIES ✳

• For anemia-induced dizziness eat iron-rich foods, including raisins, prunes, figs, spinach, beets, chard, and calf's liver at least 3 times a week.

......

• Make a tea by steeping 3 slices fresh ginger root, 1 tablespoon mint leaves, and 1 teaspoon dried licorice in 1 cup boiling water for 5 to 10 minutes. Strain, and drink 3 cups a day.

• Use 4 drops each of lavender and sandalwood essential oils as an aromatherapy treatment in an infuser, or fill a large bowl with boiling water, add the oils, cover your head and the bowl with a towel, and breathe deeply.

—————————— ✳ DAILY SUPPLEMENTS ✳ ——————————

• The B complex vitamins help with proper nervous system functioning and improve blood circulation to the brain. Vitamins C (1,000 milligrams) and E (800 IU) also improve circulation and are good antioxidants.

• Calcium (1,000 milligrams), magnesium (500 milligrams), and zinc (50 milligrams) play key roles in maintaining healthy nerve impulses.

• Omega-3 fatty acids (1,000 milligrams EPA; 800 milligrams DHA), found in fish and flaxseed oils, can improve blood circulation and reduce inflammation.

—————————— ✳ HERBAL THERAPY ✳ ——————————

• Herbs can be found in health food or vitamin stores, online, and at the offices of Chinese medicine practitioners. Herbs should be used according to individual needs; consult with a licensed practitioner for a customized formulation. To learn more about the herbs listed here, go to www.askdrmao.com.

• Traditional Chinese herbs including pinellia, atractylodis, and gastrodia are used to provide symptomatic relief for dizziness. Remember, however, to consult your physician, professional herbalist, or doctor of Chinese medicine to address the underlying cause of your dizziness.

• For anemia-induced dizziness, herbs like dong quai, ligusticum, white peony, rehmannia, and licorice are often used.

During an episode of dizziness, rigorous exercise should be avoided. Gentle walking is a good exercise to stimulate blood flow. As soon as you feel a dizzy spell coming on, step out into fresh air. Sit quietly or take a gentle walk, breathing deeply. Drink plenty of liquids. A regular regimen of moderate cardiovascular and stretching exercises can help maintain good health and proper circulation.

Here is a simple Dao In Qi Gong exercise called The Immortal Awakening from Napping that helps treat dizziness.

Lie on your back with your legs straight and feet apart. Keep your arms resting naturally next to your body, with the palms up. Bring your feet together.

Inhale, and slowly raise your head and shoulders until your shoulder blades clear the floor. At the same time, bring your palms alongside your legs and touch the outside of your thighs. Bring your chin down toward your chest and gaze at your toes. This will connect the body's energy in a circle from head to toe.

Exhale, reverse the movement, and return to the beginning posture.

Repeat 12 to 20 times twice a day.

※ ACUPRESSURE ※

• Locate the acupoint Hundred Meeting (DU-20), at the top of your head, midway between your ears. Apply gentle pressure with your index finger for 5 minutes. This point is used for improving brain and spirit functions.

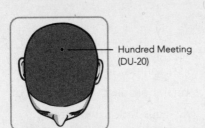

Hundred Meeting (DU-20)

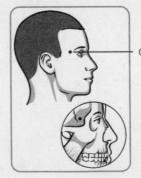

Greater Yang (Taiyang)

• Find the acupoint Greater Yang (Taiyang), in the indentation in the temples. With either the knuckles of your thumbs or the tips of your index fingers, massage in a circular motion for 5 minutes. This point is used to help clear the head of any stagnation.

AVOID

• Prescription and over-the-counter drugs that can cause dizziness. Be sure to check drug labels. Consult your physician to determine whether drug interactions play a role in your condition. Spironolactone and other antagonists of aldosterone (used for chronic heart failure, it inhibits sodium resorption in the kidneys) can react with alcohol or barbiturates and cause severe dizziness.

• Caffeine, recreational drugs, alcohol, stress, and environmental conditions such as noise and high places, as they can all cause dizziness.

• High cholesterol, low blood sugar levels, and hypertension; they should be treated properly to reduce the risk of complications, which include dizziness.

 ECZEMA

ECZEMA (FROM THE GREEK *ekzema*, meaning "to break out") is a chronic inflammation of the outer skin layer. It is an allergic condition that occurrs in bouts. During its active phase, it produces oozing, crusting blisters, redness, itching, and occasionally pain in the affected areas. As the blisters dry, moisture is lost, resulting in dry, itchy, scaly skin with the appearance of thick leathery patches. The dryness and constant itching—and scratching—may lead to ulcerations of the skin, making it prone to infections. Eczema affects more than 15 million people in the United States, particularly children under the age of five.

Eczema is exacerbated by exposure to environmental irritants such as household chemicals, laundry detergents, temperature changes, and dry weather. Food allergies and nutritional deficiencies can contribute to its development. Recent studies have linked stress and anxiety with eczema. Currently dermatologists provide palliative solutions to relieve itching—usually corticosteroids or, in severe conditions, immunosuppressant drugs.

The skin is the largest organ in your body. It is a functional part of your immune system, and it is an interface with the environment with its millions of tiny pores through which substances exit and enter the body. In Chinese medicine, the lungs govern the skin; they are responsible for the proper opening and closing of the pores and for proper nourishment of the skin. When the lung network is impaired, the skin manifests signs of the imbalance. The lung network includes the large intestine, which has the largest number of immune cells in the body. The digestive tract is responsible for removing impure substances from the body, preventing their buildup in the skin. When the bowels are sluggish, constipated, and unable to cleanse the body, toxic substances back up into the skin and show up as lesions representative of damp or toxic heat. In chronic eczema there is often an underlying condition of blood deficiency in which the blood is unable to properly nourish and moisturize the skin. This condition must be addressed.

I have seen many patients with eczema, especially children. One of my three children suffered a terrible case of eczema from one to two years of age. Imagine waking up in the morning to find your child bloody from head to toe from scratching through the night! I treated my child the same way I treat all of my patients. My approach is to first cleanse the body of toxins and residues. Then I work on improving digestive function and harmonizing the immune system to prevent allergic reactions. With strict dietary and nutritional therapies, acupuncture, oral and topical herbal preparations, and stress management, many of my patients have resolved long-standing eczema conditions. And, thank goodness, my child has been fine for seven years now—and in fact has the best skin of all of my kids.

Here are are my recommendations.

✳ DIET ✳

• What you eat eventually ends up in your skin. Many people consume foods without a second thought about what they contain. Chemicals and artificial ingredients can cause allergic reactions and irritate your immune system. Keep a diary of your meals and be attentive to your physical and emotional reactions to food. Soon you will discover whether you have allergic reactions that worsen your eczema. Avoiding problem foods can significantly reduce flare-ups.

. . . .

• Eat foods that nourish the skin. Incorporate more broccoli, dandelion green, mung beans, lentils, split peas, chickpeas, black beans, lima beans, pinto beans, seaweed, pearl barley, oats, adzuki beans, water chestnuts, winter squash, watermelon, carrots, brewer's yeast, olives, raspberries, papaya, pineapple, cherries, peaches, apples, pears, raisins, and grapes into your diet. Fish, rich in omega-3 fatty acids, can help nourish the skin. Water is essential for cleansing the body. People who drink at least 80 ounces of water a day tend to have better bowel habits and develop fewer allergic reactions.

. . . .

• Eliminate processed foods, foods containing artificial additives, bleached white flour, sugars, soft drinks, and spicy, deep-fried, and greasy foods. Stay off dairy products, eggs, shellfish, wheat, corn, tomatoes, eggplant, peanuts, most nuts, caffeine, alcohol, and citrus fruits.

ECZEMA

• Mash 1 small raw potato and apply it as poultice to the affected skin area, changing every 4 hours for 3 days, or until skin improves, to help moisturize the skin and heal the sores.

• Moisturize your skin with calendula oil twice a day.

• Boil 1 cup each of pearl barley and soaked mung beans in 8 cups of water for 1 hour. Drink 3 cups a day for 1 week, or until skin improves.

• Dissolve 1 teaspoon sea salt and 1 teaspoon borax in 1 cup of lukewarm water. Wash the affected area 2 or 3 times a day with the solution to prevent skin ulceration and infections.

• To relieve itching and to help healing, soak the affected areas in natural sulfur springs, if possible, or by adding 1/3 cup each of sulfur powder, Epsom salts, and olive oil to a lukewarm bath at home.

※ DAILY SUPPLEMENTS ※

• Supplementing with gamma-linolenic acid (GLA; 800 milligrams) can help modulate inflammatory response. Evening primrose oil and borage oil can deliver substantial amounts of GLA to help regulate the immune inflammatory response.

• Taking probiotics such as acidophilus (3 to 5 billion organisms) is helpful for removing toxic substances and supporting healthy immune response.

• Taking 15 to 30 milligrams of zinc picolinate a day can help heal skin conditions.

• Supplementing with quercetin (500 milligrams) can reduce eczema flare-ups.

- The antioxidants selenium (200 micrograms) and vitamin C (1,000 milligrams) can help heal the skin.

- Taking MSM (1,000 milligrams), a sulfur-based nutritional supplement, can reduce inflammation and help healing.

─────────────── ✳ HERBAL THERAPY ✳ ───────────────

- Herbs can be found in health food or vitamin stores, online, and at the offices of Chinese medicine practitioners. Herbs should be used according to individual needs; consult with a licensed practitioner for a customized formulation. To learn more about the herbs listed here, go to www.ask drmao.com.

- Burdock, red clover, licorice, chamomile, and calendula are traditionally used for treating eczema.

- Our Exquisite Skin Chinese herbal formula helps to support healthy skin function and reduce itching. It contains siler, caltrop, schizonepetae, astragalus, peony, dong quai, Fo-Ti, rhubarb, and licorice.

- For topical relief from itching, mix 10 drops of Tonic Oil (containing wintergreen, eucalyptus menthol, and other herbs) with fresh aloe vera gel and apply liberally and frequently.

─────────────── ✳ EXERCISE ✳ ───────────────

Stress and anxiety can trigger eczema attacks, so it is important to implement stress reduction exercises in your regular workout routine. Tai chi and qi gong are great for reducing stress and calming the emotions, in addition to their physical benefits. The General Cleansing Qi Gong is designed to help with circulation and promote opening of the pores. It should be done indoors and not too vigorously.

Sit comfortably or lie down on your back. Slow your respiration to deep, abdominal breathing. Say the word "calm" in your mind with every exhalation. In the pathways outlined below you will be visualizing your body parts, relaxing and releasing tension with every exhalation.

Starting at the top of your head, inhale, and then exhale while visualizing your scalp muscles relaxing. Say "calm" in your mind. Repeat this, saying the word as you move down through your face, throat, chest, abdomen, thighs, knees, calves, ankles, and feet. After you've relaxed your feet, visualize all the tension in your body leaving through your toes in the form of dark smoke.

Next, start at the temple region of your head. This pathway focuses on the sides and upper extremities. Inhale, then exhale while visualizing your temple muscles relaxing. Say "calm" in your mind. Repeat this, saying the word as you move down through your jaw, sides of the neck, shoulders, upper arms, elbows, forearms, wrists, and hands. Once you've completely relaxed your hands, visualize all the tension leaving your body through your fingertips in the form of dark smoke.

The final pathway begins at the back of your head. This pathway relaxes the back of your body. Repeat this breathing-visualization-word routine, as above, as you go from the back of your neck down to your upper back, middle back, lower back, back of thighs, calves, and then heels. Then focus on the acupoint Bubbling Spring (see page 328) at the soles of your feet for 1 minute.

Practice this exercise for at least 15 minutes twice a day.

--------------------------------- ✳ ACUPRESSURE ✳ ---------------------------------

• Locate the acupoint Valley of Harmony (LI-4), between your right thumb and index finger. Apply steady pressure with your left thumb until you feel soreness. Hold for 2 minutes. Repeat on the left hand.

....

• Locate the acupoint Wind Pond (GB-20), in the natural indentation at the base of your skull on either side of your neck. Press and lift up toward the base of your skull with your thumbs and lean your head back. Use the weight of your head against your thumbs for steady pressure on the acupoint. Hold for 5 minutes, breathing deeply and slowly.

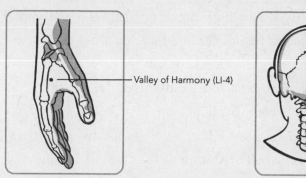

Valley of Harmony (LI-4)

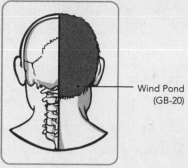

Wind Pond (GB-20)

AVOID

- Exposure to temperature changes, cold or hot water, and detergent use.

- Dehydration and constipation, and keep your skin moist.

- Alcohol, smoking, and caffeine; they are irritants that can worsen eczema.

- Stress, anxiety, and emotional turmoil, which can initiate flare-ups.

FLATULENCE

INTESTINAL GAS IS A BY-PRODUCT OF DIGESTION that produces varying symptoms in different people, including bloating, abdominal distention, belching, and the release of rectal gas. The genteel English gave us a more civilized word for gas—flatulence. Though embarrassing and uncomfortable, the production and release of intestinal gas is a normal digestive process. The fermentation and breakdown of foods by intestinal bacteria produces gas. The major causes of excessive flatulence are poor diet and improper digestion. Highly processed foods loaded with chemicals can overwhelm the digestive system, leading to a decline in function and excessive waste products, which can ferment and produce gas. A less common cause of excessive flatulence is aerophagia, or swallowing air with the food we eat.

FLATULENCE

Chinese medicine recognizes both the dietary causes of flatulence and the emotional element. Flatulence and bloating are signs of a diminished flow of liver energy, which is greatly influenced by mood and feelings. Digestive weakness and a buildup of dampness due to poor dietary habits often accompany liver stagnation. I often ask my patients about their emotional state when treating digestive disorders. My treatments focus on a balanced approach—I use herbal therapy and acupuncture to help support healthy intestinal function and promote smooth flow of energy in the liver-gallbladder network. I also educate my patients about proper eating habits.

❊ DIET ❊

• The food we eat is directly responsible for the production of intestinal gas. The speed at which we eat also has a direct effect. The faster we eat, the more air we're bound to swallow. Carbohydrates are more gas producing than fats or proteins. Eating smaller, evenly spaced meals more frequently and properly chewing your food are helpful. Foods that reduce flatulence include carrots, black pepper, coriander, chiles, cilantro, limes, lemons, and papaya. Dill, anise, parsley, cumin, caraway, turmeric, and seaweed are also helpful.

....

• Beans and legumes tend to elicit gas because they are rich in insoluble fiber; in this family focusing on split peas, lima beans, and lentils is your best bet. Beans are less gas producing if you soak them in water overnight before cooking. To further reduce gas production, cook beans with herbs and spices. Fermented soy products such as tofu or soybean are less gas producing. Yogurt and naturally fermented drinks containing lactobacillus acidophilus, a beneficial intestinal bacteria, counteract flatulence.

....

• Foods containing polysaccharides, including most beans, onions, radishes, sweet potatoes, milk and other dairy products, cashews, broccoli, cabbage, Jerusalem artichokes, oats, and yeast (found in most breads) produce excessive amounts of gas and should be avoided. Stay away from carbonated drinks, as drinking them directly causes gas. Lactose is a major source of gas especially in those who are lactose intolerant. If you do eat dairy products, take the enzyme lactase. Butter and other fatty foods containing butyric acid are responsible for the foul odor in flatulence.

—————— ❊ HOME REMEDIES ❊ ——————

• For immediate relief from gas, mix 1 teaspoon dried ginger powder with a pinch of asafetida (a resin from the ferula plant, used in pickles) and a pinch of rock salt in 1 cup of warm water, and drink.

• After meals, chew on fresh ginger slices soaked in lime juice to reduce gas production.

• Make a tea by steeping 4 or 5 sprigs of fresh mint in 1 cup of boiling water for 5 minutes. Drink after meals to reduce indigestion and bloating.

• Eat naturally fermented sauerkraut or make your own pickled vegetables by soaking sliced vegetables such as carrots, radishes, or turnips in rice vinegar. Bottle in an airtight jar, and age for at least 1 month in a dark space. Eat a few slices with each meal to help with digestion.

—————— ❊ DAILY SUPPLEMENTS ❊ ——————

• Probiotics containing 3 to 5 billion live bacterial cultures taken daily can help strengthen digestion and reduce flatulence. Use non-dairy-based probiotics if you are lactose intolerant.

• Taking 3 to 4 grams of the digestive enzyme pancreatin with each meal can help with digestion and improve absorption of vital nutrients.

• Take 2 charcoal tablets (500 milligrams) every hour until the symptoms subside.

❋ HERBAL THERAPY ❋

• Herbs can be found in health food or vitamin stores, online, and at the offices of Chinese medicine practitioners. Herbs should be used according to individual needs; consult with a licensed practitioner for a customized formulation. To learn more about the herbs listed here, go to www.askdrmao.com.

....

• Taking 3 to 5 grams of dandelion root twice daily can aid digestion by supporting liver and gallbladder function.

....

• Make tea by steeping 1 teaspoon of any of the following herbs and spices in 1 cup of boiling water: dried dill, oregano, cilantro, rosemary, sage, bay leaf, mint, basil, coriander, fennel, anise, cardamom, or turmeric. Drink after each meal to soothe and prevent bloating.

....

• Traditional Chinese herbs such as hawthorn, massa fermentata, daikon radish seed, tangerine peel, poria, ginger, and licorice are used to support healthy digestion and relieve gas.

❋ EXERCISE ❋

To help move food along the digestive tract and to improve digestion and absorption, the best exercise is walking. The energetic meridians of the digestive organs run along the large muscles of the legs, so walking stimulates energy flow within the channels and promotes digestion. Take an easy 10-minute walk after each meal. While walking, massage your abdomen with your palms in a circular motion around your navel. This helps move food through your digestive tract, avoiding prolonged accumulation.

The following is a movement from the Eight Treasures Qi Gong called Raising the Hands to Adjust the Stomach and Spleen.

Begin in a standing posture with your spine erect, feet drawn close together, and arms at your sides. Tilt your head slightly forward. Begin regular, rhythmic breathing.

Form a cup or plate with your right hand. Facing your palm toward the sky, inhale and make a large circular motion in front of you from the left to right while raising your arm above your head. Be sure to keep your palm facing the sky. As you complete this motion, move your left hand to your back with the palm facing the ground.

As your right hand reaches its highest point above your head, begin to stretch your torso, lifting your body on the balls of your feet. Exhale gently, and simultaneously push your left hand toward the ground. Be sure to push in opposite directions—your right hand pushing to the sky and the left pushing to the ground.

Repeat this movement 3 times, inhaling as your arm goes up and exhaling as you stretch.

Switch sides and repeat the exercise. Do this for 15 minutes, twice daily. The exercise helps stretch the abdominal organs, and stimulates the intestines, spleen, and stomach.

❋ ACUPRESSURE ❋

• Locate the acupoint Valley of Harmony (LI-4), in the web between your thumb and index finger on your right hand. Apply steady pressure with your left thumb until you feel soreness. Hold for 2 minutes. Repeat on the left hand.

....

• Find the acupoint Upper Great Opening (ST-37) by measuring two hand-widths or eight finger-widths below the outer indentation of your right knee next to your shinbone. Apply steady pressure with your left thumb until you feel soreness. Hold for 2 minutes. Repeat on the left leg.

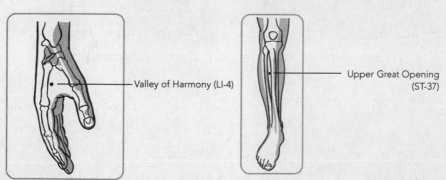

Valley of Harmony (LI-4)

Upper Great Opening (ST-37)

• Overeating and eating while anxious, as this takes the digestive energy away from the stomach, making it harder to absorb the nutrients from your food.

....

• Eating when you are stressed, angry, emotionally upset, or otherwise preoccupied with strong emotional feelings. This stagnates the energy, slows down digestion, and produces gas.

FLOATERS

THE ANNOYING, SPIDERWEB-LIKE IMAGES some people see in their field of vision are not on the surface of your eyes but inside them. Since they tend to float in and out of your vision with the movement of your eyes, they're called floaters. They're cellular debris within the vitreous fluid in the eye, a result of degeneration. Though more of a nuisance than anything else, the sudden appearance and rapid increase of floaters may signal rapidly progressing visual decline and should be addressed with your eye specialist.

In Chinese medicine, the liver stores the blood and nutrients that nourish the eye while the kidneys store the vital essence, which is necessary for good vision. Poor eating and lifestyle habits during the younger years depletes these vital substances. When combined with a buildup of metabolic and cellular waste in the form of dampness and phlegm, circulation to the sensory organs is diminished, causing malnourishment of the eyes.

I've worked with some very fine ophthalmologists on patients who have annoying floaters. With treatment, many floaters either disappear entirely or are substantially reduced. The treatment includes cleansing and detoxification protocols, herbal and nutritional therapies, acupuncture, and energy exercises like qi gong and tai chi. I instruct my patients in eye exercises and eye massage as well as appropriate lifestyle choices. Here are some of my recommendations—I hope they help you maintain good vision well into your golden years.

--- ❋ DIET ❋ ---

• Proper nutrition is essential for delivering nourishment to the eyes and for preventing a buildup of toxic waste products in the body. I recommend a wholesome, balanced diet rich in complex carbohydrates, organic sources of animal protein, and whole grains. To help nourish the kidneys, the liver, and the vital essence, eat more blood-building foods, including fresh vegetables such as spinach and beets, and dried fruits, such as raisins, figs, and prunes. Turnip tops, leeks, okra, tomatoes, lettuce, Swiss chard, cilantro, yams, carrots, cabbage, green peas, watercress, whole grains, beans (especially soybeans and mung beans), cloves, sesame seeds, and fresh fruits, including apples, peaches, pears, mulberries, blueberries, and blackberries, are all beneficial.

• Foods high in fat content, animal fats, red meat, dairy products, and spicy foods all contribute to the buildup of toxins and waste in the body and should be eliminated. Also avoid coffee and alcohol, which injure the yin essence.

--- ❋ HOME REMEDIES ❋ ---

• Alternate hot and cold eye compresses by applying a hot, moist washcloth to both eyes for 2 minutes, followed by an ice-cold washcloth for 2 minutes. Repeat 3 or 4 times a day.

• Boil 4 ounces of fresh spinach in 4 cups of water for 20 minutes. Drink this broth and eat the spinach daily to provide vital nourishment for the eyes.

--- ❋ DAILY SUPPLEMENTS ❋ ---

• Taking omega-3 fatty acids (up to 3,000 milligrams daily in capsule or liquid form) helps to promote healthy circulation and reduce inflammation.

FLOATERS

- Taking daily doses of vitamins A (200 IU), C (1,000 milligrams), and E (800 IU), beta-carotene (1,000 milligrams), and selenium (100 micrograms) can help stop the progression of macular degeneration.

- Daily use of lutein (30 milligrams), another form of beta-carotene, has been shown to help the macula.

- Chlorophyll-rich algae like spirulina, chlorella, and blue-green algae (1 to 2 grams daily) possess nutrients that are beneficial for the eyes.

❋ HERBAL THERAPY ❋

- Herbs can be found in health food or vitamin stores, online, and at the offices of Chinese medicine practitioners. Herbs should be used according to individual needs; consult with a licensed practitioner for a customized formulation. To learn more about the herbs listed here, go to www.askdrmao.com.

- Taking ginkgo biloba on a daily basis can improve circulation to the eyes.

- Make a tea by boiling 1/2 cup chrysanthemum flowers, 1/2 cup mint leaves, and 2 tablespoons cassia seeds in 4 cups of water for 15 minutes. Strain, and drink 3 cups a day to support healthy eyes by strengthening liver function and reducing inflammation.

- Grape seed extract and bilberry extract contain potent antioxidants for eye health.

❋ EXERCISE ❋

An active lifestyle is essential for preventing depletion of the vital essence and the buildup of toxic wastes in the body. I recommend a program that includes cardiovascular exercise every other day and tai chi or qi gong exercises for 30 minutes every day. The exercise called Warming Up the Eyes works directly on the eyes to improve circulation and reduce symptoms, and you can do it every day to help preserve good vision.

Sit at the front edge of a sturdy chair with your back erect, your spine stretched, and your head tilted slightly forward.

Relax and breathe deeply and rhythmically for 3 minutes to promote a feeling of relaxation and calm.

Rub your palms together with some vigor to produce heat. With light pressure, immediately place your palms on your closed eyes. Feel the warming energy from your hands bathing and penetrating your eyes. Hold for 2 breaths.

Repeat 3 times a day.

✳ ACUPRESSURE ✳

• Find the acupoint Gathering Bamboo (B-2), in the depression at the inner corner of the left eyebrow, just above the bridge of the nose. It is traditionally used to restore healthy vision. Apply steady pressure with your left index finger until you feel soreness. Hold for 2 minutes. Repeat on the right side.

• Locate the acupoint Hundred Meeting (DU-20), in the depression at the top of the head, in line with the tips of the ears. It is traditionally used to bring energy to the head area and clear heat from the liver, which can manifest as an eye disorder. Apply steady pressure with your index finger until you feel soreness. Hold for 3 minutes.

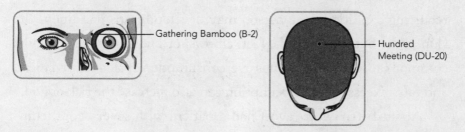

Gathering Bamboo (B-2)

Hundred Meeting (DU-20)

AVOID

• Using the computer and watching TV in the dark, watching a lot of movies, reading in poor light, and wearing sunglasses for long periods of time.

FLOATERS

• Stressful situations and emotional turmoil, which rapidly consume the vital essence and aggravate the liver.

....

• Smoking, exposure to secondhand smoke, and alcohol, which injure the kidney yin essence.

 GOUT

THE HUMAN BODY PRODUCES A SUBSTANTIAL AMOUNT of metabolic waste as a result of cellular function. One such waste product is uric acid—a by-product of protein metabolism. Waste products are normally removed from the body through the kidneys and the intestines. Gout is caused either by the overproduction of uric acid or the inability to properly excrete it, leading to a buildup of uric acid in the joints which crystallizes into gout. It usually affects middle-aged men, but postmenopausal women are also prone to gout. Symptoms often occur suddenly and develop within a matter of hours, and include excruciating pain in a single joint—often the big toe—but gout can also show up in the fingers, wrists, elbows, knees, and ankles. The affected joint may become red, swollen, hot, and stiff, perhaps accompanied by fever. In recurring conditions, the person may develop lumps just under the skin in the outer ear, hands, feet, elbows, or knees. One of the most common causes of acute gout is overconsumption of alcohol, red meat, and fats. Excess sugar consumption can also increase the risk of gout.

About fifteen years ago I had a patient with severe gout, complaining of gout attacks about two or three times a year for the previous ten years. I had him keep a diet journal for a week, and then advised him to stop eating red meat, dairy products, and acidic foods, including coffee, wine, tomatoes, citrus fruits, vinegar, and sugar. I used acupuncture and herbal therapy to help relieve his pain and inflammation. I saw him again about a year ago, and I was impressed with how he had stuck to his diet—he never experienced a relapse and looked trim and fit!

In Chinese medicine, joint pain is classified as a painful obstruction syndrome, and it is classified into heat, cold, wind, and damp subcategories based on symptoms. Treatment usually focuses first and foremost on relieving pain and then on resolving the underlying cause. Gout is classified most commonly as heat and dampness accumulation. The red, swollen joint, the sharp pain, and the accompanying heat are part of the symptoms.

Below are some simple recommendations that I suggest to my patients.

✳ DIET ✳

• Eat a diet high in fiber, favoring dark green leafy vegetables, whole grains, and fruits. Also include celery seeds, onions, leeks, shallots, chives, celery, cucumbers, green beans, asparagus, seaweed, capers, and scallions. Strawberries, blackberries, blueberries, raspberries, and black currants contain antioxidants, which can help reduce excess uric acid. Prunes, papayas, pineapple, cherries, and grapes have natural anti-inflammatory and antioxidant properties and should be eaten often.

• Ample water intake is essential for flushing excess uric acid from the system—drink at least 80 ounces of filtered room-temperature water every day.

• High-protein foods should be kept to minimum, and buy organic meat whenever possible. Eliminate foods high in the amino acid purine from your diet (purine metabolism gives rise to uric acid), including anchovies, mackerel, sardines, shellfish, herring, red meat (and gravy), mushrooms, mussels, peanuts, yeast, and sweetbreads and other organ meats. Also eliminate fried foods, processed foods, alcohol, and foods high in satu-

GOUT

rated fats, sugar, white flour, and caffeine. Avoid spicy foods, citrus fruits, and dairy products, as they can also contribute to gout.

❋ HOME REMEDIES ❋

• Eat lots of cherries and strawberries, as they contain chemicals that neutralize uric acid. Drink freshly squeezed cherry and strawberry juice, or buy unsweetened bottled cherry and strawberry juice, and drink 2 to 3 glasses a day for 1 week during a gout attack.

• Juice 3 stalks of celery with 1 bunch of dandelion green, 3 cucumbers, and 1 bunch of parsley, and combine with 1 cup aloe vera juice. Drink at least 3 glasses of the mixture a day until symptoms subside, or drink 1 glass a day as a preventive measure.

• Soak overnight, then cook 1/3 cup each of mung beans, pearl barley, and red adzuki beans in 6 cups of water for 1 to 2 hours. Eat once a day for 1 month during attacks.

❋ DAILY SUPPLEMENTS ❋

• Taking up to 5,000 milligrams of vitamin C a day can reduce uric acid levels in the blood.

• Taking folic acid (400 milligrams) can slow down the production of uric acid.

• Taking MSM (1,000 milligrams), glucosamine (1,000 milligrams), and chondroitin sulfate (400 milligrams) can reduce inflammation.

• Bromelain (500 milligrams), an enzyme found in pineapples, when taken with meals, can reduce inflammation in the joints and help improve the digestion of proteins.

✳ HERBAL THERAPY ✳

• Herbs can be found in health food or vitamin stores, online, and at the offices of Chinese medicine practitioners. Herbs should be used according to individual needs; consult with a licensed practitioner for a customized formulation. To learn more about the herbs listed here, go to www.ask drmao.com.

• Devil's claw can help to reduce inflammation and pain.

• Burdock root, colchicum, and celery seed taken as a tea infusion are useful for treating gout.

• Traditional Chinese herbs used for gout include corydalis, stephania root, apricot seeds, forsythia, gardenia, and gentian.

✳ EXERCISE ✳

Don't engage in strenuous physical activity during an acute attack of gout. Rest can help reduce stress and speed up healing. After the attack subsides, regular physical activity is important for maintaining good health and ideal weight, as obesity can increase the risk of developing gout. Focus more on stretching and improving flexibility and less on strength- and muscle-building exercises. Walking, swimming, and cycling are good choices. Tai chi and Dao In Qi Gong exercises practiced regularly normalize metabolism and support muscular and skeletal health. Below I describe a quick Dao In Qi Gong exercise called Watching Twin Flying Horses Scratching Each Other, which helps alleviate gout symptoms. Practice it regularly and you'll see the benefits.

Sit on the floor with both legs straight out in front of you. Place your arms straight behind you, with your palms on the floor. Lean your upper body back at a 45-degree angle, supported by your arms.

With the bottom of your right foot, rub the top of your left foot up and down from the ankle to the toes 36 times.

Then with the bottom of your left foot, rub the top of your right foot up and down from the ankle to the toes 36 times.

Next, with the heel of your right foot, rub the sole of your left foot from the heel to the base of the toes 36 times.

Finally, with the heel of your left foot, rub the sole of your right foot from the heel to the base of the toes 36 times.

This exercise can be done anytime, but it's particularly beneficial just before going to bed.

❋ ACUPRESSURE ❋

• Find the acupoint Kunlun Mountains (UB-60), between the outer right anklebone and the Achilles tendon in your heel. With your right thumb and index finger, pinch the point for 3 to 5 minutes. Repeat on the left foot. As you engage this acupoint you are also stimulating the Forceful Torrent (KID-3) acupoint, which is located between the inner anklebone and the Achilles tendon, just opposite Kunlun Mountains. These are kidney and bladder points, and stimulating these areas can help support the functioning of the corresponding organs, thus alleviating gout.

• You can also engage trigger points as a self-acupressure treatment. Find the trigger point by pressing around to discover the most sensitive point. Apply a small amount of vodka to the tender spot. With your thumb or middle finger rub the point, at first gently and then increasing the pressure to as much as you can tolerate, for 5 to 10 minutes.

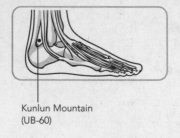

Kunlun Mountain
(UB-60)

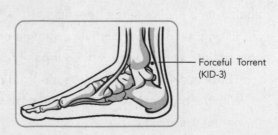

Forceful Torrent
(KID-3)

• Soak your feet in a warm Epsom salt bath every night for 15 to 20 minutes before going to bed to speed circulation of uric acid out of the feet.

AVOID

• Smoking and overindulging in alcohol, as these substances are irritants, and alcohol can cause acute gout flare-ups.

• Certain medications that can cause gout, including aspirin, immunosuppressants, diuretics, drugs used to treat Parkinson's disease, and some antibiotics. Consult your physician if you're taking any of these medications and suffering from gout.

• High doses of niacin (vitamin B₃), nicotinic acid, and vitamin A, as they can cause an attack of gout. Do not use larger-than-normal doses of these supplements unless advised to do so by your heath care provider.

 # GUM DISEASE

OVER 50 PERCENT OF AMERICANS over thirteen years old suffer from some form of gum disease. Gum disease can lead to tooth decay and, if not treated, to the complete loss of teeth. In its mild stage, gum disease is called gingivitis, which simply denotes inflammation of the gums. More severe gum disease, characterized by plaque buildup, is called periodontal disease. About 45 percent of people over sixty suffer from some form of periodontal disease. Heart attack and pancreatic cancer have been linked to periodontal disease—the bacteria that infect the gums can also irritate the walls of the arteries and induce clot formation, leading to heart disease. Infection and inflammation can also cause an increase in stomach acid production, and the bacteria can pro-

duce carcinogens such as nitrosamine in the mouth, which can increase the risk of developing pancreatic cancer.

Brushing your teeth and flossing protect against periodontal disease to some degree, but regular visits to your dentist are essential for maintaining gum health. Tooth and gum pain; red, shiny, bleeding gums; receding gums; visible plaque between the teeth; and loose teeth are all symptoms of gum disease. Severe gum disease often requires periodontal surgery, causing much grief and suffering. I have worked with dentists and periodontists on a program of gum health for patients with gum disease. The program includes a special diet to keep the oral environment alkaline, and thus unfriendly to bacteria, and simple oral rinses several times a day, coupled with massaging the gums with Tonic Oil.

The gums are an extension of the digestive system, and in Chinese medicine they reflect the condition of the stomach-spleen-pancreas network. Gum disease is caused by excess heat in the stomach due to improper diet or lifestyle or emotional stress. My treatments focus on nourishing the digestive system, cooling the heat—which translates into inflammation or infection—and educating my patients on proper diet, lifestyle, and stress management.

✳ DIET ✳

• To prevent gum disease, eat a varied diet consisting of fresh fruits, vegetables, beans and legumes, and whole grains. Drink plenty of water. Eat smaller meals, and chew your food well to allow proper enzyme secretion and healthy digestive function. Avoid overeating by eating to just 80 percent of your capacity.

• Avoid sugars, refined processed foods, and highly acidic foods, including coffee, soda, and alcohol. Reduce your consumption of spicy, greasy, and deep-fried foods.

• Nothing replaces brushing your teeth on a regular basis for preventing gum disease. Always brush before and after meals and before and after sleep. Brushing with baking soda after brushing with your toothpaste will alkalinize the gums, temporarily discouraging bacteria from developing.

• Massage Tonic Oil (available at www.askdrmao.com), consisting of essential oils of wintergreen, eucalyptus, and mint in a sesame oil base, into your gums twice a day to stimulate blood flow to the gums. The essential oils are natural antibacterial agents and are a good antidote for bad breath.

• Make your own mouthwash or rinse by mixing 1 tablespoon of food-grade hydrogen peroxide and 1 tablespoon of baking soda in a glass of warm water. Rinse first thing in the morning and before bedtime.

————————— ✳ DAILY SUPPLEMENTS ✳ —————————

• Using a folic acid mouthwash and folic acid (400 micrograms) as a supplement can prevent and heal gum inflammation.

• Vitamin C (1,000 milligrams), bioflavonoids (500 milligrams), coenzyme Q10 (50 milligrams), calcium (1,000 milligrams), and zinc (50 milligrams) supplements are helpful in fighting gum disease.

• Fish oil and flaxseed oil contain a rich supply of anti-inflammatory omega-3 essential fatty acids (1,000 milligrams EPA; 800 milligrams DHA), which are good for preventing and treating gum disease.

————————— ✳ HERBAL THERAPY ✳ —————————

• Herbs can be found in health food or vitamin stores, online, and at the offices of Chinese medicine practitioners. Herbs should be used according to individual needs; consult with a licensed practitioner for a customized formulation. To learn more about the herbs listed here, go to www.askdrmao.com.

GUM DISEASE

- Bloodroot, caraway, echinacea, sage oil, peppermint, menthol, and myrrh in their essential oil forms are good for treating gum disease.

- Traditional Chinese herbs used for treating gum inflammation include coptidis, skullcap, anemarrhena, gypsum, peony, and rehmannia.

- Herbs used as a preventive include lotus, mulberry, cassia seed, chrysanthemum, hawthorn, and mint.

--------------------------------- ✳ EXERCISE ✳ ---------------------------------

Physical activity helps maintain good digestion and can reduce stress, anxiety, and excessive emotions, all of which can cause heat to build up in the stomach. A daily fitness program consisting of 30-minute daily walks and a regular practice of qi gong or tai chi will promote a healthy digestive system, which benefits the gums. The following is part of the Eight Treasures Qi Gong practice known as Pushing Down the Fierce Tiger. It works to strengthen the teeth, improve circulation to the gums, and improve oral health.

In a quiet, comfortable environment, preferably outdoors, stand with your feet shoulder-width apart, knees slightly bent, spine erect, tailbone tucked in, and head tilted slightly forward. Place your arms palms down on your lower abdomen just below the navel, one hand on top of the other.

Begin with rhythmic, slow, and relaxed breathing. Inhale deeply but softly, and imagine the breath extending all the way down to the lower abdomen, about two finger-widths below the navel. Exhale gently and softly. Stay in this position for 7 breath cycles, relaxing and calming your mind.

Now begin the exercise—you will be moving the energy from the inner part of your legs up into your lower abdomen. Then, in a brisk but gentle move, you'll push it back down to the ground with your teeth gently clenched.

On an inhale, bend forward, and extend your arms to the inner part of your lower legs. Begin massaging the inner part of your leg in a tight circular motion, starting at your lower leg and moving up to your knee, inner thigh, groin, and into the lower abdomen.

Exhale, and with your palms facing down push the energy briskly down toward the ground, bending your knees to accommodate the motion. Remember to keep your spine erect and your upper body straight.

Repeat the exercise 3 times a day. Return to the starting posture and stand for 1 minute in quiet meditation after completing the exercise.

✳ ACUPRESSURE ✳

• Find the acupoint Nectar Receptor (REN-24), in the depression at the center of the lower chin about a finger-width below the lower lip. Apply steady pressure with your index finger until you feel soreness. Hold for 1 minute.

. . . .

• Find the acupoint Three Yin Crossing (SP-6), four finger-widths above the right inner anklebone, in the depression near the bone. Apply steady pressure with your thumb until you feel soreness. Hold for 3 minutes. Repeat on the left leg.

. . . .

• Engaging the combination of these points can help reduce inflammation of the gums.

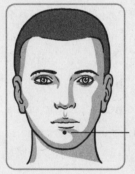

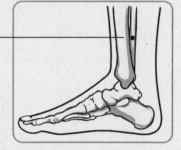

Three Yin Crossing (SP-6)

Nectar Receptor (REN-24)

AVOID

• Smoking and using chewing tobacco, as they can cause gum disease and oral cancer.

. . . .

• Sugar, which is the worst culprit for tooth decay and gum disease.

GUM DISEASE

HAIR LOSS

THE AVERAGE PERSON HAS MORE THAN 100,000 hair follicles in the head alone, each capable of producing at least twenty hair strands in a lifetime. Hair growth is affected by the hormonal system, in particular the androgenic (male) hormones, which include testosterone and a derivative of testosterone called DHT. Normally a person loses about 100 hairs each day, which are replaced within days. As we age, our hormone levels fluctuate and begin to decline, which reduces the stimulus to the hair follicles and results in hair loss. Hair loss affects both men and women, though it is more pronounced in men. There are many types of hair loss, or alopecia, in addition to those related to age. A type of hair loss known as alopecia areata occurs in patches, primarily affecting the head. Less common are drug-induced (chemotherapy) hair loss and genetic hair loss. Entire industries exist to help ease the emotional and social impact of baldness; purported solutions range from invasive surgical procedures to miracle drugs and ointments.

In Chinese medicine, hair loss is attributed primarily to the decline of the vital kidney essence as a result of overindulgence during youth. Stress, physical and emotional strain, an unhealthy lifestyle (including excessive sexual activity), and alcohol deplete the vital essence. This is often complicated by blood deficiency in the patient, as in cases of patchy hair loss resulting from pregnancy and giving birth, the mother being severely depleted of her vital essence and blood. I've had the gratifying experience of helping many patients recover from hair loss, whether the result of chemotherapy, radiation treatment, stress, or menopause. One of my patients who had extensive radiation to her scalp for brain cancer was told by her radiologist that her hair follicles had been permanently damaged. I'm happy to report that she now has a full head of hair. She even wrote about her experience, and she included a photograph that we published in our *Tao of Wellness* newsletter.

My approach to hair loss is to help replenish the vital essence by administering herbal remedies and advising my patients on proper lifestyle, diet, and exercise. I also incorporate topical remedies and acupuncture to stimulate circulation and the hair follicles. In general, alopecia responds well to topical remedies and acupuncture.

❋ DIET ❋

• Diet must be focused on replenishing kidney essence and nourishing blood. In addition to organic vegetables, grains, and fruits, you should favor walnuts, sesame seeds, sunflower seeds, pumpkin seeds, beets, beet tops, mushrooms, mulberries, blueberries, raspberries, blackberries, cranberries, apples, pears, peaches, black beans, mung beans, and other beans and legumes. Add organic lamb, chicken, and deep-sea fish to your diet for quality protein.

....

• Eliminate processed foods, artificial additives, bleached flour, sugars, soft drinks, and spicy, deep-fried, and fatty foods.

❋ HOME REMEDIES ❋

• Massage the affected area on your scalp with fresh ginger juice. Wait 10 minutes, then tap the affected area with the bristles of a stiff toothbrush for 3 minutes, stimulating the scalp. Do this twice daily for 1 month. It promotes circulation and decreases oily deposits that block follicles.

HAIR LOSS

• Apply aloe vera juice directly from the stem of the plant to the affected area twice daily for 1 month.

• Practice handstands, shoulderstands, or headstands for 1 to 2 minutes every day. This will increase blood flow to your scalp.

───────────── ⁂ DAILY SUPPLEMENTS ⁂ ─────────────

• Methysulfonylmethane (MSM; 1,000 milligrams) is a building block of strong hair.

• Biotin (500 micrograms) and vitamin B complex are essential nutrients for hair growth. Vitamin E (800 IU) increases oxygen uptake and zinc may stimulate hair growth by enhancing hormonal function.

• Vitamin C (1,000 milligrams) together with bioflavonoids improves circulation to the scalp, while silica aids hair growth and strengthens hair.

• The amino acids L-methionine (500 milligrams), L-cysteine (500 milligrams), and glutathione (600 milligrams) improve the overall quality, texture, and growth of hair.

───────────── ⁂ HERBAL THERAPY ⁂ ─────────────

• Herbs can be found in health food or vitamin stores, online, and at the offices of Chinese medicine practitioners. Herbs should be used according to individual needs; consult with a licensed practitioner for a customized formulation. To learn more about the herbs listed here, go to www.ask drmao.com.

• Evening primrose (300 milligrams GLA), flaxseed, and fish oils (1,000 milligrams omega-3) are good for preventing damage to the hair and hair follicles. They are usually taken in capsule form.

• Ginkgo biloba (120 milligrams daily) improves circulation to the scalp, green tea (300 milligrams polyphenol content) provides antioxidant benefits, and saw palmetto (320 milligrams) blocks DHT and prevents hair loss.

• Traditional Chinese herbs used to prevent hair loss include Chinese arborvitae (flat fir leaves), eclipa, Chinese foxglove, black cohosh, vitex, ginger, and sesame.

❋ EXERCISE ❋

Regular physical exercise is important for maintaining proper circulation to the scalp. Excessively strenuous exercise is not recommended, as it will deplete vital energy. Stress-reduction exercises and meditation can help regulate your energy and strengthen your essence. I recommend a Dao In Qi Gong exercise called Gentle Rainfall Experience, which promotes blood circulation to the scalp and hair follicle, to all my hair-loss patients. Do the exercise twice a day for best results.

Sit comfortably at the edge of a stiff chair, or cross-legged on a soft pillow.

With the tips of every finger (including the thumbs) gently tap your head all over, stimulating the scalp for about 1 minute. Use light force at the beginning and gently increase to moderate strength.

Massage the scalp with both hands, moving the scalp gently and then more vigorously for 2 to 3 minutes.

Straighten the fingers of your right hand, and with the palm side of the fingers gently tap all over the scalp 36 times. Then do the same with your left hand another 36 times.

❋ ACUPRESSURE ❋

• Locate the acupoint Forceful Torrent (KID-3), between your right ankle-bone and right Achilles tendon. Pinch the point with your right thumb and index finger and hold for 3 to 5 minutes. Repeat on the left foot.

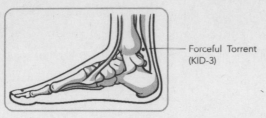

Forceful Torrent
(KID-3)

• Use a stiff toothbrush or the tips of your fingers to tap the balding area with moderate strength for 5 minutes twice a day to help invigorate blood circulation.

AVOID

• Chemicals, food additives, and pesticides, as they may interfere with healthy hormonal functions, potentially injuring the hair follicles.

• Stress and exhaustion, which damage the vital essence and deplete the kidney energy.

• Certain gout medications, antiarthritis medications, and antidepressants, as they can cause hair loss. Check with your physician for alternatives.

HEADACHE

MOST PEOPLE GET OCCASIONAL HEADACHES as a result of catching a cold, staying up too late, or drinking too much, enduring the consequences the next morning. One in six Americans experiences chronic headaches, which can be caused by sinus problems, muscle tension, eyestrain, jaw clenching, a virus, or allergies. Headaches can be experienced at the front of the head, the temples, the back of the head near the neck, and the top of the head. Factors that worsen headaches include poor eating habits, stress, and lack of sleep. Headaches can occur during the day or in the evening, while you are active or at rest. In complicated cases like migraines or neurological headaches, the headache may be accompanied by sensitivity to light and sound, nausea, and vomiting. (Migraine headaches are addressed on page 408.)

According to Chinese medicine, pain is the body's signal that there is a blockage of energy and blood. Causes of the stagnation include developing a cold, depression, or trauma to the energy meridian as a result of physical injury. By identifying the underlying cause of the headache, I deliver targeted therapies to my patients, including acupuncture for pain relief, herbal medicine for inflammation and muscle spasms, diet therapy to eliminate allergies, and meditation to reduce stress and tension.

Below I've summarized my favorite home remedies for headaches. Note that headaches may be caused by severe medical conditions like glaucoma and brain hemorrhages. If you experience severe, debilitating headaches that don't respond to over-the-counter medication, or if you wake up in the middle of the night with excruciating head pain, visit your physician or the emergency room immediately.

❋ DIET ❋

• Energy and blood flow rely heavily on what we consume on a regular basis—the foods we eat eventually end up in our blood and meridians in the form of energy. Proper eating habits can help maintain a good flow of energy and blood to the head, preventing headaches. Eat wholesome foods free of preservatives, additives, and other artificial ingredients. Artificial colors and preservatives such as sulfites in wines and dried fruits can cause headaches. Add a good amount of fiber-rich foods, including whole grains, green leafy vegetables, parsley, chrysanthemum flowers, mint, green tea, onions, ginger, pearl barley, carrots, prunes, buckwheat, peach kernels (eaten like raw nuts), and almonds. Eat regularly, more frequently, and in smaller quantities. Do not eat on the run or while under stress. Do not eat late at night or lie down immediately after eating.

• Avoid greasy and fried foods. When oils are heated they produce chemicals that can cause headaches. Spicy, stimulating foods and heavy starchy foods should be avoided as well. Drinking coffee or other caffeinated beverages can raise blood pressure and cause headaches, although some-times caffeine can temporarily relieve headaches. Giving up coffee abruptly can cause withdrawal headaches at first. Drinking alcohol can also cause headaches.

―――――――――― ✳ HOME REMEDIES ✳ ――――――――――

• Make a rice porridge by simmering 1 cup of white rice with 2 chopped green onions, 1 garlic clove, and 5 slices of ginger in 6 cups of water for 20 minutes, keeping the pot covered. The spices will make you sweat and boost your immune system, which helps to fight virus and bacteria. This porridge is also good for treating high blood pressure, PMS, and ten-sion headaches.

• Make a tea by boiling 5 prunes, 1 tablespoon green tea, and 2 table-spoons chopped fresh mint in 3 1/2 cups of water for 15 minutes. Strain, and drink 3 cups a day until the headache subsides. You may also eat a handful of prunes 3 times a day until the headache subsides.

• Make fresh carrot juice and drink a glass every 4 hours until the headache subsides. Also put carrot juice in a small squirt bottle, and squirt a little car-rot juice into the left, right, or both nostrils, depending on where the headache is located.

• Put 5 drops of lavender essential oil in 1 cup of warm water. Soak a small towel in the water, and then wring it dry. Place it on your forehead as a compress to alleviate a headache.

―――――――――― ✳ DAILY SUPPLEMENTS ✳ ――――――――――

• Magnesium (500 milligrams) and calcium (1,000 milligrams) can help con-trol muscle spasms and can help relieve tension headaches.

• The amino acid 5-HTP (100 milligrams), fish oil (1,000 milligrams EPA; 800 milligrams DHA), vitamin B_2 (riboflavin; 400 milligrams), chromium (200 micrograms), folic acid (800 micrograms), and vitamin C (1,000 milligrams) can be helpful for temporary relief of headaches.

• Niacin (vitamin B_3; 500 milligrams) is useful for treating acute headache attack. Take 3 times a day when you have a headache.

─────────── ✳ HERBAL THERAPY ✳ ───────────

• Herbs can be found in health food or vitamin stores, online, and at the offices of Chinese medicine practitioners. Herbs should be used according to individual needs; consult with a licensed practitioner for a customized formulation. To learn more about the herbs listed here, go to www.ask drmao.com.

• Make a tea by boiling 2 tablespoons each of chrysanthemum flowers, cassia seeds, and mint leaves in 4 cups of water for 15 minutes. Strain, and drink 3 cups a day until the headache subsides. These herbs help clear the sinuses and reduce the pressure in the head.

• Feverfew has been used since ancient times for treating headaches, and some studies show that it may help reduce the frequency and severity of headaches.

• Traditional Chinese herbs used for headaches include mint, ligustici, angelica, notopterygii, siler, schizonepetae, green tea, and licorice.

─────────── ✳ EXERCISE ✳ ───────────

I recommend avoiding vigorous exercise during headache episodes, as exercise may worsen the condition. Taking a walk in fresh air will help stimulate blood flow and increase oxygenation to the head. Gentle walking can nip the headache in the bud before it starts—as soon as you feel a headache coming on, step out into the fresh air and go for a 10-minute walk, breathing deeply and vigorously. A regular regimen of moderate cardiovascular and stretching exercises can help maintain good health and

HEADACHE

proper circulation. Daily meditation practice and tai chi exercises can also help. Here is a simple visualization meditation called White Light Meditation that I teach my patients.

Sit or lie down comfortably. Clear your mind, relax your body, and breathe deeply and slowly.

Inhale, and visualize a white light or clear mountain spring water entering your body at the top of your head and flowing down to your abdomen.

Exhale, and visualize the white light or water continuing its downward course from your abdomen to the bottom of your feet, where it drains out.

Repeat the breathing cycle and visualization for 10 minutes. Do this meditation often as necessary—it often brings on a quick reduction in symptoms.

❊ ACUPRESSURE ❊

• Locate the acupoint Wind Pond (GB-20), in the natural indentation at the base of your skull on either side of your neck. Press and lift up toward the base of your skull with your thumbs and lean your head back. Use the weight of your head against your thumbs for steady pressure on the acupoint. Hold for 5 minutes, breathing deeply and slowly.

• Find the acupoint Greater Yang (Taiyang), in the indentation of the temples. Stimulate the point with the knuckles of your thumbs or the tips of your index fingers. Massage in a circular motion for 5 minutes.

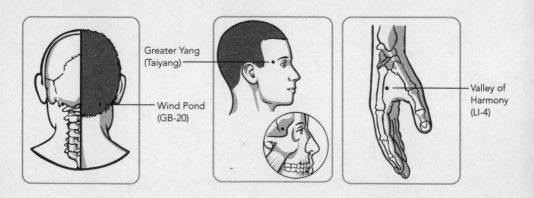

Greater Yang (Taiyang)

Wind Pond (GB-20)

Valley of Harmony (LI-4)

• Find the acupoint Valley of Harmony (LI-4), in the web between the thumb and index finger on your right hand. Apply steady pressure with your left thumb until you feel soreness. Hold for 2 minutes. Repeat on the left hand.

• You may wish to check out whether there are any physical imbalances in your spine, neck, or jaw, as these imbalances can exacerbate headaches. Proper structural adjustments may be helpful—consult a chiropractor or an osteopath.

AVOID

• Some medications that cause headaches, including birth control pills, antihistamines, vasodilators (such as nitroglycerin), isosorbide dinitrate, antiarrythmic agents (such as quinidine), digoxin, and ergotamine. Hormone therapy can also cause headaches. Consult your physician for alternatives.

• Caffeine, recreational drugs, and alcohol. Lack of sleep is another major cause of common headaches. The common cold and neck injuries also may cause headaches.

• High blood pressure and blood sugar fluctuations; they should be regulated and controlled, as both of these conditions can cause headaches.

HEARING LOSS

AN UNFORTUNATE FACT: THE AVERAGE PERSON starts losing hearing in his or her twenties. The loss is so gradual that most people don't notice until it affects their lives. Even when they need to use the highest volume on the television, some people don't recognize or admit that they have a hearing problem. The gradual deterioration of hearing is primarily a result of the environmental, lifestyle, and dietary choices we make during our youth. The popularity of digital audio players is cer-

HEARING LOSS

tainly adding to the problem. Continued exposure to loud environments, inadequate sleep and rest, overindulgence, and being overworked place an enormous amount of strain on the body. Combined with a poor diet, including increasing amounts of chemical and artificial ingredients in our food, our bodies begin to fail as a result of toxic buildup. For example, there is a link between high blood cholesterol and loss of hearing. Genetic, physical, and other disease factors may also be involved. Some childhood illnesses, such as measles, mumps, and chronic adenoid inflammations (inflammation of the tonsils), can lead directly to hearing loss.

Chinese medicine recognizes a link between hearing loss and the underlying essence of the person. Prolonged overindulgence and being overworked during youth deplete the body's vital essence, causing deficiencies—especially of the kidney-bladder network. Depleted kidney energy can lead to a premature decline in hearing. Strong emotions such as anger and frustration can aggravate the liver energy, which rises to the head and ears, producing hearing impairment and tinnitus (ringing in the ears). Ménière's disease, an inner ear condition, often corresponds to a rise in liver energy. Acute loss of hearing is often associated with external pathogens such as the viruses that cause colds, flu, ear infections, and shingles.

I've worked with a number of ear, nose, and throat specialists on hearing-related problems in patients ranging from three to ninety-three years old. My treatments focus on fortifying the underlying essence, strengthening the vital energy of the kidneys, and opening blocked sensory orifices. I often use acupuncture with electrostimulation to increase neurological function and circulation within the ears, while using herbal therapy to reduce inflammation and swelling and to promote healing.

• A balanced diet of smaller and more frequent meals with ample amounts of complex carbohydrates and organic animal proteins is a good start. Adding more warming foods, such as organic chicken and lamb, can help strengthen the kidney yang energy. Scallions, sesame seeds, fish, baked tofu, soybeans, walnuts, eggs, lentils, black beans, lotus seeds, ginger, and cinnamon bark are also helpful.

• Avoid cold and raw foods and icy beverages, as the coldness may constrict the eustachian tubes, causing poor drainage from the inner ears. Maintain a diet low in saturated fats, and eliminate fried and greasy foods. Avoid processed meats and dairy products, as they have a tendency to increase mucus production. Protein deposits similar to those in milk have been found in the inner ear of patients with partial hearing loss.

━━━━━━━━━━ ❋ HOME REMEDIES ❋ ━━━━━━━━━━

• Ear irrigation can remove excess wax buildup, which can be a cause of diminished hearing. Ear wax kits with specific instructions are available at some pharmacies. You may also want to visit your ear, nose, and throat specialist if the problem becomes severe.

• Make a tea by boiling together 1 heaping tablespoon each of dried oregano, cilantro, rosemary, sage, and cinnamon, plus 3 slices of fresh ginger in 4 cups of water for 15 minutes. Cover the pot to prevent steam from escaping as it boils. Strain, and drink 3 cups a day for at least 3 weeks.

• Make a bone marrow soup with organic sheep's bones or calves' bones. Cook 3 pounds bones in a large pot filled with 8 cups water with 1/3 cup each of black beans, kidney beans, and adzuki beans, 2 diced carrots, 2 diced celery stalks, 1 sliced onion, and 1/2 cup dried seaweed. Season with 1 teaspoon each turmeric, cumin, and black pepper. Do not use salt.

HEARING LOSS

• Ear, nose, and throat specialists will sometimes recommend up to 300 milligrams of niacin (vitamin B₃) to increase blood flow to the microcapillaries of the inner ear, which feed the auditory nerve. Taking niacin can cause a heat flush lasting for about 30 minutes.

• N-acetylcysteine (NAC; 500 milligrams) may help prevent hearing loss—this is especially useful for people who are constantly exposed to loud noise.

• Taking folate (folic acid; 400 micrograms) on a daily basis has been shown to slow hearing loss.

• Carotenoids (1,000 milligrams) and vitamins A (200 IU), C (1,000 milligrams), and E (800 IU) can reduce the risk of noise-induced hearing loss.

———————————— ❊ HERBAL THERAPY ❊ ————————————

• Herbs can be found in health food or vitamin stores, online, and at the offices of Chinese medicine practitioners. Herbs should be used according to individual needs; consult with a licensed practitioner for a customized formulation. To learn more, go to www.askdrmao.com.

• Ginkgo biloba can help stabilize hearing loss by increasing capillary blood circulation.

• Hawthorn berry activates blood flow and can be helpful in preventing hearing loss.

• Traditional Chinese herbs used to support healthy hearing include rehmannia, wild yam, schizandra, Asian cornelian, and magnetite.

———————————— ❊ EXERCISE ❊ ————————————

Exercise is important for stimulating blood circulation, maintaining healthy immunity, and preventing colds and flu. I recommend a daily regimen of qi gong and tai chi combined with moderate cardiovascular exercise.

I often use Dao In Qi Gong exercises to help support healthy hearing function in my patients. Immortal Beating the Heavenly Drum and Immortal Sounding the Heavenly Bell exercises work best—do these exercises daily for optimum results.

To perform the Immortal Beating the Heavenly Drum exercise, sit comfortably at the tip of a sturdy chair with your spine erect, arms on your legs, and head tilted slightly forward.

Begin breathing slowly and rhythmically, inhaling deeply and gently and exhaling slowly.

Cover both ears with your palms, with the fingers of each hand pointing toward each other at the back of the head.

Inhaling, place your index fingers on top of your middle fingers and then snap them off, striking the back of the head on the depressions located behind the ears at the base of the skull, where the Wind Pond (GB-20) acupoints are located. Repeat continuously, with about one strike per second.

On an exhale, continue striking the Wind Pond points with your index fingers while bending forward at the waist. Tilt your head down.

Continue breathing and striking for 20 to 30 seconds, until you've struck the points 36 times.

Conclude the exercise by rising back to the sitting position on your last exhalation.

To perform the Immortal Sounding the Heavenly Bell exercise, begin by sitting comfortably at the tip of a sturdy chair with your spine erect, arms on your legs, and head tilted slightly forward.

Begin breathing slowly and rhythmically, inhaling deeply and gently and exhaling slowly.

While holding your palms over both ears, create a tight seal and repeatedly clench your teeth firmly: 9 times focusing on the front of your mouth, 9 times focusing on the left side, 9 times focusing on the right side, and 9 times focusing on the back of your mouth, for a total of 36 times. Inhale each time you bite down, and exhale when you relax your jaw.

Conclude with restful breathing for 1 minute. This is a great exercise for maintaining the health of the mouth, teeth, and auditory canal.

• Find the acupoint Forceful Torrent (KID-3), in the depression between the inner anklebone and the Achilles tendon of the right foot. Apply steady pressure with your right thumb until you feel soreness. Hold for 2 minutes. Repeat on the left foot.

• Locate the acupoint Listening Palace (SI-19), directly in front of the right ear canal, in the depression formed when the mouth is slightly open. Apply steady pressure with your index or middle finger until you feel soreness. Hold for 2 minutes. Repeat on the left side.

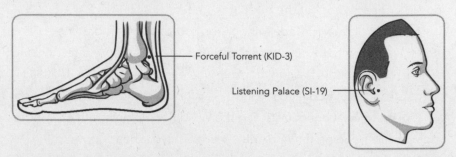

Forceful Torrent (KID-3)

Listening Palace (SI-19)

AVOID

• Antibiotics such as aminoglycosides, gentamicin, and tobramicin, which have been shown to cause hearing loss, usually temporary, but occasionally permanent. Consult your physician.

• Aspirin overuse, which has been linked to acute hearing loss.

• Some diuretics, such as furosemide (Lasix), in high doses and some antihypertensive drugs, such as a combination of bisoprolol and hydrochlorothiazide (Ziac), which can cause hearing loss. Consult your physician.

• Loud noise, by wearing earplugs to concerts and turning down the volume on the television.

HALF OF ALL AMERICANS SUFFER FROM HEMORRHOIDS at least once during their lifetime. Most people don't seek medical treatment, but pain in your behind that prevents you from sitting comfortably is no laughing matter. Hemorrhoids are similar to varicose veins in the legs, except now we're talking about veins in the rectum, which cause swelling, inflammation, and pain. Symptoms include anal pain, itching, and bleeding during and after bowel movements. In severe cases the veins can protrude through the rectum and become infected. The most common cause of hemorrhoids is weakness of the rectal muscles. Chronic constipation and straining can also bring on hemorrhoids or make an existing condition worse. Obesity, pregnancy, sedentary lifestyle, and improper diet are some of the other causes.

In Chinese medicine, a variety of factors play a role in the development of hemorrhoids. Heat accumulation in the large intestine combined with a lack of fluids leads to constipation. The heat also causes swelling and inflammation of the rectum and puts excess strain on the rectal muscles and veins. A poor diet—especially one lacking adequate fiber—and emotional stress take a toll on the spleen-pancreas-stomach network, which is charged with keeping the muscles, tendons, and sphincter tissues strong. Under constant strain, the weakened tissues develop blood and energy blockages, resulting in hemorrhoids.

My father's favorite advice to his patients with hemorrhoids was to eat a yam a day. I give out the same advice to my patients, with great efficacy. I also use acupuncture therapy to help reduce the pain and swelling, and herbal therapy—both oral and topical—to restore healthy bowel movements. I also educate my patients on dietary and lifestyle changes to prevent recurrence. In severe cases, surgery may be necessary to repair the tissue.

HEMORRHOIDS

Here is some of the advice that I give to my patients. If you experience prolonged, severe bleeding from your rectum, see a proctologist immediately.

❊ DIET ❊

• The best way to ensure a happy and healthy rectum is to maintain a high-fiber diet rich in bran, whole grains, fruits, and leafy vegetables. Eat regularly, more often, and in smaller quantities. Favor cucumbers, water chestnuts, buckwheat, black fungus (an Asian mushroom also known as wood ear), tangerines, figs, plums, prunes, guavas, bamboo shoots, mung beans, winter melon, nuts and seeds (such as black sesame seeds, almonds, and apricot seeds), bananas, squash, tofu, and fish. Drink plenty of water, as adequate hydration can help soften the stools and help reduce straining.

• Avoid spicy foods, alcohol, smoking, greasy or deep-fried foods, and foods containing preservatives and artificial colors and sweeteners.

❊ HOME REMEDIES ❊

• Eat a yam or sweet potato a day to keep the hemorrhoids away.

• In acute cases, apply an ice compress to help temporarily constrict the blood vessels, stop the bleeding, and reduce swelling.

• Take a sitz bath by dissolving 1/2 cup of Epsom salts in a warm water bath and soaking for 15 minutes once a day for a month, or until condition clears.

• Clean the hemorrhoids with warm water and rub with witch hazel, every hour.

• Apply fresh vera aloe gel to the affected area to stop the itching and reduce inflammation.

❊ DAILY SUPPLEMENTS ❊

• Bioflavonoids (500 milligrams) can help strengthen the vein walls and prevent hemorrhoids.

- Vitamin C (1,000 milligrams) tones the bowel wall tissue.

- Vitamin E (1,000 IU) is an antioxidant that promotes tissue healing.

——————————— ❋ HERBAL THERAPY ❋ ———————————

- Herbs can be found in health food or vitamin stores, online, and at the offices of Chinese medicine practitioners. Herbs should be used according to individual needs; consult with a licensed practitioner for a customized formulation. To learn more about the herbs listed here, go to www.ask drmao.com.

- Bilberry extract can reduce the inflammation and pain from hemorrhoids.

- Butcher's broom can help ease inflammation. It constricts the small vessels, which can reduce pain. It can also be used as a suppository or in cream form for topical use.

- Horse chestnut can strengthen the vascular walls.

- Traditional Chinese herbs to support rectal health include sophorae, schizonepetae, rehmannia, scrophulariae, ophiopogonis, and biota.

——————————— ❋ EXERCISE ❋ ———————————

Adequate physical activity is important for avoiding constipation. Thirty minutes a day of walking, cycling, or swimming can help maintain regular bowel habits. Moderate exercise also helps to maintain a calm, stress-free lifestyle. Meditation and energy exercises can help as well. The third sequence of the Eight Treasures Qi Gong practice, Raising the Hands to Adjust the Stomach and Spleen, performed 10 minutes every day, can help strengthen your digestive and elimination systems, promoting good bowel habits and preventing hemorrhoids.

Begin in a standing posture with your spine erect, feet drawn close to-

HEMORRHOIDS

gether, and arms at your sides. Tilt your head slightly forward. Begin regular, rhythmic breathing.

Form a cup or plate with your right hand. Facing the palm toward the sky, inhale and make a large circular motion in front of you from the left to right while raising your arm above your head. Be sure to keep your palm facing the sky.

As you do this movement with the right hand, move your left hand to your back with the palm facing the ground.

As your right hand reaches its highest point above your head, begin to stretch your torso, lifting your body on the balls of your feet. Exhale gently. Simultaneously push your left hand toward the ground. Be sure to push in opposite directions—your right hand pushing to the sky and the left pushing to the ground.

Repeat this movement 3 times, inhaling as your arm goes up and exhaling as you stretch.

Switch sides and repeat the exercise.

This exercise helps stretch the abdominal organs and stimulates the intestines, spleen, and stomach.

To help move the bowels and prevent constipation, follow the instructions for self-massage in the section on constipation (page 249).

❊ ACUPRESSURE ❊

• Find the acupoint Valley of Harmony (LI-4), at the web between your right thumb and index finger. Apply steady pressure with your left thumb until you feel soreness. Hold for 2 minutes. Repeat on the left hand.

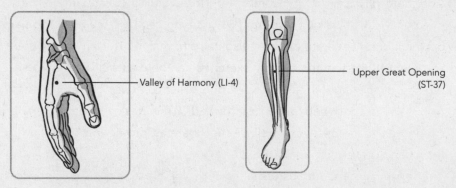

Valley of Harmony (LI-4)

Upper Great Opening (ST-37)

• Find the acupoint Upper Great Opening (ST-37) by measuring 2 hand-widths or 8 finger-widths below the outer indentation of your right knee next to your shinbone. Apply steady pressure with your left thumb until you feel soreness. Hold for 2 minutes. Repeat on the left leg.

AVOID

• Alcohol and coffee, as they tend to deplete fluids in the bowels and cause inflammation, worsening the condition.

• Foods that irritate the intestinal tract, including MSG, preservatives, and additives.

• Smoking, which can worsen hemorrhoids.

HIGH BLOOD PRESSURE

HIGH BLOOD PRESSURE, OR HYPERTENSION, is a condition in which blood pressure is chronically elevated. According to the National Institutes of Health, blood pressure readings of 140/90 mmHg and higher on recurring measurements is considered hypertension. Persistent hypertension is one of the highest risk factors for stroke, heart attack, heart failure, and arterial aneurysm. It is a leading cause of chronic kidney failure. Essential or primary hypertension has no specific causes; it's associated with genetics, environment, diet, and lifestyle factors, including salt intake, stress, and lack of exercise. Secondary hypertension is a result of other underlying—often serious—conditions such as tumors and kidney or liver disorders. Some medications, such as oral contraceptives, can also cause elevated blood pressure.

According to Chinese medicine, diet and emotions play key roles

HIGH BLOOD PRESSURE

in hypertension. The Western-style diet is perhaps the primary contributing cause of essential hypertension, according to research. People living in rural areas of China, Brazil, and Africa show no signs of essential hypertension, even with advanced age. Hypertension in Chinese medicine is related to imbalances of the kidney and liver organ systems. If the kidneys fail to regulate the water energy and balance the liver, the liver fire energy rises and causes hypertension. My treatments focus on strengthening the kidney system and regulating the liver by soothing and cooling its fire energy. I've also found that teaching my patients meditation practices has enabled the majority of them to control their blood pressure and keep it in check.

I have a number of patients who suffer from "white coat" syndrome—their blood pressure shoots up when they visit the doctor's office but drops outside of these encounters. I use acupuncture and herbal and dietary therapies to support healthy blood pressure. I also believe in empowering my patients with simple practices such as stress-release meditation, which they can use to gain control over their blood pressure during stressful times—like having their blood pressure measured at their doctors' offices. One of my patients was able to bring down her blood pressure from 150/98 mmHg to 124/82 mmHg over a three-month period while also overcoming an anxiety condition.

Here are some of my favorite remedies for maintaining good cardiovascular health and clean arteries. Do not stop your blood pressure medication on your own—always consult with your physician before making any changes to your treatment plan.

❋ DIET ❋

• Eat wholesome foods, with no preservatives, additives, or pesticides. Eat smaller meals more frequently. Consume more leafy green vegetables, whole grains, celery, tofu, spinach, garlic, bananas, sunflower seeds, honey, mung beans, bamboo shoots, seaweed, vinegar, tomatoes, water chestnuts, corn, apples, persimmons, peas, buckwheat, jellyfish (soak and cook), watermelon, hawthorn berries (make tea), eggplant, plums, mushrooms, lemons, lotus root, chrysanthemum flowers and cassia seeds (make tea), pearl barley, peach kernels (eaten raw like nuts), ginger, sprouted vegetables, wheat bran, and green tea. Spices including fennel, oregano, black pepper, basil, and tarragon contain active ingredients beneficial for treating hypertension. Drink at least six 8-ounce glasses of room temperature water a day.

....

• Avoid excessive salt, fried and greasy foods, spicy stimulating foods, and simple carbohydrates like sugar and white flour. MSG and other preservatives should also be avoided. Alcohol, coffee, and tobacco should be avoided. Cheeses and aged, cured meats should also be avoided, as they promote plaque buildup.

❊ HOME REMEDIES ❊

• Drink an 8-ounce glass of fresh celery juice 3 times a day for 1 to 3 months, until blood pressure is normal. This is one of the most common Chinese folk remedies for lowering blood pressure, and it works despite the sodium content of the celery.

....

• First thing upon waking, on an empty stomach, drink 8 ounces of warm water mixed with 1 tablespoon apple cider vinegar and 1 teaspoon honey. Drink this regularly. The honey ensures regularity of the bowels, and is helpful because constipation may aggravate high blood pressure. The vinegar alkalizes the body and lowers blood pressure as well.

....

• Eat 2 fresh cucumbers every day for 2 weeks, or until blood pressure improves. Since cucumber is a natural diuretic, it will help hydrate your body and lower blood pressure.

....

HIGH BLOOD PRESSURE

• Make a tea by boiling 1/4 cup fresh mint leaves, 1/4 cup dried chrysanthemum flowers, and 2 tablespoons cassia seeds in 5 cups of water for 20
minutes. Strain. Drink 3 cups a day.

• Sleep on a pillow stuffed with mung beans, lentils, and split peas—they
help to draw the fire from the head and lower blood pressure.

─────────────── ❋ DAILY SUPPLEMENTS ❋ ───────────────

• Magnesium (600 milligrams), calcium (1,000 milligrams), Zinc (25 milligrams) and essential fatty acids such as gamma-linoleic acid and omega-
3 fatty acids (1,000 milligrams EPA) are essential. Magnesium is a
vasodilator and helps regulate calcium levels.

• Vitamin B complex helps lower blood pressure. B_6 (200 milligrams) acts as
a diuretic, while niacin (50 milligrams) relaxes the blood vessels.

• Taking coenzyme Q_{10} (15 milligrams) 3 times a day can reduce blood
pressure.

• Beta carotene (500 milligrams) taken every other day can reduce incidence of coronary and vascular events.

• Folic acid (200 micrograms) taken daily can improve blood flow to the
capillaries.

─────────────── ❋ HERBAL THERAPY ❋ ───────────────

• Herbs can be found in health food or vitamin stores, online, and at the offices of Chinese medicine practitioners. Herbs should be used according
to individual needs; consult with a licensed practitioner for a customized
formulation. To learn more about the herbs listed here, go to www.ask
drmao.com.

• Hawthorn berries (150 milligrams) have traditionally been used to support
healthy blood pressure levels.

• A traditional Chinese herbal formula called gastrodia gambir is used to support healthy blood pressure. It contains gastrodia, gambir vine, abalone shell, gardenia, skullcap, motherwort, cyathulae, eucommia, loranthus, polygoni, and poria.

❊ EXERCISE ❊

Physical exercise is essential for promoting circulation and strengthening heart function. Sedentary life inhibits circulation. Doing moderate cardiovascular exercise every day for at least 30 minutes will help reduce hypertension. Effective moderate exercise includes walking briskly (3 to 4 miles per hour), general calisthenics, racket sports such as table tennis, swimming (with moderate effort), cycling (at a moderate speed of 10 miles per hour or less), canoeing, and rowing (at a speed of about 2 to 4 miles per hour). I've also taught many of my patients the following simple stress-release meditation to help control their stress and blood pressure.

Sit comfortably or lie down on your back. Slow your respiration to deep, abdominal breathing. Say the word "calm" in your mind with every exhalation. You'll be visualizing the relaxation of a specific body part and releasing tension with every exhalation. Trace the following 3 pathways outlined below.

Start at the top of your head. Inhale, and then exhale and visualize your scalp muscles relaxing. Say "calm" in your mind. Repeat, saying the word as you move into each body part, down through your face, throat, chest, abdomen, thighs, knees, calves, ankles, and feet. After you've relaxed your feet, visualize all the tension leaving your body through your toes in the form of dark smoke.

Start at the temple region of your head. This path focuses on the sides and upper extremities. Inhale, and then exhale and visualize your temple muscles relaxing. Say "calm" in your mind. Repeat, saying the word as you move into each body part, down through your jaws, the sides of your neck, shoulders, upper arms, elbows, forearms, wrists, and hands. Once you've relaxed your hands, visualize all the tension leaving your body through your fingertips in the form of dark smoke.

HIGH BLOOD PRESSURE

The final pathway begins at the back of your head. This path relaxes the back of your body. Repeat the breathing-visualization-word routine, as above, as you go from the back of your neck to your upper back, middle back, lower back, back of the thighs, calves, and heels. Then focus on the acupoint Bubbling Spring (KID-1; see illustration below) on the soles of your feet, for 1 minute.

Practice this sequence for at least 15 minutes twice a day.

❈ ACUPRESSURE ❈

• Locate the acupoint Winding Gulch (LI-11), in the depression at the outer part of the right elbow crease, between the elbow tendon and the bone. The point is best located when the arm is bent at 90 degrees with the palm facing the abdomen. Apply steady pressure with your thumb until you feel soreness. Hold for 5 minutes. Repeat on the left arm.

• Find the acupoint Bubbling Spring (KID-1), on the sole of the right foot between the bones of the second and third toes, two-thirds of the distance from the heel to the base of the second toe, just below the ball of the foot in a natural indentation. Apply heavy pressure with your thumb for 5 minutes. Repeat on the left foot.

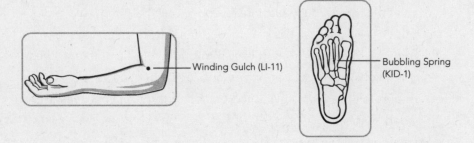

Winding Gulch (LI-11)

Bubbling Spring (KID-1)

AVOID

• Sedentary life and stress, as they not only increase the risk of heart problems but also cause other disorders, such as obesity and diabetes, complicating the condition.

- Over-the-counter drugs containing ibuprofen (such as Motrin and Advil) as they can raise blood pressure.

- Smoking and exposure to secondhand smoke, as it can lead to hardening of the arteries.

HIGH CHOLESTEROL

HIGH BLOOD CHOLESTEROL, OR HYPERCHOLESTEROLEMIA, is a condition in which elevated levels of cholesterol are present in the blood. It is not a disease but a metabolic dysfunction, which means that it can contribute to many other serious diseases—most notably by affecting the heart and cardiovascular system, resulting in conditions including angina, heart attack, stroke, and atherosclerosis (hardening of the arteries). There are two types of cholesterol: high-density lipoprotein (HDL), the good cholesterol that protects against heart disease, and low-density lipoprotein (LDL), the bad cholesterol that contributes to plaque buildup in the arteries. Although there are no outward symptoms of elevated cholesterol, it slowly clogs up the arteries and its impact can be devastating over time. Aside from a genetic predisposition to high cholesterol, the most common causes of elevated cholesterol are diet and lifestyle.

Chinese medicine recognizes that diet and emotions play a key role in high cholesterol. Cholesterol is viewed as a result of the accumulation of dampness and mucus as a result of impaired function of the digestive system, most notably of the spleen, stomach, liver, and pancreas. Western medicine similarly recognizes that cholesterol is either consumed and absorbed through the digestive tract or produced by the liver. Metabolic and hormonal conditions like diabetes and menopause can also contribute to elevated cholesterol levels.

HIGH CHOLESTEROL

With a correct diagnosis and treatment with acupuncture, herbs, diet, and exercise, I've helped many patients reduce their blood cholesterol levels.

A woman recently came in with a cholesterol reading of 405. Her HDL was 56, her LDL was 349, and her triglyceride reading was 312. She was forty-eight years old and experiencing menopausal symptoms—she had missed her period for the previous four months and had gained weight around her belly. Upon close examination, she also showed signs of insulin resistance. Her cells were not responding to insulin, thereby allowing glucose to build up in her blood, and much of it was converted to fat storage in her belly. I called her internist and we put together a comprehensive program including a high-fiber and low-cholesterol diet, daily cardiovascular exercise, and acupuncture and herbal therapies to balance her digestive and hormonal functions.

She agreed to go on statin drugs, which block cholesterol production by the liver, for two months. She had an ultrasound taken of the carotid arteries in her neck and a calcium plaque scoring CT scan of her heart to see if any plaque had built up. To her relief, both scans were clear. After two months her cholesterol dropped to 252 and her HDL/LDL/triglyceride levels improved, although they weren't yet in normal range. However, the level of liver enzymes in her blood was rising—a potential side effect of the statin drug—so her internist took her off the drug. We continued with the dietary and lifestyle regimen and the Eastern medical therapies. Three months later, her cholesterol had dropped to 178 with the HDL at 97 and LDL at 81. As a nice bonus, her period came back and she lost twenty-three pounds. She has remained off the medication and continues to be vigilant about diet and exercise.

Here are some of my favorite home remedies to help lower cholesterol and maintain good cardiovascular health. Always work with your physician to formulate a holistic program for healthy cholesterol.

———————————————— ✳ DIET ✳ ————————————————

• Eat wholesome foods containing no preservatives, additives, pesticides. Eat smaller meals more frequently. Favor leafy green vegetables, whole grains, celery, tofu, spinach, garlic, sunflower seeds, mung beans, bamboo shoots, oats, barley, rye, legumes (peas, beans), apples, prunes, blueberries, carrots, Brussels sprouts, broccoli, yams, buckwheat, jellyfish (soak and cook), watermelon, hawthorn berries (make tea), eggplant, mushrooms, lemons, lotus root, chrysanthemum flowers and cassia seeds (make tea), pearl barley, peach kernels (eat raw like nuts), ginger, sprouted vegetables, wheat bran, and green tea. Various spices, including fennel, oregano, black pepper, basil, and tarragon, have active ingredients beneficial for lowering cholesterol.

• Avoid deep-fried, fatty foods, simple carbohydrates including sugars and white flour, sodium, MSG and other preservatives, trans fats, and saturated fats. Coffee and tobacco should be avoided. Cheeses and aged cured meats should also be avoided, as they promote plaque buildup.

———————————— ✳ HOME REMEDIES ✳ ————————————

• Eating 3 apples a day for 3 months can lower your cholesterol by at least 20 points, according to a Finnish study on nutrition and heart disease.

• Eat homemade orange marmalade, including the rind, to lower LDL cholesterol. A USDA study has shown that compounds called polymethoxylated flavones (PMFs), found in the pigment of orange and tangerine peel can work to reduce bad cholesterol (LDL) without altering the level of good cholesterol (HDL).

• Drinking 1 cup of green or black tea daily may lower LDL cholesterol and triglycerides.

─────────── ❋ DAILY SUPPLEMENTS ❋ ───────────

• Coenzyme Q_{10} (50 milligrams) increases oxygen supply to the heart muscle. Statin drugs can block the production of coenzyme Q_{10} in the body and cause muscle pain, so supplementation is a must.

• Taking beta carotene (1,000 milligrams) supplements can help reduce the incidence of coronary and vascular events.

• Taking folic acid (400 micrograms) can improve blood flow to the capillaries, feeding the heart muscle.

• Supplementing with soluble fiber can help absorb and excrete excess fat from the digestive tract, and thereby reduce cholesterol absorption.

• Supplementing with red yeast rice (1,200 milligrams) can help lower cholesterol, its action being similar to that of statin drugs.

─────────── ❋ HERBAL THERAPY ❋ ───────────

• Herbs can be found in health food or vitamin stores, online, and at the offices of Chinese medicine practitioners. Herbs should be used according to individual needs; consult with a licensed practitioner for a customized formulation. To learn more about the herbs listed here, go to www.askdrmao.com.

• Taking artichoke leaf extract can help lower cholesterol.

• White willow bark, which aspirin is derived from, helps prevent abnormal clumping and clotting of blood platelets.

• Drink 3 cups of Internal Cleanse tea a day. This tea contains chrysanthemum, hawthorn, cassia, lotus, mulberry, and peppermint, traditional Chinese herbs that help support healthy cholesterol.

Physical exercise is essential for promoting circulation and strengthening heart function. Sedentary life inhibits circulation. A good way to reduce cholesterol and to stimulate circulation is to do moderate cardiovascular exercise every day for at least 30 minutes. I suggest walking briskly (3 to 4 miles per hour), general calisthenics, racket sports such as table tennis, swimming (with moderate effort), cycling (at a moderate speed of 10 miles per hour or less), canoeing, or rowing (at a speed of about 2 to 4 miles per hour).

I also recommend a simple walking exercise called Merry-Go-Around Circle Walk for people with health conditions that preclude them from exercising vigorously.

In a quiet outdoor setting—a park or yard—find a tree with at least five feet of clear space around the trunk in all directions. If you were to draw a circle around the tree, its diameter would be around 10 to 12 feet, though larger or smaller circles are also fine. Perform the following walking exercise for 15 minutes twice a day.

First, walk clockwise around the tree, and with each completed circle, change the position of your arms by slightly raising or lowering your hands in front or at the sides of your trunk.

Halfway through, reverse the circles, walking counterclockwise around the tree, and again, with each completed circle, change the position of your arms by slightly raising or lowering your hands in front or at the sides of your trunk.

❋ ACUPRESSURE ❋

• Find the acupoint Foot Three Miles (ST-36), four finger-widths below the kneecap on the right leg. Apply moderate pressure with your right thumb until you feel soreness. Hold for 5 minutes. Repeat on the left leg. This is traditionally used to improve digestion and the metabolism of fats.

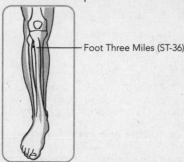

Foot Three Miles (ST-36)

HIVES

URTICARIA, OR HIVES, IS A COMMON SKIN CONDITION in which red, itchy eruptions appear on the skin. They vary from small goose pimples to large raised welts, and they may appear suddenly anywhere on the body. Hives are caused by the release of histamines in the skin tissue in response to foreign irritants either ingested or in physical contact with the skin. Chemicals, pesticides, household cleaning products, soaps, shampoos, perfumes, pet dander, and insect bites are a few of the many irritants that can cause hives. Strong emotions, stress, and some foods can also produce allergic reaction in the skin. Although uncomfortable, hives cause no permanent damage. Common symptoms include severe itching, redness, and swelling, and there may be a severe burning sensation just beneath the skin. Symptoms can last anywhere from twenty-four hours to several weeks or occasionally can become chronic and last for months. However, hives can be a medical emergency when accompanied by any difficulty breathing, or swelling in the throat.

The energetic meridians run through the body just under the surface of the skin. When hives appear, causing itching, in Chinese medicine it is described as wind invading the skin and the meridian channels. Redness and swelling indicate heat and/or toxins combined with the wind pathogen. Proper treatment focuses on resolving the underlying triggers involving dietary or lifestyle alterations to eliminate irritants or eliminating the pathogen that causes the allergic reaction. Every spring I see a number of patients with hives caused by an immune system that is hypersensitive to pollen in the air. These patients often exhibit sinus allergies as well. I use special herbal preparations—both topically and orally—to immediately reduce the itching. Then I use acupuncture, work with the patient to eliminate potential food and environmental allergens, and use stress-release techniques to get rid of the hives.

❊ DIET ❊

• The most common cause of hives is a food or chemical allergen. Pay attention to your diet—keep a food log to determine which foods cause hives, and eliminate them from your diet. Eat a wholesome diet rich in organic animal protein and fresh fruits and vegetables, making sure they are thoroughly washed. Keep your diet on the bland side and avoid spices. Favor leafy greens, broccoli, dandelion greens, mung beans, black beans, pearl barley, adzuki beans, millet, quinoa, beets and beet tops, cabbage, carrots, and yams. Corn silk, water chestnuts, winter melon, and watermelon are also good. Apples, pears, chrysanthemum flowers, papaya, Chinese black dates, plums, black sesame seeds, hawthorn berries, mulberries, and blueberries should be incorporated into your diet as well. Drink at least eight glasses of water a day.

• Eliminate foods that contain potential irritants, including processed foods, artificial flavorings, additives, and preservatives, pesticides and herbicides, all dairy products, refined sugar and flour, and shellfish. Tomatoes, eggplant, bell peppers, mangoes, and strawberries are irritants for many people. Chocolate, alcohol, soft drinks, and spicy and deep-fried foods can cause allergies as well.

❊ HOME REMEDIES ❊

• Take a sea salt bath or rub sea salt on the affected area for temporary relief of itching.

• An oatmeal or bran bath can also provide relief from itching. Boil 1 cup of oatmeal or bran in 4 cups of water for 15 minutes. Pour into bath and soak in it for 20 minutes.

• Make a mint and dandelion tea and apply as a topical wash, repeating until condition improves. Boil 1 cup each of fresh mint and dandelion greens in 10 cups of water for 20 minutes. Strain, and use the liquid as a wash.

• Apply aloe vera gel directly from the plant to the affected area to help with healing and stop itching.

❊ DAILY SUPPLEMENTS ❊

• Acidophilus (3 to 5 billion organisms) and evening primrose oil (450 milligrams GLA) contain beneficial anti-inflammatory properties.

• Taking Vitamin B complex can help prevent production of histamines.

• Taking quercetin (500 milligrams) can help to reduce hive breakouts.

❊ HERBAL THERAPY ❊

• Herbs can be found in health food or vitamin stores, online, and at the offices of Chinese medicine practitioners. Herbs should be used according to individual needs; consult with a licensed practitioner for a customized formulation. To learn more about the herbs listed here, go to www.ask drmao.com.

• Nettle or stinging nettle can be used to relieve allergies.

• Traditional Chinese herbs such as uncaria or cat's claw, burdock, siler, schizonepetae, liquidambar, sophora, and cnidium are used to stop itching and relieve hives.

• A cleansing and detoxification program using diet (including vegetable juice and broth) and herbs can help reduce the allergic load of the body.

✳ EXERCISE ✳

Regular physical exercise is important for maintaining proper circulation to the skin. I also recommend a qi gong exercise called the Dragon Dance, which can help with circulation and promote the opening of skin pores, eliminating toxins and wind in the channels. Do this exercise indoors for 15 minutes, twice daily, and not too vigorously.

This exercise resembles a belly dance—it is a wriggling rhythmic dance of the torso, which burns energy and promotes fat burning in the abdomen.

In a comfortable, quiet place, stand with your feet together and ankles touching, or as close together as you can get them. Place your hands over your head, with palms together and fingers pointing up. You'll be keeping your palms together during the entire exercise.

Inhale, and push your waist out to the right while keeping your head and upper torso straight. Simultaneously move your right elbow to the right so that it rests at shoulder height.

Exhale, and push your waist out to the left while keeping your head and upper torso straight. Simultaneously move your left elbow to the left so that it rests at shoulder height.

Repeat this movement several times. Every time you move your waist to the right, bend your knees a little more, lowering your entire body as you squat, keeping your upper torso and head straight. And as you lower your body, move your hands lower, keeping your palms together and fingers pointing up. When your arms reach your chest, turn your fingers toward the ground and continue the movement.

When your arms reach your knees, you should be squatting. Continue the movements, now rising with each right movement until you reach a standing position. When your arms reach your chest, switch the direction of your fingers so that they're pointing up again.

Throughout this exercise your hands should make an S-shaped move-

HIVES

ment and your body should do a rhythmic belly dance. Remember to in-hale on the rightward movement and exhale to the left.

Do this exercise during the day on an empty stomach. Begin slowly, then start to increase speed and vigor, warming up the whole body but not to the point of perspiration.

─────────────── ❊ ACUPRESSURE ❊ ───────────────

• Find the acupoint Sea of Blood (SP-10), two thumb-widths above the top inner corner of the right kneecap when the knee is slightly bent. Apply steady pressure with your right thumb until you feel soreness. Hold for 2 minutes. Repeat on your left knee. This point is used to treat itching caused by hives.

• Locate the acupoint Winding Gulch (LI-11), in the depression at the outer part of the left elbow crease, between the elbow tendon and the bone. The point is best located when the arm is bent at 90 degrees with the palm fac-ing the abdomen. Apply steady pressure with your right thumb until you feel soreness. Hold for 3 minutes. Repeat on the right arm. This helps clear heat and reduce inflammation, as well as detoxify the body.

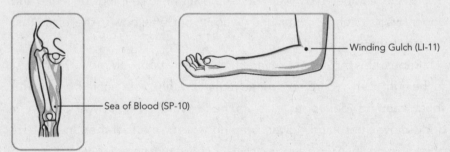

Winding Gulch (LI-11)

Sea of Blood (SP-10)

──────────────────── AVOID ────────────────────

• Stress and emotional upsets, as they can trigger hive outbreaks.

• The antidiabetic sulfonylurea glimepiride (Amaryl), as it can induce an al-lergic reaction, manifesting as hives. Consult your physician for alternatives.

- Certain medications, such as aspirin and penicillin, as well as certain perfumes, cosmetics, soaps, and detergents, as they may also trigger hives. Consult your physician.

INCONTINENCE

AFFECTING MORE THAN 13 MILLION AMERICANS—mostly the elderly and women—incontinence is simply the inability to control urination. Incontinence may be induced by stress (coughing, laughing, sneezing), overflow (constant leaking of urine), or the inability to hold urine, with the sudden urge to urinate. The underlying causes of incontinence include hormonal deficiencies in women, chronic urinary tract infections, an enlarged prostate or weakened or damaged nerves from prostate surgery in men, and even some medications. Exercise, lifestyle modifications, biofeedback, and self-training are often prescribed, in combination with medications and external devices such as absorbent underwear, catheters, or urethral plugs.

In Chinese medicine, incontinence is often attributed to weakness of kidney energy. The vital energy in the kidney-bladder network is depleted because of aging, and this depletion is hastened in individuals with chronic degenerative diseases, excessive strain, excessive sexual activity, and sometimes in women from pregnancy.

A male patient of mine suffered from incontinence after the removal of his prostate to treat prostate cancer. He began aggressive acupuncture treatment two to three times a week within two weeks after his surgery. He went from wearing a diaper for the first three weeks to a pad for the next three weeks. About eight weeks after we began treatment, he was able to go all day without any incontinence. As an extra bonus his erectile function returned to about 80 percent after three months of acupuncture and herbal therapy.

INCONTINENCE

✳ DIET ✳

• Diet should include foods that strengthen the kidney-bladder network. Favor warming energy foods, including organic chicken and lamb, scallions, sesame seeds, saltwater fish, baked tofu, soybeans, walnuts, lentils, black beans, kidney beans, lotus seeds (cook like beans), ginger, cinnamon, and chives. Hawthorn berries (make tea), cranberries, raspberries, and blueberries contain bioflavonoids that are beneficial to the bladder.

• Avoid all sugars, soft drinks, and sweetened juices. Cold and raw foods should also be avoided. Eliminate caffeine, alcohol, and artificial sweeteners.

✳ HOME REMEDIES ✳

• Cook up a lamb stew to help strengthen the kidneys and restore fire energy in the belly. Place 2 pounds organic lamb chops into a pot with 6 cups of water, making sure you cut the bone so the marrow is exposed. Add 1/3 cup each of presoaked black beans, adzuki beans, and navy beans, along with 1/2 cup each of chopped yams or sweet potatoes, turnips, and onions. Bring to a boil and simmer, covered, for 2 hours, adding water as needed so it doesn't dry out. Season with salt and pepper to taste.

• Eat 1 cup of fresh, dried, or frozen and thawed raspberries every day for 2 to 3 weeks to strengthen the kidney-bladder network function.

• Drink 3 cups of cinnamon and ginger tea daily. Steep 1 teaspoon of each in 3 cups of boiling water for 5 minutes.

✳ DAILY SUPPLEMENTS ✳

• Taking vitamin C (1,000 milligrams) and cranberry extract (400 milligrams) helps reduce the chances of bacterial infections in the urinary tract, a known cause of incontinence.

• Taking beta-carotene (800 milligrams) supplements can help improves immune function and promote mucus membrane health. Zinc (50 milligrams) also supports immune function.

• Calcium (1,000 milligram) and magnesium (500 milligrams) taken together can work to improve muscle function.

❈ HERBAL THERAPY ❈

• Herbs can be found in health food or vitamin stores, online, and at the offices of Chinese medicine practitioners. Herbs should be used according to individual needs; consult with a licensed practitioner for a customized formulation. To learn more about the herbs listed here, go to www.ask drmao.com.

• Horsetail, plantain, and marshmallow are good herbal remedies for incontinence.

• Black raspberry and bearberry are natural astringents, good for bladder health.

• Traditional Chinese herbs used for incontinence include morinda, cibotium, psoralea, Chinese dodder seeds, astragalus, schizandra, Asian cornelian cherries, and Cherokee rosehip.

❈ EXERCISE ❈

Tai chi or qi gong exercises are great additions to any exercise regimen. Practicing qi gong can enhance kidney function and strengthen the bladder and rectal sphincter muscles. I often recommend a movement section from the Eight Treasures Qi Gong practice called The White Crane Guards the Plum Flower, specifically targeting the kidney energies to help deal with incontinence.

In a quiet, comfortable environment, preferably outdoors, stand with your feet shoulder-width apart, knees slightly bent, spine erect, tailbone tucked in, and head tilted slightly forward. Drape your arms at your sides and relax your shoulders.

Being breathing with a rhythmic, slow, and relaxed breath, inhaling deeply and softly, imagining the breath extending all the way down to your

INCONTINENCE

lower abdomen and into your rectal area. As you inhale, tighten your sphincter muscles in your rectum and bladder.

Exhale gently and softly, and relax your sphincter muscles. Stay in this position for 7 breath cycles. Relax and calm your mind.

Now begin the exercise: On an inhale, bend and raise your right knee to your chest. Grab your knee with your right hand and your ankle with your left hand. Pull your knee as close to your chest as you can. You should now be standing on your left leg. Tighten your sphincter muscles in your rectum and bladder.

On an exhale, relax and let your knee drop slightly away from the chest. Keep holding your knee and ankle with both hands. Relax your sphincter muscles. Repeat 10 times, then switch sides and do the exercise with your left leg 10 times.

Return to a standing position and do a quiet meditation for 1 minute, regulating your breath.

❋ ACUPRESSURE ❋

• Find the acupoint Gate of Origin (REN-4), four finger-widths below the navel on the lower abdomen. Apply steady pressure with your index finger until you feel soreness. Hold for 3 minutes.

• Find the acupoint Forceful Torrent (KID-3), in the depression between the inner anklebone and the Achilles tendon of the right foot. Apply steady

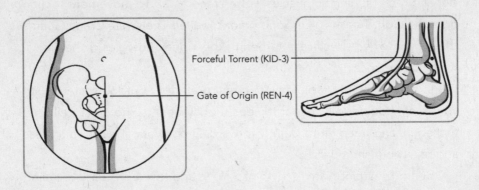

Forceful Torrent (KID-3)

Gate of Origin (REN-4)

pressure with your right thumb until you feel soreness. Hold for 2 minutes. Repeat on the left foot.

• These points benefit the urinary system and strengthen the kidneys.

—————————————— AVOID ——————————————

• Alcohol, coffee, and smoking, as they irritate the bladder and the urethra.

• Cold temperatures, overstrain, and excessive sexual activity weaken the kidney-bladder network and thus worsen incontinence.

INDIGESTION AND HEARTBURN

"OH, I ATE TOO MUCH!" Most of us have regretfully uttered these words more often than we'd like. The resulting indigestion or heartburn is often experienced as pain, a burning sensation in the stomach or chest, abdominal bloating, gurgling, distention, and belching. Indigestion is caused and made worse by overeating, especially fatty, rich, or spicy foods, alcohol, coffee, and acidic foods such as tomatoes and citrus fruits. Eating while stressed, on the run, or late at night also can cause indigestion. Heartburn can accompany indigestion, as the excessive food and liquid in the stomach churns up stomach acid, which spills up into the esophagus and irritates the lining. Over time chronic heartburn can develop into gastritis or esophagitis, much more serious conditions in which the lining of the stomach or esophagus erodes and ulcerates. The regurgitation of acids is also called gastroesophageal reflux disease, commonly referred to as GERD. Chronic acid reflux can lead to cancer of the esophagus.

Chinese medicine sees three main causes of indigestion. First, poor diet damages the spleen-pancreas-stomach network. Second, emotional

INDIGESTION AND HEARTBURN

turmoil stresses the liver-gallbladder network, slows down the digestive process, and potentially causes hiatal hernia by pulling the stomach upward into the diaphragm. Third, pathogens in a postnasal mucus drip or food-borne microbes can invade the stomach, causing upheaval. My approach to patients with GERD is diet change—from rich and spicy foods to simple, bland, alkaline, easy-to-digest foods—and stress release with meditation, exercise, and massage. If I suspect pathogens as the cause of the GERD, I'll address the sinuses and mucus drip, and I'll work to clear out the pathogens. Acupuncture can provide quick symptom relief and restore the natural flow of the intestinal tract, while herbal remedies support a healthy esophageal and stomach lining and normal gastric juice production.

 ❋ DIET ❋

• Eat slowly and in small amounts more frequently—you should leave the table only three-quarters full. Chew each bite thoroughly—remember that digestion begins in the mouth and that your stomach doesn't have teeth. Eat plenty of fresh fruits, vegetables, and whole grains. Favor enzyme-rich foods, including papayas, mangoes, sweet potatoes, yams, figs, brown rice, oats, pearl barley, daikon radish, apples, parsley, coriander, mint, dill, rosemary, ginger, bay leaf, fennel, dill, oregano, cilantro, sage, and anise.

• Avoid acidic foods, such as tomatoes, coffee, tea, wine, citrus fruits, vinegar, pineapple, rich sauces, cream, greasy and fried foods, processed foods, refined sugars and flour, and alcohol. Intake of dairy products and wheat should be reduced.

• Eat with mindfulness—savor and be grateful with each bite and do not eat while stressed, angry, or preoccupied. Don't watch television or read the newspaper while you eat, as the distraction takes energy away from the digestive system and makes its job that much harder.

❋ HOME REMEDIES ❋

• Juice 1 large or 2 small white russet potatoes. Discard the pulp, mix the juice with an equal amount of hot water, and drink on an empty stomach first thing in the morning.

....

• Juice 1 medium daikon radish. Discard the pulp, mix the juice with an equal amount of hot water, and drink once a day after eating.

....

• For heartburn, dissolve 1 teaspoon baking soda in an 8-ounce cup of warm water and sip for immediate relief.

....

• Make a tea by boiling 1 tablespoon licorice root in 3 1/2 cups of water for 15 minutes. Strain, and drink 1 cup after each meal 3 times a day for 2 weeks. Licorice is neutralizing and helps with digestion.

❋ DAILY SUPPLEMENTS ❋

• When your body is deficient in digestive enzymes, it compensates by increasing acid production. Supplemention with the enzymes bromelain (450 milligrams), amylase (1,500 units), and lipase (1,000 units) can help with the digestion of protein, starch, and fat and can also relieve symptoms of stomach upset or heartburn.

....

• Vitamin A (200 IU) is important for maintaining the health of the mucous membranes, which line the esophagus and the stomach.

....

• Taking lecithin supplements (500 milligrams) three times a day can help ease heartburn and indigestion, especially for people who have a low tolerance for oily and fatty foods.

❋ HERBAL THERAPY ❋

• Herbs can be found in health food or vitamin stores, online, and at the offices of Chinese medicine practitioners. Herbs should be used according

to individual needs; consult with a licensed practitioner for a customized formulation. To learn more about the herbs listed here, go to www.ask drmao.com.

• Dandelion root and gentian root can help aid digestion by supporting the liver and gallbladder.

• Chamomile and slippery elm help to settle the stomach and protect the mucous membrane from assaults.

• Traditional Chinese herbal therapy for indigestion includes rhubarb root, bitter orange, coptidis, skullcap, poria, alisma, licorice, and atractylodis.

✳ EXERCISE ✳

Walking is the best exercise for helping food move along the digestive tract, and for improving digestion and absorption. The energetic meridians of the digestive organs run along the large muscles of the legs, so walking stimulates energy flow within the channels and promotes digestion. Take an easy 10-minute walk after each meal and massage your abdomen with your palms in a circle around your navel as you walk. This helps move food through your digestive tract, avoiding prolonged accumulation.

✳ ACUPRESSURE ✳

• Find the acupoint Middle Core (REN-12), about midway between your navel and the lower tip of your sternum. It is used in acupuncture for balancing digestive function. With your index and middle fingers, apply mild pressure for 5 minutes. Then with the palm of your hand make small concentric circles rubbing the point in clockwise direction for 5 minutes.

• Find the acupoint Inner Gate (P-6), three finger-widths above the wrist crease, between the two tendons on the inside of the left forearm. It is used to settle the stomach and reduce acid. Apply moderate pressure with your right thumb. Hold for 5 minutes. Repeat on the right arm.

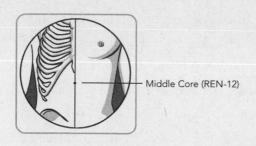
Middle Core (REN-12)

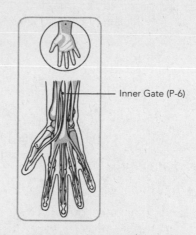
Inner Gate (P-6)

AVOID

• Lying down immediately after eating. Lying down enables the acid to reflux from the stomach into the esophagus. During a flare-up, avoid lying flat on your back when you sleep—instead prop up your head and upper body with pillows at a 45-degree angle.

• Certain drugs, including antidepressants and sedatives, as they can worsen heartburn. Talk to your doctor about alternatives.

• Smoking, as nicotine is a muscle relaxant and can relax the esophageal opening in the stomach, making it easier for acid to spill into it.

❧ INSECT AND OTHER BITES ❧

THERE IS SIMPLY NO WAY AROUND IT—humans eat to survive and bugs bite to survive. It's humans versus bugs and, unfortunately, we lose most of the time. A bug bite is at minimum an annoyance, at worst life threatening. Fleas, mosquitoes, gnats, fire ants, wasps, bees, ticks, mites, and spiders all bite. The moment of the bite itself is rarely painful, but the body's reaction can cause symptoms of pain, itching, redness, swelling, and in some cases a serious allergic reaction called

INSECT AND OTHER BITES

anaphylactic shock—which can cause breathing difficulties and requires immediate medical attention. Some insects carry diseases such as malaria or dengue fever (mosquitoes) and Lyme disease (ticks). If you think you have any of these diseases, consult an infectious disease specialist immediately. Scorpion, centipede, and poisonous snake bites can be deadly and should be dealt with immediately by going to the emergency room. The most common bites are from mosquitoes, causing itching, and bees, causing pain. Prevention is the easiest way to avoid insect and other bites, but once you are bitten, if there is no serious allergic reaction, the approach is to relieve the symptoms with topical remedies.

In Chinese medicine, most bites are seen as a fire toxin. In severe cases the fire toxin produces pain, burning, and redness in the skin. There is a wealth of topical and oral herbal Chinese remedies to relieve the itching, burning, and pain caused by such bites.

Here are some of my favorite remedies.

❋ DIET ❋

• A cleansing diet works to detoxify the body from toxins and reduce allergic symptoms from bites. Drink plenty of water to help flush out the toxins, and eat fluid-rich foods such as clear soups, vegetable broths and juices, melons, other fruits, and juicy vegetables including cucumber, jicama, and beets. To prevent bug bites, include more garlic, onions, and spice in your diet.

• Avoid overeating and heavy fats, red meat, and shellfish. Sweets and sugars can further aggravate the immune response, potentially worsening the condition and prolonging the suffering.

❋ HOME REMEDIES ❋

• Remove stinger, if any, and clean the area with water. Place an ice pack on the affected area for temporary relief of itching and swelling.

• Cut 2-inch-round slices from a fresh eggplant and place on top of the bite for 5 to 10 minutes to draw out the toxins and soothe the irritation. You can also use cucumber skin in the same way.

• Mash 1 cup fresh dandelion greens into a poultice or puree in a blender with 1/2 cup aloe vera gel, and apply to the bite to help soothe skin irritation. Dandelion greens can also be made into a tea by boiling 1 cup fresh dandelion greens for 20 minutes in 3 1/2 cups water, then straining and drinking the liquid. Drink 3 cups a day.

• Apply honey to bug bites to soothe them and prevent infection.

• For prevention, try not to provoke insects—remember that this is their world, too, and they will defend their territory. Live and let live.

• Do not wear a lot of perfume or brightly colored or floral-patterned clothing outdoors, as bugs and bees might mistake you for a flower. ·

• Use natural and organic insect repellent, such as those including lemongrass, citronella, and lavender. Wear protective clothing and be cautious when eating outdoors, especially when drinking sweet beverages.

———————————— ❊ DAILY SUPPLEMENTS ❊ ————————————

• Vitamin C (1,000 milligrams) is helpful as an antioxidant and toxin neutralizer.

• Vitamin B_5 (300 milligrams, 3 times a day) is also helpful as a detoxifier.

• Bromelain (1 gram of powder mixed with a little water into a paste), applied topically, can help with the redness, irritation and inflammation.

• Taking quercetin (500 milligrams) or other bioflavonoids (1,000 milligrams) is useful to protect against allergic reactions on the skin.

❋ HERBAL THERAPY ❋

• Herbs can be found in health food or vitamin stores, online, and at the offices of Chinese medicine practitioners. Herbs should be used according to individual needs; consult with a licensed practitioner for a customized formulation. To learn more about the herbs listed here, go to www.askdrmao.com.

• Lemon balm, stinging nettle, turmeric, and licorice root are effective in treating insect bites.

• Oil of turmeric and eucalyptus, lavender, and lemongrass oils are natural insect repellents.

• Apply tea tree oil to bites every 2 to 3 hours to relieve itching and speed up healing.

• Traditional Chinese herbs used to relieve bites and stings include typhonium, oldenlandia, lithospermi, lobelia, smilacis, and bletilla rhizome.

❋ EXERCISE ❋

A meditation called the General Cleansing Qi Gong can help with circulation and promote opening of the pores. Do this indoors and not too vigorously.

Sit comfortably or lie down on your back. Slow your respiration to deep, abdominal breathing. Say the word "calm" in your mind with every exhalation. You'll be visualizing the relaxation of a body part and releasing tension with every exhalation. Trace the following 3 pathways outlined below.

Start at the top of your head. Inhale, and then exhale and visualize your scalp muscles relaxing. Say "calm" in your mind. Repeat this, saying the word with each body part as you move down through your face, throat, chest, abdomen, thighs, knees, calves, ankles, and feet. When you've relaxed your feet, visualize all the tension in your body leaving through your toes in the form of dark smoke.

Next, start at the temple region of your head. This path focuses on the sides and upper extremities. Inhale, and then exhale while visualizing your temple muscles relaxing. Say "calm" in your mind. Repeat this, saying the word with each body part as you move down through your jaw, the sides of your neck, shoulders, upper arms, elbows, forearms, wrists, and hands. Once you've relaxed your hands, visualize all the tension leaving your body through your fingertips in the form of dark smoke.

The final pathway begins at the back of your head. This pathway relaxes the back of your body. Repeat the breathing-visualization-word routine, as above, as you go from the back of your neck to your upper back, middle back, lower back, back of thighs, calves, and heels. Then focus on the acupoint Bubbling Spring (KID-1), on the soles of your feet, for 1 minute.

Practice this meditation for at least 15 minutes, twice daily.

※ ACUPRESSURE ※

• Find the acupoint Valley of Harmony (LI-4), at the web between your right thumb and index finger. It is used here to reduce itching and inflammation, as well as to detoxify the body. Apply steady pressure with your left thumb until you feel soreness. Hold for 2 minutes. Repeat on the left hand.

• Locate the acupoint Wind Pond (GB-20), in the natural indentation at the base of your skull on either side of your neck. It activates immune functions and expels toxins. Press and lift up toward the base of your skull with your thumbs and lean your head back. Use the weight of your head against

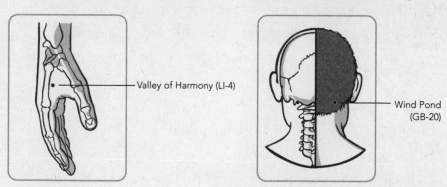

Valley of Harmony (LI-4)

Wind Pond (GB-20)

your thumbs for steady pressure on the acupoint. Hold for 5 minutes, breathing deeply and slowly.

AVOID

• Scratching the skin, as scratching can cause secondary infections, thereby worsening the condition.

••

• Alcohol, chocolate, caffeine, nicotine and sugar; they are irritants and can aggravate the condition.

 INSOMNIA

WE'VE ALL SUFFERED FROM OCCASIONAL SLEEPLESSNESS. When the turning and tossing in bed become more frequent, and begin to affect energy and mental clarity during the day, sleeplessness is called insomnia. Insomnia includes difficulty falling asleep or staying asleep, early-morning awakening, and unrefreshing sleep. These kinds of poor sleep patterns affect almost two out of three Americans—that's a lot of people lying awake at night! People who suffer from insomnia tend to complain of memory problems, lack of concentration, depression, and the inability to be effective at work.

As it becomes a chronic condition, insomnia can increase the risk of developing cardiovascular disease, gastroesophageal reflux disease (GERD), chronic pain, stress and anxiety, depression, and alcohol and drug abuse. Likewise, these same conditions can be the causes of lying awake at night. Other contributing factors include pregnancy, menopause, and sleep apnea—a condition in which one stops breathing and awakens gasping for air throughout the night. Insomnia can also be one of many symptoms of a neurological disease that requires medical attention.

In Chinese medicine, nighttime is yin time—or, simply, when the body takes care of itself instead of your desires. Proper sleep is required for your body to repair itself and regenerate. To reach deep, restful sleep, your spirit and heart must be calm and your liver and spleen networks must work together to process nutrients.

Excessive worry, anxiety, and depression all affect the delicate balance of the liver, spleen, and heart, causing disturbances to the spirit and activating the mind. Once the mind is active, it becomes harder to fall asleep. No wonder infomercials do so well in the middle of the night!

Insomnia is one of the most common conditions I see. Typical of my patients with insomnia was a woman in her late forties who was perimenopausal and complaining of hot flashes, night sweats, and difficulty falling and staying asleep. She also felt depressed and anxious. After treating her with acupuncture and herbal therapies for four months, her hot flashes and night sweats disappeared. Her sleep improved dramatically, although occasionally she still had a hard time falling asleep, so I taught her a stress-release meditation to do before bedtime to help calm her anxiety. She is now sleeping like a baby.

Here's some advice that may help you sleep like a baby, or a log—whichever your prefer.

❋ DIET ❋

• Choose wholesome foods with no preservatives, additives, or artificial flavors or colors. Food coloring can cause hyperactivity in children. Do not eat anything for at least three hours before bedtime. Include ample leafy green vegetables, whole grains, and low-acidic food in your diet. Eat plenty of asparagus, avocados, apricots, bananas, broccoli, brown rice, figs, salmon, soy products, mulberries, basil, dill, and all types of squash. Since carbohydrates tend to make us sleepy, eating a grain-based meal for dinner can be helpful. A cup of warm milk rich in the amino acid tryptophan before bed can also be helpful.

INSOMNIA

• Avoid coffee, soft drinks, tea, chocolate, candy, or dessert, drinks with artificial sweeteners, foods with preservatives and MSG, spicy foods, and hard-to-digest foods.

❋ HOME REMEDIES ❋

• Eat 1 cup of plain yogurt an hour before bedtime. It contains a rich supply of tryptopham an amino acid essential in the production of helpful neurochemicals to aid sleep.

• Soak your feet in a hot Epsom salt bath for 15 minutes before bedtime to produce a relaxation response.

• Keep a journal at night to empty thoughts from your mind before bedtime and take the burdens off of your mind for a more peaceful sleep.

• Meditate for 15 minutes before bedtime to settle your mind.

❋ DAILY SUPPLEMENTS ❋

• Calcium (1,000 milligrams), magnesium (500 milligrams), phosphorus (800 milligrams), potassium (25 milligrams), and vitamin B complex and E (800 IU) supplementation can help improve sleep.

• The amino acid compounds 5HTP (200 milligrams) and inositol (1,000 milligrams) act as precursors to neurotransmitters for sleep.

• Supplementing with melatonin (1 gram) can help counter insomnia.

❋ HERBAL THERAPY ❋

• Herbs can be found in health food or vitamin stores, online, and at the offices of Chinese medicine practitioners. Herbs should be used according to individual needs; consult with a licensed practitioner for a customized formulation. To learn more about the herbs listed here, go to www.ask drmao.com.

• Drink valerian or passionflower tea before bedtime every night for 1 month, or until sleep improves.

• Traditional Chinese herbs used for peaceful sleep and relaxation include oyster shell, chamomile flower, ziziphus, Chinese senega, curcuma, lily bulb, bamboo shavings, China root, and licorice.

❊ EXERCISE ❊

People with regular exercise routines have fewer episodes of insomnia, and those who suffer from insomnia often are not very physically active. Exercise promotes sleep and improves sleep quality by altering brain chemistry. Exercising moderately for 20 to 30 minutes 3 times a week, combined with meditation or tai chi in the evening, will not only help you fall and stay asleep but will also increase the amount of time you spend in REM sleep. For some people exercise alone is sufficient for overcoming sleep problems. Exercise in the morning or afternoon but not close to bedtime. Below is a stress-release meditation that I teach my patients. (Many people report falling asleep to this meditation as I narrate it on a CD. I try to take that as a compliment.)

Sit comfortably or lie down on your back. Slow your respiration to deep, abdominal breathing. Say the word "calm" in your mind with every exhalation. You'll be visualizing the relaxation of a body part and releasing tension with every exhalation. Trace the following 3 pathways outlined below. First, start at the top of your head. Inhale, and then exhale and visualize your scalp muscles relaxing. Say "calm" in your mind. Repeat this, saying the word with each body part as you move down through your face, throat, chest, abdomen, thighs, knees, calves, ankles, and feet. When you've relaxed your feet, visualize all the tension in your body leaving through your toes in the form of dark smoke.

Next, start at the temple region of your head. This pathway focuses on the sides and upper extremities. Inhale, then exhale and visualize your temple muscles relaxing. Say the word "calm" in your mind. Repeat this, saying the word with each body part as you move down through your jaw, the sides of your neck, shoulders, upper arms, elbows, forearms, wrists, and hands. Once you've relaxed your hands, visualize all the tension leaving your body through your fingertips in the form of dark smoke.

The final pathway begins at the back of your head. This path relaxes the back of your body. Repeat the breathing-visualization-word routine, as above, as you go from the back of your neck to your upper back, middle back, lower back, back of thighs, calves, and heels. Then focus on the acupoint Bubbling Spring (KID-1), on the soles of your feet, for 1 minute.

Practice this meditation for at least 15 minutes twice daily, and once before bedtime.

------------------- ❋ ACUPRESSURE ❋ -------------------

• Find the acupoint Inner Gate (P-6), three finger-widths above the wrist crease, between the two tendons on inside of the left forearm. Apply moderate pressure with your right thumb. Hold for 5 minutes. Repeat on the right arm. This may help calm the spirit, and therefore improve sleep.

....

• Locate the acupoint Gate of Spirit (H-7), on the palm side of your left hand at the end of the wrist crease below the little finger. Apply moderate pressure with your right thumb. Hold for 5 minutes. Repeat on left hand. This strengthens the heart–small intestine network and calms the spirit, thus aiding sleep.

....

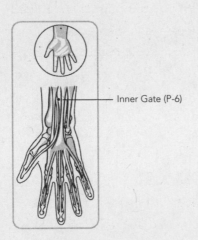

Inner Gate (P-6)

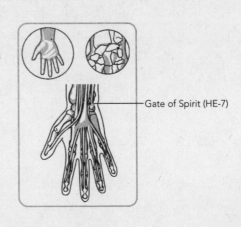

Gate of Spirit (HE-7)

• It is especially beneficial to do accupressure on these acupoints an hour before bedtime.

❧ IRRITABLE BOWEL SYNDROME ❧

DO YOU EXPERIENCE ON-AND-OFF CONSTIPATION and diarrhea, abdominal bloating and pain, and excessive gas as a reaction to stress? And perhaps heartburn, fatigue, headache, faintness, back pain, palpitations, and general weakness? If you find yourself nodding your head, join the estimated 20 million Americans who suffer from irritable bowel syndrome, or IBS. This is a functional or movement disorder of the bowel rather than a structural problem. It's most often present in people with a history of stress, anxiety, drug abuse, or emotional problems. It is more common in women than men. Symptoms can show up unexpectedly, and though it is not considered life threatening, it can become debilitating and can affect quality of life to a great degree.

Chinese medicine classifies IBS as stagnant liver energy overacting on the digestive system or the spleen-pancreas-stomach network. Stress and emotional disturbances can greatly contribute to stagnant liver en-

IRRITABLE BOWEL SYNDROME

ergy. Couple that with poor dietary habits, and you've got a digestive system prone to functional breakdowns. To my patients with digestive disorders I often ask, "What's eating you up inside?" I might also ask, "What feelings are you swallowing and not expressing, causing gut-wrenching sensations?" The answers usually validate the Chinese medical view that emotional suppression is one of the main causes of IBS.

One of my patients, a thirty-five-year-old woman, is a perfect example of the many IBS patients I've seen. She suffered from chronic abdominal bloating, gas, and irregular bowel movements that alternated from tight to loose. She was always tired and had difficulty concentrating. Her menstrual period was slightly irregular and she also suffered from PMS—premenstrual syndrome—with mood swings that caused anxiety and depression. I determined that the causes of her IBS were a poor diet and inability to cope with emotional stress. I put her on a strict diet rich in fiber, and eliminated sugar, coffee, alcohol, and raw vegetables. I treated her with acupuncture and herbal therapy to balance her digestive tract and modulate her nervous system. I also referred her to a hypnotherapist to work on her stress-coping skills. After about three months of treatment, she was virtually symptom free, and has continued to be symptom free for the past three years.

Here is some advice that I give to patients with IBS. Consult your physician if you experience constant abdominal pain and diarrhea with blood in your stool.

———————————— ✳ DIET ✳ ————————————

• Eating a high-fiber diet keeps the bowels moving properly and balances the intestines. Favor well-cooked and tender vegetables such as potatoes, yams, beets, carrots, celery, cucumbers, lettuce, mushrooms, green peppers, squash, zucchini, spinach, Swiss chard, green peas, and other dark green leafy vegetables, nuts and seeds, including almonds, ground flaxseed and soy nuts. Drink plenty of room-temperature water and freshly squeezed fruit and vegetable juices. Be sure to eat more often and in small quantities, and keep a food diary to determine which foods might trigger the symptoms. And pay attention to food labels, as many foods contain hidden chemicals and artificial sweeteners, which can irritate the intestinal lining and aggravate IBS.

• Wheat, corn, dairy, and carrageenan-containing products are among the most common symptom-provoking foods, as are peanuts, red meat, sugar and other sweets, refined and processed foods, corn, soybeans, most legumes, coffee, caffeine, oranges, alcohol, hot sauce, spicy foods, fried foods, fatty foods, rich foods, and salty foods.

• Eat your food slowly, chewing and salivating well. Eat in a relaxed atmosphere. Do not read or watch television while eating, and do not eat when stressed, angry, or depressed.

❋ HOME REMEDIES ❋

• Eat a cup of high-fiber cereal for breakfast every morning, including: oat bran, brown rice, psyllium husks, flaxseed meal, or hemp seeds. Substitute almond milk or rice milk for cow's milk.

• Eat a sweet potato or yam every day—the fiber and carotenoids are helpful for maintaining regular bowel movements

• Make a fiber-rich soup that includes a cup each of diced potato, carrot, squash, pumpkin, parsnip, daikon radish, okra, and beet. Put the vegetables into a pot and cover with water. Boil for 30 to 40 minutes. Blend the soup, and eat a bowl every day for a month, or until symptoms subside.

❋ DAILY SUPPLEMENTS ❋

• Taking acacia fiber (2 to 4 grams) or psyllium (2 to 4 grams) can provide relief for IBS.

IRRITABLE BOWEL SYNDROME

• Probiotic supplements containing lactobacillus acidophilus (3 to 5 billion organisms) and lactobacillus bifidus (bifidobacteria) can dramatically increase the natural gut bacteria, reducing inflammation and helping the healing process.

• Peppermint oil (0.2 milliliter entere-coated capsules) can help with digestion and relieve symptoms of IBS.

• Taking 2 tablespoons of an oil rich in essential fatty acids, such as fish oil, flax oil, evening primrose oil, black currant oil, or walnut oil can help to reduce inflammation.

• Pectin (1 to 2 grams), found in apples, is an excellent bulking agent, and can improve bowel function.

❋ HERBAL THERAPY ❋

• Herbs can be found in health food or vitamin stores, online, and at the offices of Chinese medicine practitioners. Herbs should be used according to individual needs; consult with a licensed practitioner for a customized formulation. To learn more about the herbs listed here, go to www.askdr mao.com.

• Make a tea by boiling 1 tablespoon each of dried chamomile, valerian, ginger, and peppermint in 4 cups of water for 20 minutes. Strain, and drink a cup after each meal every day.

• Goldenseal can be used to support healthy bowel function.

• Traditional Chinese herbs used to treat IBS symptoms include magnolia bark, tangerine, ginger, siler, white peony, poria, polyporus, cinnamon, atractylodis, jujube, and licorice.

✴ EXERCISE ✴

Daily exercise is one of the most effective treatments for staying fit and strengthening your muscles. Start your morning or end your day with a brisk 30-minute walk. Stress-reduction meditations and qi gong exercises are also helpful. Following is a Dao In Qi Gong self-massage to help reduce abdominal pain and bowel irregularities. Perform the massage for 10 to 15 minutes twice daily, or anytime for immediate symptom relief.

Lie in bed on your back with a pillow under your knees, making sure you're comfortable. If you'd like, apply a small amount of peppermint oil to your hands to help stimulate energy and blood flow in the abdomen. Lie on your back and bend your knees slightly to a comfortable position.

Begin a circular massage of the abdomen with both palms moving together: Starting from the lower right side and with moderate pressure, rub your abdomen in small clockwise circles with your palms. Keep making small circles as you slowly traverse the abdomen around the navel.

When you reach the lower left abdomen lift your arms and begin again from the lower right abdomen. Repeat for the remaining time.

✴ ACUPRESSURE ✴

• Find the acupoint Foot Three Miles (ST-36), four finger-widths below the kneecap on the right leg. Apply moderate pressure with your right thumb until you feel soreness. Hold for 5 minutes. Repeat on the left leg. This point is often tender in people suffering from IBS.

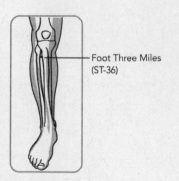

Foot Three Miles (ST-36)

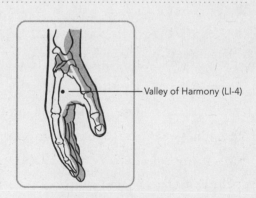

Valley of Harmony (LI-4)

IRRITABLE BOWEL SYNDROME

• Find the acupoint Valley of Harmony (LI-4), at the web between your right thumb and index finger. Apply steady pressure with your left thumb until you feel soreness. Hold for 2 minutes. Repeat on the left hand.

AVOID

• Caffeine, alcohol, and sorbitol (an artificial sweetener), as they can irritate the intestines.

....

• Some anti-inflammatory drugs containing ibuprofen (such as Advil), aspirin, and some prescription drugs (including Naprosyn, Voltaren, and Feldene), which can erode the lining of the small intestine and colon. Consult your physician for alternatives.

....

• Dairy products containing lactose, which is hard to digest and irritates the bowel lining.

JET LAG

THE HUMAN BODY LONG AGO DEVELOPED an internal clock that harmonizes biological functions, such as sleeping and waking up, with regular environmental changes, such as the sun rising and setting. The daily, cyclical changes that occur in us follow the energy rotation of the universe. The cycles known as the circadian rhythm—which regulate your body's natural cycles, such as appetite, sleep, and mood—are controlled mainly by light. If you travel over large distances to the east or west, you'll cross through different time zones, but your internal clock will want to continue on its usual schedule. This conflict creates the condition we call jet lag. Symptoms can include fatigue, lightheadedness, sleep disruption, cognitive problems (such as loss of short-term memory), inability to concentrate, and digestive irregularities, including diarrhea and constipation. Although not referred to as jet lag, these symptoms are also common in people who work night shifts.

Since ancient times, Chinese medicine has recognized the existence of a bioenergetic clock. Within this clock, energy is the fullest in certain organ networks at certain times of the day. (See Chapter 6 for more details.) For example, the spleen-pancreas-stomach network is at its peak energy from 7:00 to 9:00 A.M. Eating breakfast is critical because the body digests and absorbs nutrients best in the morning. Chinese medicine practitioners have long believed that respect for nature's cycles brings health, and violation of its rhythms leads to disease. Biochemical changes occur when humans transgress the natural behavior patterns associated with the division of night and day. When the body's rhythm is off kilter, energy flow becomes disorderly, and body functions fall out of balance. The key to reducing the symptoms of jet lag is to restore energy flow and to quickly return balance to the body's circadian rhythm.

I've helped many patients prevent and recover from jet lag through acupuncture, herbal therapy, exercise, meditation techniques, and light exposure. Often acupuncture will immediately induce the brain to release endorphins, resetting the autonomic nervous system, which regulates many of the rhythmic functions of the body. Herbs, timing and selection of food, and exercise are critical in supporting internal consistency. I also ask my patients who travel across time zones to get as much natural light as possible by not wearing sunglasses and by working or sitting near windows. Many of them are now happy travelers because they suffer from little or no jet lag.

❋ DIET ❋

• I encourage eating foods rich in B vitamins, which help the functioning of the neurological system. These include parsley, broccoli, beets, turnips, mustard greens, brewer's yeast, bananas, endive, spinach, collard greens, Swiss chard, bell peppers, lentils, fish, strawberries, peppermint, eggs, asparagus, royal jelly, and mung beans. Foods rich in tryptophan, including nuts, beans, and fish, are also useful. Drink plenty of water, as dehydration is one of the most common results of prolonged travel. Drink at least 80 ounces of room-temperature water a day.

• Avoid dairy products; cold, raw foods; greasy, fatty foods; and spicy foods.

• Avoid alcohol and caffeine, as they can dehydrate you and worsen the condition, and deplete the body's yin.

❊ HOME REMEDIES ❊

• Take an Epsom salt bath for 15 to 20 minutes before bedtime.

• Add 2 drops of rosemary oil to 1 cup of warm water and drink in the evening 2 hours before bedtime.

• Get outdoors or be near windows to expose your eyes to light, not necessarily the sun, during the daytime and wear an eye mask to sleep.

❊ DAILY SUPPLEMENTS ❊

• Melatonin helps regulate the human biological clock and reduces jet lag. Take 3 to 5 milligrams in the evening. Start the night before your trip and continue for 2 or 3 consecutive nights.

• The amino acid tyrosine (150 milligrams) improves alertness and cognitive function; take it in the morning.

• Vitamin B complex is helpful for supporting healthy nervous system function.

❊ HERBAL THERAPY ❊

• Herbs can be found in health food or vitamin stores, online, and at the offices of Chinese medicine practitioners. Herbs should be used according to individual needs; consult with a licensed practitioner for a customized formulation. To learn more about the herbs listed here, go to www.ask drmao.com.

• Drink a tea made from licorice and goji berries to help support kidney and adrenal functions, which are critical for supporting healthy neurochemical balance. Make tea by boiling 1 teaspoon licorice and 1 tablespoon goji in 3 1/2 cups of water for 30 minutes. Strain, and drink 3 cups daily.

• Valerian and chamomile teas are good for relaxing and regulating sleep. They are best taken at night.

• Essential oils of lavender, geranium, and rosemary are useful for treating jet lag. Massage them into the Inner Gate acupressure points (P-6) or your temples.

• Traditional Chinese herbal therapy for symptoms of jet lag includes ginseng, jujube, longan, biota, reishi mushroom, wheatberries, poria, and lily. These herbs are used to nourish heart yin and calm irritability.

❋ EXERCISE ❋

Physical activity is important for mitigating jet lag. Be sure to remain active in the days before travel. Do some stretching exercises while you're in the air. Upon arrival, take a walk outdoors. Expose yourself to sunlight until the evening to inhibit release of the hormone melatonin, which plays an important role in the biological clock. This way, melatonin will naturally release after sundown.

The following is a simple Dao In Qi Gong exercise to help with jet lag, called Immortal Imitating the Lazy Tiger Stretching. Do this exercise when you get to your destination and for a a few days after arrival to help regulate your body's natural rhythms.

Lie on your stomach in a push-up position with your arms bent, hands under your shoulders, and your chin tilted up.

Inhale and straighten both arms, raising your torso and lifting your chin up while your legs rest on the floor.

Exhale, and with your arms straight, move your body back, bending your knees until your buttocks are over your feet.

JET LAG

Inhale and move forward with your arms straight, returning to the same position as when you first raised your torso off the ground.

Repeat for a total of 3 times.

Next, on an exhale, move your body halfway back and place your forearms on the floor. You should now be resting on your knees and forearms, as if you were crawling.

Move off your knees and onto the balls of your feet.

Inhale, and with your legs straight, raise your buttocks up, bending your body to form an inverted V. Your head should be between your elbows.

Exhale and lower your body, keeping your legs straight and allowing your head to move forward until your body is parallel to the floor. Lift your chin up and don't let your legs touch the floor.

Repeat the steps in the two previous paragraphs for a total of 3 times.

Inhale, and with your legs straight, raise your buttocks up, bending your body to form an inverted V again.

Exhale, placing your head on the floor between your elbows. Slowly shift your weight onto your head.

Place your hands over your tailbone and clasp your hands with your palms up. Remain in this position for about 10 seconds, breathing naturally.

Move your hands down by your shoulders, with your palms on the floor.

Inhale and straighten your arms, raising your body and keeping your legs straight.

Bending your knees, lower your body into a crawling position. You should be on your knees, with your hands and feet remaining in the previous position.

Exhale, and with your arms straight, move your body back, bending your knees until your buttocks are over your feet.

Move your hands slightly forward.

Inhale and shift onto the balls of your feet, and, straightening your arms and legs, raise your body to form an inverted V.

Exhale, and while keeping your legs straight, bend your elbows to lower your body so that it's parallel with the floor in a low push-up position. Then straighten your elbows, arch your back, and raise your upper body. Lift your chin and look up.

Inhale and bend your elbows, lowering your head and upper body, and returning to a low push-up position. Then, straightening your arms, raise your buttocks up to form an inverted V. Rise as high as you can.

Repeat the steps in the previous two paragraphs for a total of 3 times. If you find yourself losing your breath, take frequent breaks.

❋ ACUPRESSURE ❋

• Find the acupoint Inner Gate (P-6), three finger-widths above the right wrist crease, between the two tendons on the inside of the forearm. Apply steady pressure with your left thumb or index finger until you feel soreness. Hold for 1 minute. Repeat on the left arm.

• Find the acupoint Foot Three Miles (ST-36), four finger-widths below the kneecap on the right leg. Apply moderate pressure with your thumb until you feel soreness. Hold for 5 minutes. Repeat on the left leg.

• Engaging both of these points helps calm the mind, regulate sleep, and increase qi.

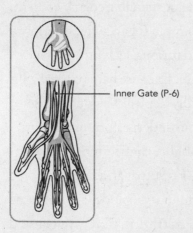
Inner Gate (P-6)

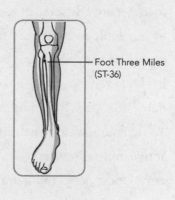
Foot Three Miles (ST-36)

AVOID

• Alcohol and caffeine, as they severely deplete the yin of the body and can cause dehydration.

JET LAG

> • Sleeping pills, as they slow down your body's ability to adjust to the new time zone. Consult your physician for alternatives.

LOW ENERGY

ARE YOU OFTEN TIRED AFTER THE SIMPLEST ACTIVITIES? Do the days drag on until you reach home, only to slump on the couch and crash, unable to enjoy your daily activities? If so, you are suffering from low energy. Energy normally fluctuates according to daily rhythms, which vary from person to person. In general, we have more energy in the morning and wind down toward the evening. However, many people suffer from chronic low energy and fatigue. They start the day tired and end the day tired. The causes of low energy are numerous. But first and foremost, low energy is often a result of stressful living in our modern world. Coping with stressful situations requires a lot of energy, leaving the average person drained and at times depressed. Poor diet also contributes to low energy. Instead of eating foods with a sustainable energy content, most people eat too many foods made of simple sugars, which supply a rapid burst of energy, but burn out fast and furious, leaving us depleted. Lack of exercise is the final nail in the coffin. Exercise helps us deal with daily stresses; without it, the body is rapidly depleted of vital energy.

Immune system malfunction—either an underperforming or hyperactive immune system—can also cause fatigue, contributing to low energy. Underperforming immunity is often a result of an acute or chronic viral or bacterial infection. Hyperactive immunity includes autoimmune inflammatory disorders such as rheumatoid arthritis, fibromyalgia, and lupus. And the functional decline of organs that occurs with diseases like congestive heart failure, emphysema, hepatitis, kidney disease, hypothyroidism, and anemia can leave patients tired and exhausted.

Energy is qi. The level and quality of a person's qi define how he or she feels. Chinese medicine recognized the concept of vital energy thousands of years ago and has developed a full understanding of the essential functions and role of qi in health and wellness. As a result, very effective means of addressing low energy have been developed. Once we've figured out the underlying cause of the fatigue, I work with internists to create a treatment plan specific to each patient's needs. Treatment usually consists of acupuncture and herbal therapy for three months or more, depending on the condition. I then counsel each patient on a dietary, lifestyle, and mind-body exercise regimen. In the more than twenty years that I've been working with patients with low energy, I've helped the majority of my patients overcome their fatigue.

Here are some simple steps to work on regaining your vitality.

✳ DIET ✳

• For sustained vitality and energy, the foods you consume must be wholesome, organic, and packed with essential vitamins, minerals, and nutrients. A balanced diet based on organic whole foods with fresh vegetables, whole grains, nuts, seeds, legumes, and moderate amounts of organic animal protein is best. The foods you eat must also be easily digested and absorbed. Dark green leafy vegetables, such as kale, broccoli, spinach, dandelions, collard greens, carrot tops, Brussels sprouts, and beet tops, and various mushrooms, including shiitake, maitake, white, black, and reishi, contribute to a healthy immune system. Pearl barley, bitter melon, squash, pumpkin, pumpkin seeds, yams, mung beans, black beans, and water chestnuts are also beneficial, as they nourish the organs and provide vital nutrition.

• Nuts, including pistachio nuts, almonds, hazelnuts, pine nuts, lotus root and seeds, and loquat help strengthen digestion. Green tea and daikon radish are good for digestion, too.

• Berries are rich in antioxidants and can also help remove toxic residues from the system, which is often the cause of chronic fatigue and low energy. Try blueberries, blackberries, raspberries, cranberries, goji berries, hawthorn berries, and cherries.

....

• Foods rich in essential fatty acids, including olive oil, sunflower oil, and omega-3 fatty acids obtained from deep-sea fish, can help improve cellular function. Chlorella, spirulina, wheat grass juice, and barley grass juice all contain chlorophyll and play key roles in energy metabolism and immune system.

....

• Water is important for properly flushing the system and hydrating the cells to prevent buildup of toxic waste products. Drink at least eight glasses of room-temperature water a day. Do not skip breakfast; always eat a nutritious breakfast including a high-quality protein like eggs, fish, or beans. Eat a snack at midmorning and another one at midafternoon to help you sustain your energy and prevent low blood sugar from setting in. Nuts, seeds, fruits, or a bean dip like hummus are good choices. Lunch should consist of vegetables and chicken or other protein sources but stay away from starchy foods. Dinner should be no later than 7:00 P.M., and keep it light, with dairy-free soups, vegetables and whole grains.

....

• Avoid all forms of processed sugar, including sodas, sweetened juices, and pastries. Sugar is extremely damaging to your energy levels, as the initial rush is followed by a spectacular crash, something we've all seen in children.

....

• Most dairy products should be avoided, as they tend to produce mucus and can cause digestive problems. They also contain lots of sugar in the form of lactose.

....

• Alcohol, coffee, deep-fried and fatty foods, and cold, raw foods should also be avoided, as they can injure the spleen and stomach and impair digestion.

—————————————— ✳ HOME REMEDIES ✳ ——————————————

• Make your own trail mix—include almonds, pine nuts, walnuts, dried cranberries, prunes, and raisins, or any other combination of nuts, seeds, and dried fruits that are high in antioxidants, essential fatty acids and fiber to help sustain energy over a long period of time.

• Make a tea or broth from any combination of the following herbs and spices: dill, oregano, cilantro, rosemary, sage, bay leaf, peppermint, ginger, garlic, parsley, cinnamon, onions, chives, garlic, and leeks. These herbs and spices contain volatile oils that stimulate your senses and increase alertness. Boil 1 tablespoon of the herb or spice in 3 1/2 cups of water for 15 minutes. Strain, and drink 3 cups daily.

• Jump rope for 5 minutes every hour throughout the day and drink a glass of water afterward to increase circulation and oxygenation and remove toxins from your body more frequently.

❊ DAILY SUPPLEMENTS ❊

• Chlorella (3 grams), spirulina (500 milligrams), kelp (100 milligrams), and other forms of chlorophyll are high-quality protein sources that enhance long-term energy.

• Vitamins B_3 (100 milligrams), B_6 (200 milligrams), and B_{12} (50 milligrams) are essential for energy metabolism. Vitamin C (1,000 milligrams) is also a good energy stimulator and helps reduce toxic cellular waste.

• L-carnitine (200 milligrams), coenzyme Q_{10} (50 milligrams), and lecithin (2 grams) promote energy metabolism, while chromium picolinate (300 micrograms) helps to balance blood sugar.

HERBAL REMEDIES

• Herbs can be found in health food or vitamin stores, online, and at the offices of Chinese medicine practitioners. Herbs should be used according to individual needs; consult with a licensed practitioner for a customized formulation. To learn more about the herbs listed here, go to www.askdrmao.com.

• Ginseng has been known as the king of energy tonics throughout history in Asia. Research studies have confirmed its energy-enhancing properties.

LOW ENERGY

• Gotu kola, ashwagandha, and damiana are herbs used to promote energy.

• Chinese medicine uses herbs such as astragalus root, ginseng root, ginger, licorice root, goji berry, red jujube, codonopsis, Chinese gooseberry, and schizandra berry to support abundant energy.

EXERCISE

To have energy, you must promote its flow within your body. Exercise actually helps increase the energy metabolism pathways, making more energy available to you and improving your mood. I recommend a daily 30-minute cardiovascular exercise routine combined with stretching and flexibility training. Many of my patients learn qi gong exercises to help them gather, store, and properly use energy. Dao In Qi Gong, a qi gong exercise for energy metabolism, has been practiced for thousands of years by the Taoist masters of China. With these exercises and proper diet and lifestyle, these ancient masters were able to prolong their lives and enjoy abundant energy. The fourth movement of the practice, called Immortal Tightening the Body Like a Bow, is included here to help get you started.

Lie on your back with your legs straight and arms at your side.

Bring your hands up and cross them over your chest, with your palms facing your chest.

Inhale, and slowly raise your torso and both your legs, keeping them straight, so that your body forms a V. At the same time, touch your toes with your fingers. Your tailbone should be the only part of your body touching the floor.

Exhale, and slowly return to the beginning posture.

Repeat for a total of 3 times.

Gradually work toward being able to hold yourself in the raised position for 1 minute. Repeat 3 times daily.

ACUPRESSURE

• Find the acupoint Arm Three Miles (LI-10), on the outer part of the right forearm, three finger-widths below the elbow crease on a line between the outer corner of the elbow crease and the tip of the index finger when the arm is bent at the elbow. Apply steady pressure with your left thumb until you feel soreness. Hold for 1 minute. Repeat on the left arm.

• Find the acupoint Foot Three Miles (ST-36), four finger-widths below the kneecap on the right leg. Apply moderate pressure with your right thumb until you feel soreness. Hold for 5 minutes. Repeat on the left leg.

• Regular stimulation of these points helps strengthen the body's resistance to stress, enhances immunity, and strengthens the vital organs.

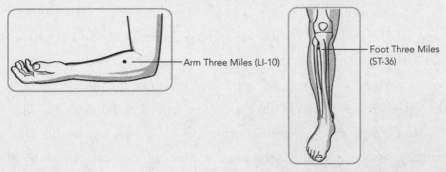

Arm Three Miles (LI-10)

Foot Three Miles (ST-36)

AVOID

• Smoking and taking drugs, as they are notorious for depleting the vital qi and weakening the body. Excessive sexual activity and physical and mental strain should also be avoided, as they drain the vital essence of the kidneys, leaving the body weak.

• Stress, emotional upset, and other negative emotions, which are damaging to the vital qi and reduce your immunity. Remain optimistic and keep a positive attitude.

LOW IMMUNE FUNCTION

THE HUMAN BODY HAS EVOLVED an amazing mechanism for protecting you against external pathogens and self-inflicted harm. Under normal conditions, the immune system is called upon to combat an invader only when it's needed. It's like the National Guard coming to the rescue during times of grave danger—whether it's a threat from the outside or a disaster on the inside. Unfortunately, as a result of the increasing stress, inadequate nutrition, environmental toxins, and lack of exercise that characterize our modern lifestyle, the immune system is always on high alert. And just like the guardsmen, after constant and prolonged battle, the immune system gets fatigued and burned out. At this point, two troubling scenarios can occur. In some people, the immune system becomes overwhelmed and loses its ability to distinguish between the body and a foreign organism. It begins attacking organs, tissues, and cells, giving rise to such autoimmune conditions as lupus, arthritis, or asthma. In the second scenario, the immune system capitulates and become too weak to respond in sufficient force to an invading substance or organism, leaving you vulnerable to infections and disease.

In Chinese medicine, immunity relies on several key factors. The kidney essence or vitality serves as the source of all energy in the body and supplies the necessary fuel for all metabolic functions. The spleen-pancreas-stomach network or the digestive system is responsible for absorption and distribution of vital nutrients in the body. The lungs govern the defensive energy and are responsible for protecting you from external pathogens. The liver manages neurological responses and promotes flow of energy. These organs must work in unison for the body's immunity to function properly. An unhealthy lifestyle can damage the kidney essence, and a poor diet combined with stress and emotional turmoil can injure the digestive and absorption system. Chronic infections and inflammation injure the energy reserves of the body, as in the HIV virus. These factors combine to create the complex condition of low immune function.

The most common immune-deficiency condition I see involves chronic fatigue syndrome, which is typically the result of chronic viral infections that leave the patient with weakened immunity. I've worked with immunologists to pinpoint the specific cause of the low immune function, and the majority of our immune-deficiency patients have returned to their normal activities after undergoing acupuncture and herbal therapies, immune-boosting dietary changes, lifestyle modifications, and mind-body exercises. Prolonged immune deficiency can lead to cancer and other degenerative diseases. In some cases, intravenous immunoglobulin (IVIG) therapy may be needed to maintain basic immune function. Always consult your physician and ask to be monitored if you learn that you have low immune function.

❊ DIET ❊

• Immune-boosting foods include cruciferous vegetables such as broccoli, cauliflower, Brussels sprouts, and cabbage; mushrooms such as shiitake, maitake, wood ear, and reishi; root vegetables such as carrots, yams, sweet potatoes, and radishes; grains such as brown rice, oats, quinoa, and amaranth; and fruits such as blueberries, cranberries, and raspberries.

• Certain herbs and spices, such as oregano, cilantro, rosemary, sage, peppermint, ginger, garlic, chives, onions, and turmeric, can perk up the immune system.

• Avoid sugar, as it is damaging to the immune system. This includes sodas and sweetened juices. Most dairy products should be avoided, as they tend to produce mucus. Excess mucus indicates an allergic response, which distracts the immune system and lowers its effectiveness in combating infections. Alcohol, coffee, deep-fried and fatty foods, and cold or raw foods should also be avoided or greatly reduced.

❊ HOME REMEDIES ❊

• Sunbathing for 20 to 30 minutes a day before 10 A.M. and after 3 P.M. can be helpful for your immune system. The UV rays can stimulate skin immunity and inhibit bacterial activity.

• Dry brushing your body daily can activate lymph circulation, which helps to clear out toxic debris and stimulate immunity.

• Cook up an immune broth consisting of 10 shiitake mushrooms (soaked first if using dried), 1/2 cup seaweed (any kind), 1 chopped head cabbage, 2 diced squash (any type), 2 diced carrots, 10 slices ginger, 3 sprigs oregano, and 1 chopped onion in 6 cups chicken stock. Boil for 30 minutes. Eat at least 1 large bowl every day.

• Make an immunity-boosting trail mix with dried blueberries, goji berries, Brazil nuts, and pine nuts for a treat rich in antioxidants, carotenoids, and selenium, which are critical for healthy immune function.

❊ DAILY SUPPLEMENTS ❊

• Supplementing with probiotics such as acidophilus (3 to 5 billion organisms) can help restore intestinal immunity.

• Deficiencies of vitamins A (200 IU), C (1,000 milligrams), E (800 IU), B_6 (30 milligrams), B_{12} (100 micrograms), and folic acid (400 micrograms) may result in significantly impaired immune function. Minerals that support immune function include zinc, iron, and selenium.

• Bovine colostrum (10 grams) contains immunoglobulin and other immune-stimulating factors.

• Thymus extract (200 milligrams) can help support healthy immune function.

• Royal jelly (1,000 milligrams) and bee propolis (80 milligrams) can stimulate immune function.

❊ HERBAL THERAPY ❊

• Herbs can be found in health food or vitamin stores, online, and at the offices of Chinese medicine practitioners. Herbs should be used according

to individual needs; consult with a licensed practitioner for a customized formulation. To learn more about the herbs listed here, go to www.ask drmao.com.

....

• Traditional Chinese herbs used to boost immunity include ginseng, astragalus, atractylodis, ligustrum, schizandra, white peony, bupleurum, rehmannia, Chinese cucumber, andrographis, and licorice.

....

• Cat's claw, pau d'arco, tea tree oil, echinacea, goldenseal, and St.-John's-wort are also used to support healthy immune function.

⁂ EXERCISE ⁂

Exercise is essential for maintaining immune function, not to mention its contributions to general wellness, mental clarity, and stress reduction. I recommend a daily 30-minute cardiovascular exercise combined with stretching and flexibility training. I've also advised many of my patients to learn immune-balancing meditation, tai chi, and qi gong exercises. The Self-Healing Qi Gong exercise is simple and helps strengthen the body, support the vital organs, support healthy immunity, and balance the hormonal functions. It consists of five practices, one for each organ network. Below are directions for the Hungry Tiger Lung Network Qi Gong, which targets the lungs and supports immune function. Practice this exercise daily.

Begin in a standing position with your feet shoulder-width apart. Bend down at the waist and touch the floor with your palms stretched shoulder-width apart. Bend your knees slightly. This should create an upside-down V—your buttocks should be pointing up while your feet and palms are firmly planted on the floor.

Inhale gently and deeply while focusing your attention on your perineum, the area between the genitals and the anus. Imagine the inhalation is drawing air in through the perineum.

As you exhale, start to bend your knees as you begin to transfer your weight backward onto your legs. In a sweeping downward and forward motion, bring your chest close to the floor, ending in a modified push-up posture. Your legs should be straight and slightly above the floor, your back arched up starting from the waist, your hands pushing against the floor directly below your shoulders, your arms straight, and your eyes looking forward (not down or up). As you exhale, focus your attention on the center of your palms, imagining the exhalation going out through the palms into the ground.

As you inhale again, focus on the perineum and return to the starting upside-down V position.

Repeat the exhale-inhale steps above 5 times, and work your way up to 10 times or more.

───────────────── ✳ ACUPRESSURE ✳ ─────────────────

• Find the acupoint Arm Three Miles (LI-10), on the outer part of the left forearm, three finger-widths below the elbow crease on a line between the outer corner of the elbow crease and the tip of the index finger when the arm is bent at the elbow. Apply steady pressure with your right thumb until you feel soreness. Hold for 1 minute. Repeat on the right arm.

· ·

• Find the acupoint Foot Three Miles (ST-36), four finger-widths below the kneecap on the right leg. Apply moderate pressure with your right thumb until you feel soreness. Hold for 5 minutes. Repeat on the left leg.

· ·

• Regular stimulation of these points helps strengthen the body's resistance to stress, enhances immunity, and strengthens the vital organs.

· ·

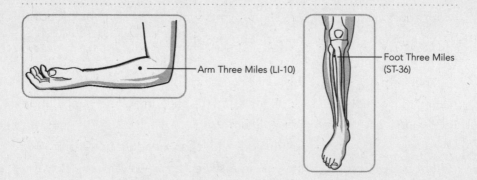

Arm Three Miles (LI-10)

Foot Three Miles (ST-36)

• The Chinese therapeutic massage Tui Na is makes an excellent addition to a treatment protocol. Ask your acupuncturist for a recommendation.

LOW LIBIDO

APPETITE IS NOT RESERVED JUST FOR FOOD. Sexual appetite is a normal physiological desire and can be an indicator of the mental and physical health of a person. Sexual libido typically peaks around the mid-twenties for both men and women and then generally declines at a steady rate with aging and reduced growth hormone. However, nearly 43 percent of women and 31 percent of men complain of low sexual drive during middle age. For women, emotional issues, childbirth, breastfeeding, onset of menopause, stress, weight gain, relationship conflicts, headaches, back pain, and inability to reach orgasm are among the causes for declining interest in sex. Certain drugs, hormonal imbalances, and clinical depression can also cause low libido. For men, low libido is often related to underlying disorders including thyroid problems, pituitary gland tumors, depression, and impotence—which, by itself, doesn't cause low libido but does psychologically interfere with a man's confidence and interest in sex. There are no simple solutions for rekindling sexual fire, although entire industries have sprung up touting instant fixes. The road back to a healthy libido varies greatly

LOW LIBIDO

from person to person and is also gender dependent. For most men, physical fitness and activity can increase their testosterone levels and give them confidence. For most women, getting reconnected with their emotions, feeling connected with their partner, and feeling desirable are essential to restoring libido.

In classical Chinese medicine, sexual desire is the function of the fire or yang energy of the kidney-adrenal network. (Each organ system has a yin/yang or water/fire aspect. The yin aspect represents the physical organ while the yang aspect represents the function of the organ system.) When the yang energy wanes or is obstructed by negative emotions or dampness (mucus) as a result of dietary or lifestyle factors, there is insufficient 'fire' to get the sexual sparks flying. Also, the heart network, which houses the spirit, must be in synchrony and must provide the physical attraction and emotional connection necessary for stoking the fire in the belly. At my wellness center, we work with many infertility patients and postmenopausal women. Low libido is an issue that gets top priority. My approach is to boost kidney-adrenal fire by supporting hormonal function and aligning the heart and kidney networks—the mind and the body, so to speak. I use acupuncture and herbal therapies, and I offer dietary advice and personal life coaching to help my patients reconnect with their sexuality. I also work with endocrinologists and psychotherapists as needed. In most cases, my patients have been satisfied with the results.

Here I share with you some simple suggestions.

❈ DIET ❈

• Libido-enhancing foods are typically warming and pungent in nature and taste and can help motivate the yang or body's fire energy. Garlic, onions, scallions, leeks, chives, ginger, cinnamon, fennel, cardamom, anise, turmeric, cayenne pepper, black pepper, and horseradish fall under this category. Lentils, black beans, kidney beans, adzuki beans, sesame seeds, walnuts, yams, sea cucumber, blueberries, raspberries, cranberries, and organic sources of animal protein from shrimp, eggs, lamb, and chicken also are helpful.

• Because of their high concentrations of essential omega-3 fatty acids, deep-sea and cold-water fish, such as halibut, salmon, sardines, and shellfish, combined with fish eggs or roe, can increase libido by improving overall sexual health. A little wine can also help warm the flow of yang energy, but amounts should be moderated, as too much can cause temporary impotence.

• Avoid dairy products and cold and raw foods. They tend to promote buildup of dampness in the body, which can impair circulation to the sex organs.

• A special note on food: How you prepare and eat foods is as important as what you eat. In today's fast-paced world, most people have abandoned traditional family dinners and romantic evening meals for the sake of expediency. Revisit your dining habits. Remember how sensual your first dinner date was, or the first time you treated your partner to a romantic candlelit dinner. These energetic qualities can have a powerful effect on our emotions and can instantly arouse sexual desire.

❋ HOME REMEDIES ❋

• Eat a clove of vinegar-pickled garlic daily for 1 month. Buy pickled garlic at health food stores or Middle Eastern markets, or make your own: Fill a glass jar with peeled cloves of garlic and pour in white vinegar. Add 1 teaspoon salt and seal the jar (airtight). Age in a dark space for 1 month.

• Boil 1 chopped onion, 1 chopped leek, 3 chopped stalks chives, 10 slices fresh ginger root, and 1 teaspoon each of turmeric and cayenne in 4 cups of canned chicken stock for 30 minutes. Eat at least one bowl a day.

LOW LIBIDO

• A sulfur bath or hot spring soak can be helpful for restoring kidney-adrenal energy and promotes circulation.

———————————— ❋ DAILY SUPPLEMENTS ❋ ————————————
• Taking DHEA (1 milligram) and L-arginine (500 milligrams) helps increase vitality and sexual desire.

• Vitamin C (1,000 milligrams) with bioflavonoids (500 milligrams), vitamin E (800 IU), and zinc (50 milligrams) are beneficial for circulation.

• Essential fatty acids such as those found in fish oil, flaxseed oil, or evening primrose oil, along with zinc, can provide hormonal support.

———————————— ❋ HERBAL THERAPY ❋ ————————————
• Herbs can be found in health food or vitamin stores, online, and at the offices of Chinese medicine practitioners. Herbs should be used according to individual needs; consult with a licensed practitioner for a customized formulation. To learn more about the herbs listed here, go to www.askdrmao.com.

• Horny goat weed is a Chinese herb that has traditionally been used to rekindle sexual desire in both men and women.

• Ginkgo biloba can increase blood supply to the brain and sexual organs.

• Korean ginseng can enhance sexual desire and potency.

• Other herbs used for low libido in Chinese medicine include psoralea, goji berry, cordyceps, eucommia, deer antlers, cinnamon bark, Chinese dodder, wild yam, morinda, and Asian cornelian.

———————————— ❋ EXERCISE ❋ ————————————
Physical activity has been proven clinically to improve sexual health. Thirty minutes of walking or jogging daily can be combined with tai chi or qi

gong exercises for good results. Kegel-type exercises can help strengthen the lower pelvic muscles and help prevent prostate problems in men and incontinence in women. Here I share with you a special Dao In Qi Gong exercise known as Immortal Imitating Peacock Turning and Looking at Tail Feathers, which will help increase the circulation of energy and blood to the sexual organs.

Begin in a semi-sitting position on the floor with your right leg straight out behind you forming a straight line down from the center of your body, your left leg bent up under your abdomen, and your left foot under your left buttock. Keep your arms straight and slightly wider than your shoulders with your hands on the floor. Keep your upper body straight and look straight ahead.

On an exhale, bend at both elbows, lowering your torso down to touch your left thigh. Then twist to the left, placing your right ear over your left hand, looking back at your left foot.

Inhale, and return to the beginning posture.

Exhale, and bend both elbows, lowering your torso down. Then twist to the right, placing your left ear over your right hand, looking back at your right foot.

Inhale, and return to the beginning posture.

Repeat the steps above for a total of 3 times.

Now repeat the exercise on the other side. Begin in a semisitting position on the floor with your left leg straight out behind you forming straight line down from the center of your body, your right leg bent up under your abdomen, and your right foot under your right buttock. Keep your arms straight and slightly wider than your shoulders with your hands on the floor. Keep your upper body straight and look straight ahead.

Exhale, and bend both of your elbows, lowering your torso down to touch your right thigh. Then twist to the right, placing your left ear over your right hand, looking back at your right foot.

Inhale, and return to the beginning posture.

Exhale, and bend both elbows, lowering your torso down. Then twist to the left, placing your right ear over your left hand, looking back at your left foot.

Inhale, and return to the beginning posture.

Repeat the steps above for this side for a total of 3 times.

Throughout the exercise move slowly, gently, and gracefully with rhythmic motion and intentional control. Do the exercise twice daily.

──────────────── ✳ ACUPRESSURE ✳ ────────────────

• Find the acupoint Restore Flow (KID-7), three finger-widths above the inner anklebone of the right foot. Apply pressure with your right thumb until you feel soreness. Hold for 3 minutes. Repeat on the left foot.

. . . .

• Find the acupoint Between Extremes (REN-3), one finger-width above the pubic bone. Apply pressure with your index finger until you feel soreness. Hold for 3 minutes. Make sure to empty your bladder before stimulating this point.

. . . .

• These points have traditionally been used to treat urinary problems, kidney weakness, prostate problems, and impotence.

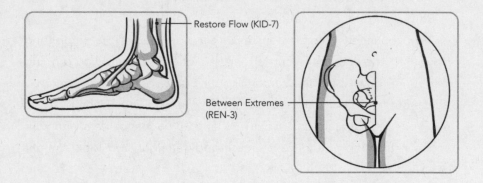

Restore Flow (KID-7)

Between Extremes
(REN-3)

─────────────────── AVOID ───────────────────

• Over-the-counter medications for colds and allergies, including antihistamines and decongestants, which can worsen the condition. Ask your doctor for alternatives if you suffer from low libido.

. . . .

• Sitting for prolonged periods of time and physical inactivity, as they also contribute to stagnant libido.

• Smoking, which depletes zinc, a mineral critical for healthy hormonal production and function.

LOWER BACK PAIN

EIGHT OUT OF TEN ADULTS IN AMERICA have or will soon experience back pain. Most commonly, lower back pain is attributed to strain and injury. The wear and tear of living eventually weaken the skeletal structure, causing bone loss or a displaced disk, and affecting our agility, stability, and strength. This is compounded by poor diet, sedentary lifestyle, and obesity. As we age we lose calcium from our bones, which can lead to osteopenia or osteoporosis. Our backs become more sensitive to strain and can go out with the slightest awkward movement or physical strain. Lower back pain can range from mild discomfort to debilitating. Pain, stiffness, radiating pain to the buttocks and lower legs, inability to stand or sit for prolonged periods, weakness, and fatigue are just some of the symptoms of lower back problems.

Bones, the skeletal structure, and particularly the lower back, are part of the kidney-bladder network, according to Chinese medicine. Kidney energy tends to diminish as we age, more rapidly with unhealthy diet, excessive physical and mental strain, overindulgence in drugs and alcohol, and excessive sexual activity. Weakness of the kidney network can result in lower back pain as well general weakness, fatigue, and other symptoms of premature aging. Replenishing kidney energy is difficult; it's a slow process, but it is essential to preserve kidney energy. Fortunately, through qi gong exercises, herbs, and a proper

LOWER BACK PAIN

diet and lifestyle, you can slow down kidney depletion and even re-generate certain aspects of kidney energy.

Lower back pain is one of the most common problems we treat at the Tao of Wellness. We use acupuncture and bodywork to reduce pain, and I work with my patients to identify and eliminate lifestyle and dietary factors that drain the kidney energy. I use herbs to support the healing process, ease inflammation, and relax muscle spasms. I also offer tailored stretching and strengthening exercises for the spine, abdomen, and lower back that don't put the patient at risk of reinjury.

Here are some of my recommendations.

──────────────── ❋ DIET ❋ ────────────────

• Eat a healthy, well-balanced diet rich in vegetables and fruits, whole grains, and organic animal protein. The skeletal structure has additional nutritional requirements, as the bones are made of calcium and other minerals. Foods high in calcium and vitamin D (required to enhance calcium absorption) include broccoli, chestnuts, clams, dark green vegetables, saltwater fish (such as flounder, salmon, and sardines), shrimp, mussels, and soybeans. Kidney beans, black beans, garlic, onions, kale, tempeh, pineapple, grapes, mulberries, anise seeds, cinnamon, cloves, almonds, walnuts, and prunes are also beneficial for the bones.

• Avoid carbonated soft drinks, alcohol, and smoking. Yeast and sugars, especially processed, bleached sugars, should be eliminated as well. Salt in small quantities can help strengthen the bones, but it should be used in moderation.

──────────────── ❋ HOME REMEDIES ❋ ────────────────

• For acute back injury, apply an ice pack to the painful area 2 or 3 times a day for 15 to 20 minutes at a time for the first 24 to 48 hours.

• Take a hot Epsom salt bath for 20 minutes a day until the pain is substantially reduced.

• Make a natural anti-inflammatory nonalcoholic cocktail by mixing equal parts of unsweetened black cherry juice with dark grape juice. Drink 3 to 6 glasses daily until the pain has eased.

• Make a calcium broth by making an oxtail or thighbone stew cooked with onions, garlic, tomatoes, and ginger to strengthen bones and stimulate bone growth. Drink a large bowl of the broth daily for 1 month.

❋ DAILY SUPPLEMENTS ❋

• The enzyme bromelain (500 milligrams) found in pineapple, is a natural anti-inflammatory and can help ease muscle and joint pain.

• Vitamin B complex and folate (400 micrograms) can be depleted from stress and pain, so supplementation can help ease symptoms.

• Glucosamine (1,000 milligrams), chondroitin sulfate (400 milligrams), and MSM (1,000 milligrams) taken together can help support healthy bones and joints.

• Calcium (1,000 milligrams), combined with magnesium citrate (500 milligrams), vitamin D (400 IU), and boron (3 milligrams), can help strengthen the bones.

❋ HERBAL THERAPY ❋

• Herbs can be found in health food or vitamin stores, online, and at the offices of Chinese medicine practitioners. Herbs should be used according to individual needs; consult with a licensed practitioner for a customized formulation. To learn more about the herbs listed here, go to www.ask drmao.com.

- Turmeric, white willow bark, and valerian work in conjunction to alleviate inflammation and pain.

. . . .

- Black haw, wild yam, and Jamaican dogwood are good muscle relaxants, and devil's claw and St.-John's-wort have anti-inflammatory and analgesic properties.

. . . .

- Traditional Chinese herbs used for back pain and back health include angelica root, red peony, eucommia, siler, notoginseng, gastrodia, clematis, corydalis, myrrh, frankincense, rehmannia, and achyranthes.

❋ EXERCISE ❋

Research conclusively shows that exercise early in life builds bone mass and strengthens the skeletal structure, helping to prevent injury. Regular exercise as we age can slow the progress of degenerative bone disorders. I recommend a combination of weight-bearing exercises in the form of 30-minute daily walks, moderate weight training to strengthen muscles and bones, and tai chi or qi gong to build endurance and flexibility.

During a bout of acute back pain, exercise may be difficult or too painful. Until you are mobile, bed rest is best. I recommend Dao In Qi Gong exercises, which are gentle, less stressful on the body, and great for loosening up the back. The movement called Immortal Imitating Butterfly Opening Its Wings is specifically targeted to the lower back. Practice this exercise regularly, upon waking and before bed.

Lie on your back with your knees slightly bent and arms at your sides. Relax and breathe gently, rhythmically, and deeply, inhaling into the lower abdomen and exhaling fully. Stay in this position until your breath is calm and you are relaxed.

Inhale, and bend your left knee, folding your left leg up to your chest.

Exhale, and clasp your bent leg with both hands, interlacing your fingers above the kneecap. Your body should be relaxed, with your head remaining on the floor.

Inhale, and gently and slowly raise your head to meet your left knee. Reach as far as you feel comfortable—do not overreach or push yourself.

Exhale, and slowly lower your head. Your left leg should remain in the bent position, clasped by your hands.

Repeat the steps above for a total of 3 times.

Inhale and straighten your knee so that your leg is straight up, perpendicular to the floor.

Exhale and slowly lower the straightened leg to the floor. Return to the beginning posture.

Repeat the exercise with your right leg. Inhale and bend your right knee, folding your right leg up to your chest.

Exhale, and clasp the bent leg with both hands, interlacing your fingers above the kneecap. Your body should be relaxed with your head remaining on the floor.

Inhale, and gently and slowly raise your head to meet your right knee. Reach as far as you feel comfortable—do not overreach or push yourself.

Exhale, and slowly lower your head. Your right leg should remain in the bent position, clasped by your hands.

Repeat the steps above for a total of 3 times.

Inhale, and straighten your knee so that your leg is straight up, perpendicular to the floor.

Exhale, and slowly lower the straight leg to the floor. Return to the beginning posture.

Now you'll do the movement with both legs together: Inhale, and bend both knees, folding both legs up toward the chest.

Exhale, and clasp your bent legs with both hands, interlacing your fingers at the knees. Your body should be relaxed, with your head remaining on the floor.

Inhale, and gently and slowly raise your head to meet the knees. Reach as far as you feel comfortable—do not overreach or push yourself.

Exhale and slowly lower your head. Your legs should remain in the bent position, clasped by your hands.

Repeat the steps above for a total of 3 times.

Inhale, and place your hands on top of your kneecaps. Straighten your knees so that your legs are straight up, perpendicular to the floor.

Exhale, and bend your knees, keeping your hands on your kneecaps.

Inhale, and straighten your legs so that they're again perpendicular to the floor.

Exhale, and gently lower your legs to the ground. Return to the beginning posture.

❋ ACUPRESSURE ❋

• Find the acupoint Forceful Torrent (KID-3), in the depression between the inner anklebone and the Achilles tendon of the right foot. Apply steady pressure with your right thumb until you feel soreness. Hold for 3 minutes. Repeat on the left foot.

• Find the acupoint Balance the Core (BL-40), located in the middle of the crease behind the knee of the right leg. Apply pressure with your right middle finger until you feel soreness. Hold for 3 minutes. Repeat on the left leg.

• Engaging the combination of these points is good for strengthening the kidneys and alleviating back pain.

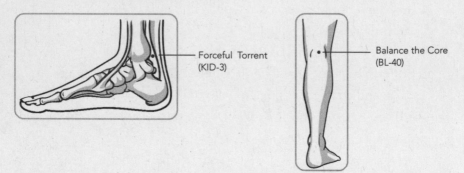

Forceful Torrent (KID-3)

Balance the Core (BL-40)

AVOID

• Smoking and excessive use of coffee and alcohol, as they can deplete the body of vital nutrients needed for bone health. Coffee consumption can cause calcium to be excreted through the urine, and nicotine reduces blood flow to the spine.

• High doses of vitamin A (including retinol-A and the medication Acutane used for acne), which can speed up bone loss and weaken the back.

• Steroids, thyroid medication, blood thinners, diuretics, and aluminum-containing substances, which can deplete bone mass and speed up osteoporosis. Consult your doctor about alternatives.

• Stress, worry, and tension, as they tighten the back muscles.

• Excess sexual activity.

MEMORY LOSS

MEMORY IS AN INTRICATE AND COMPLEX FUNCTION of the brain. It requires millions of neurons to operate in perfect harmony. As we age, we experience memory glitches in which spontaneous memory loss occurs, such as when you can't recall something that is at the tip of your tongue—a senior moment, yikes! Aging causes neuron loss, which can affect your memory of recent events. You might forget where you left your keys, or the name of a person you just met. More serious, non-aging-related memory loss might manifest as forgetting how to do things that you've done many times before or being unable to learn new things. Progressive memory loss is a serious condition. Causes of memory loss include depression, dementia, Alzheimer's disease and other neurodegenerative brain disorders, side effects from certain drugs, stroke, trauma, and alcoholism.

In Chinese medicine, memory depends heavily on the kidney-adrenal network and the spleen-pancreas-stomach network. The kid-

MEMORY LOSS

ney network stores your life essence and the spleen network supplies energy for daily living through healthy digestive processes, producing vital nutrients and distributing energy to the brain and other organs. As we age, our kidney essence is depleted. Combine aging with a weakened digestive system, and the brain receives less and less of its essential nutrients. Lack of physical and mental exercise also prevents nourishment from reaching the brain.

I regularly treat patients suffering from memory loss. One patient, a woman about fifty years came old, came to see me, complaining of dramatic short-term memory decline and other symptoms. She was going through menopause and she decided, in consultation with her gynecologist, not to go on hormonal replacement therapy (HRT) because of a family history of breast cancer. I approached her treatment by fortifying the underlying vital life essence and bolstering the digestive system to help with proper nutrient absorption and delivery. After a three- to four-month course of acupuncture and herbal therapy, she reported substantial improvement in her memory, and her menopausal symptoms improved as well. I also instructed her in memory exercises and qi gong practice.

--------------------------------- ✳ DIET ✳ ---------------------------------

• A regular and balanced diet rich in essential amino acids, omega-3 fatty acids, minerals, and vitamins will help to ensure a vibrant and sharp memory. Make sure to eat some form of protein, such as nuts, seeds, beans, legumes, or animal products, with each meal. Foods to favor include yams, squash, snow peas, pumpkin, potatoes, parsley, mushrooms, lotus root, ale, celery, beets, bamboo shoots, bell peppers, apples, Chinese dates, hawthorn berries (make tea), papaya, pineapples, raspberries, oats, pearl barley, adzuki beans, black beans, chestnuts, lotus seeds, sesame seeds, and black walnuts. Fish, especially deep-ocean fish, are a good source of the essential oils that our cells need for healthy function.

• Avoid excessive fatty, fried, and processed foods, dairy products, chocolate, caffeine, carbonated beverages, and alcohol. Do not overeat, as overeating stalls the energy at the center of the body, preventing it from nourishing the brain.

------------------------------ ❋ HOME REMEDIES ❋ ------------------------------

• Make Dr. Mao's Anti-Aging Brain Mix by mixing together 1 cup walnuts, 1/2 cup pine nuts, 1/4 cup sesame seeds, 1/2 cup pumpkin seeds, 1/3 cup dried goji berries, 1/2 cup dried apricots and 1/2 cup dried blueberries. Pack in a sealed container or zipper-lock bag to preserve freshness. Eat a small handful in between meals daily as a snack. The essential fatty acids and rich carotenoids and antioxidants in the nuts and fruit will nourish and support your brain and prevent low blood sugar.

• Drink green tea daily, as green tea prevents an enzyme found in people with Alzheimer's disease from forming and is also rich in polyphenols, antioxidants that help prevent premature brain aging.

• Make a tea or broth from any of the herbs and spices below, which are rich in volatile oils and B vitamins and act as natural brain boosters. Steep 1 teaspoon of any of the following in combination or by themselves in boiling water for 5 minutes: dill, cloves, oregano, cilantro, rosemary, sage, fennel, anise, cardamom, garlic, onions, ginger, leeks, scallions, peppers, chives, cinnamon, basil, and coriander. Drink a cup when you need to concentrate or find your focus waning.

------------------------------ ❋ DAILY SUPPLEMENTS ❋ ------------------------------

• Phosphatidylserine (PS; 300 milligrams), a compound made by the body from the amino acid serine, can help lower the stress response and promotes the release of neurotransmitters in the brain. Its role in reversing age-related dementia and memory loss is well documented in Europe.

• L-carnitine (500 milligrams) has been studied for its potential to enter the brain and help delay the onset of Alzheimer's and other memory-loss conditions.

• Microalgae from lakes and oceans, such as blue-green algae, spirulina, and chlorella (1 to 3 grams), are easy-to-digest, high-protein and high-energy supplements that support healthy brain function.

• The amino acid compound GABA (250 milligrams), consisting of glycine, taurine, L-glutamine, L-phenylalanine, and L-tyrosine can be helpful when taken daily.

❋ HERBAL THERAPY ❋

• Herbs can be found in health food or vitamin stores, online, and at the offices of Chinese medicine practitioners. Herbs should be used according to individual needs; consult with a licensed practitioner for a customized formulation. To learn more about the herbs listed here, go to www.askdrmao.com.

• Gingko biloba supplements can help strengthen learning, thinking, retention, and recall.

• Gotu kola can help improve cerebral circulation.

• Taoist masters of ancient China used reishi or ganoderma mushrooms daily to support healthy mental function.

• To support healthy brain function, you can try our family formula Enduring Youth, which contains: Chinese yam, goji berry, schizandra berry, Asian cornelian, China root, cistanches, sweet flag, Chinese senega, dipsacus, anise, Chinese foxglove, and other herbs.

❋ EXERCISE ❋

The best way to keep your brain sharp is to exercise it. Incorporate mind-stimulating games into your daily life. Listen intently and memorize names, shopping lists, and daily activities—this keeps your mind working and stimulated. Puzzles and memory games are also helpful. Regular cardiovascular exercise is a natural way of improving circulation to the brain and can help improve memory by 20 to 30 percent. When you feel tired, take a 15-minute power nap. During sleep our body regenerates, so a good night's sleep is crucial for mental energy.

I also recommend Dao In Qi Gong exercises to help you lead a long and healthy life. One of my favorite Dao In moves, Immortal Beating the Heavenly Drum, stimulates the brain and improves circulation to the head. Practice this exercise once in the morning and once in the evening, but not immediately before bed, for optimum results.

Sit comfortably at the tip of a sturdy chair with your spine erect, arms on top of your legs, and head tilted slightly forward.

Begin breathing slowly and rhythmically, inhaling deeply and gently and exhaling slowly.

Cover both ears with your palms, with the fingers of each hand pointing toward each other at back of your head.

Inhaling, place your index fingers on top of your middle fingers and then snap them off, striking the back of your head on the depressions located behind the ears at the base of the skull, where the Wind Pond (GB-20) acupoints are located. Repeat continuously, with about one strike per second.

Exhaling, continue striking the Wind Pond points with your index fingers while bending forward at the waist. Tilt your head down.

Continue breathing and striking for 20 to 30 seconds, until you've struck the points 36 times.

Conclude the sequence by rising back to the sitting position with your last exhalation.

✳ ACUPRESSURE ✳

• Locate the acupoint Hundred Meeting (DU-20), at the top of your head, midway between your ears. Apply gentle pressure with your index finger for 5 minutes. This point is traditionally used for improving brain and spirit functions.

• Locate the acupoint Forceful Torrent (KID-3), on the inside of your left ankle between the Achilles tendon and the anklebone. Pinch the point with your right thumb and index finger using moderate pressure for about 5 minutes. Repeat on the other foot. This acupoint is traditionally used to strengthen the kidney system, and it also has anti-aging benefits.

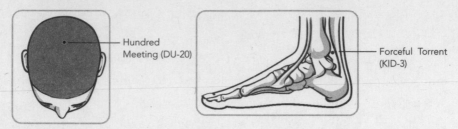

Hundred Meeting (DU-20)

Forceful Torrent (KID-3)

MENOPAUSE

THE FEMALE REPRODUCTIVE CYCLE begins during the teen years and declines around the fifth decade of life. The ovaries gradually reduce their production of female hormones, such as estrogen, as a natural biological process. The end result of this decline is the cessation of menstruation. Known as menopause, this process affects every woman, though some experience a higher degree of discomfort than others. Without the beneficial effects of estrogen, women are at a higher risk of developing medical conditions such as cardiovascular and degenerative bone disorders. As estrogen production declines, the body's hormonal balance is lost, resulting in menstrual irregularities, hot flashes, night sweats, mood changes, and memory impairment. Some women may also experience cold hands and feet, insomnia, loss of skin elasticity, weight gain, and urinary and vaginal changes. Western medicine has traditionally recommended hormone replacement therapy (HRT), with both estrogen and progesterone. However, after some results of the landmark Women's Health Initiative were published in 2002, the use of HRT dropped significantly, and breast cancer rates dropped dramatically the following year. Studies are still in progress, but experts believe that reduced HRT use resulted in the lower occurrence of estrogen-sensitive breast cancer.

Estrogen and other hormones represent the yin, or the substance aspect, of the body. Hormones are primarily associated with the essence of the kidney-bladder network. The decline of the kidney essence over time affects the formation of blood, bones, and body fluids, producing symptoms of dryness, aging, and bone degeneration. Chinese medicine has long recognized that the human body is highly regenerative. By providing the right nutritional foundation and supporting glandular functions, all biological substances—including hormones—can be naturally restored without replacement. This is a basic tenet of the Taoist art of longevity. The key to dealing with bodily decline is to address it early, during perimenopause, before menopause sets in. With an appropriate diet, lifestyle, and exercise regimen, and by using acupuncture and herbal therapy to support healthy glandular function, the passage through menopause can be smooth and even empowering.

A patient who came to see me about five years ago for mood disorders is representative of the many women I see who are going through menopause. She had been put on antidepressants and antianxiety drugs

MENOPAUSE

by her psychiatrist but was still having symptoms. She wanted to get off the medication. I never recommend that a patient go off any medication without checking with the prescribing physician, so I called up her psychiatrist and worked out a therapeutic program that he agreed with. As I began treating her, I noticed that she had started to show perimenopausal symptoms. Within two months, she developed hot flashes, insomnia, palpitations, anxiety upon waking, and weight gain, and her mood took a turn for the worse. I knew that unless we turned our attention toward regeneration, her mood wouldn't improve. As I worked on her menopause issues with acupuncture and herbal therapies, I spoke to her about the concept of Second Spring. Menopause is a pivotal junction in a woman's life. The loss of childbearing capability can represent freedom for a woman for the first time to live her life as she wants to. Typically the first half of a woman's life is devoted to family and does not belong to her. By menopause many women's familial responsibilities have been substantially fulfilled, making it an opportune time for a woman to reestablish her personal and sexual identity. The process can be very empowering. I counseled my patient on changing her diet, lifestyle, and even career choices. She is now past menopause and has lost most of the weight she gained, is symptom free, and is happily pursuing a new career. Moreover, she has been off the psychotropic drugs for more than two years, with the blessing of her psychiatrist.

The following suggestions are those that I give my patients who are nearing or going through menopause.

❋ DIET ❋

• Diet should include ample leafy green vegetables for their mineral content; nuts, seeds, and their oils; rich supplies of essential fatty acids; lean protein sources including fish, egg whites, shellfish, and poultry; and beans and legumes for their abundant supply of natural phytoestrogens—Mother

Nature's hormonal supplement. Eat a large variety of foods to ensure the broadest nutritional support.

....

• Stop smoking and eliminate alcohol, dairy products, coffee, sugar, deep-fried, fatty foods, and processed, refined foods.

———————— ✳ HOME REMEDIES ✳ ————————

• Make your own trail mix, including almonds, sunflower seeds, walnuts, dried cranberries, prunes, and goji berries, or any other combination of nuts, seeds, and dried fruits. Their high content of antioxidants, essential fatty acids, and fiber helps provide nutritional support during menopause, and they are good for memory too.

....

• Cook up some Second Spring Chili, with beneficial phytoestrogen-rich beans and legumes: 1/2 cup each soy, black, kidney, navy, and adzuki beans, with 1 can tomato paste, 4 cups chicken stock, 4 cups water, 1 teaspoon turmeric, 5 chopped garlic cloves, and 1 chopped onion. Cook for 2 hours and add water as needed. Feel free to adapt the recipe to use your favorite beans, vegetables, and spices.

....

• Make a juice from cucumbers, celery, watermelon, and apples to relieve hot flashes.

———————— ✳ DAILY SUPPLEMENTS ✳ ————————

• Essential fatty acid supplements, including fish oils (1,000 milligrams EPA; 800 milligrams DHA), evening primrose oil (450 milligrams GLA), flaxseed oil, and borage oil are helpful for reducing symptoms of menopause.

....

• Vitamin B complex and vitamins C (1,000 milligrams), and E (800 IU) can help you cope with the changes, especially mood swings, of menopause.

....

• Vitamin D (800 IU), calcium (1,000 milligrams), magnesium citrate (500 milligrams), boron (10 milligrams), and zinc (50 milligrams) can help support bone health during menopause.

MENOPAUSE

• DHEA (1 gram) is a precursor nutrient for the production of hormones in the body.

⁑ HERBAL THERAPY ⁑

• Herbs can be found in health food or vitamin stores, online, and at the offices of Chinese medicine practitioners. Herbs should be used according to individual needs; consult with a licensed practitioner for a customized formulation. To learn more about the herbs listed here, go to www.askdrmao.com.

• Black cohosh, red clover, evening primrose oil, saw palmetto, and valerian are herbs used to help cope with menopausal symptoms.

• A tea made from motherwort, mulberry, sesame, zizyphus, and Chinese senega supports healthy menstruation and calms the spirit.

• A formula from our family medical tradition called Passages Plus helps provide support for my menopausal patients. It includes herbs traditionally used in Chinese medicine for healthy hormonal function, such as wild yam, rehmannia, dong quai, epimedium, fermented soybean, conch shell, zizyphus, gardenia, alisma, peony root, and other Chinese herbs.

⁑ EXERCISE ⁑

Regular physical exercise has been clinically proven to alleviate the symptoms of menopause. I recommend a 30-minute walk every day combined with the Eight Treasures Qi Gong mind-body exercise. One section of the practice that I often use with my patients, known as The White Crane Strengthens Its Vital Force, helps strengthen vital energy and support menopausal changes. Do the sequence twice daily for optimum results.

In a quiet, comfortable environment, preferably outdoors, stand with your feet shoulder-width apart, knees slightly bent, spine erect, tailbone tucked in, and head tilted slightly forward. Drape your arms at your sides, with your shoulders relaxed.

Begin with rhythmic, slow, and relaxed breathing. Inhale deeply but softly, and imagine the breath extending all the way down to the lower abdomen, about two finger-widths below the navel. Exhale gently and softly. Stay in this position for 7 breath cycles, relaxing and calming your mind.

Now, begin the exercise: On an inhale, raise your arms to your head, placing your palms behind your head and interlocking your fingers.

Exhale, and bend forward at the hips while gently pushing your head down with your interlocked hands. As your head reaches the lowest point, move your hands over your head and extend them to the ground in front of you, keeping your fingers interlocked.

Push your extended hands down toward your feet, touching the tops of your feet.

Inhale, and grasp the backs of your ankles with both hands, pulling your bent upper torso toward your legs. Touch your nose to one knee, if possible.

Exhale, release your grip on your ankles, and gently rise up with your hands in front of you and your palms facing the ground.

Repeat the above sequence 3 times.

This exercise should be gentle, smooth, and rhythmic. Don't overstretch or force the movement. If you're unable to touch your nose to your knee, just bend as far as you can.

✳ ACUPRESSURE ✳

• Find the acupoint Forceful Torrent (KID-3), in the depression between the inner anklebone and the Achilles tendon of the right foot. Apply steady pressure with your right thumb until you feel soreness. Hold for 2 minutes.

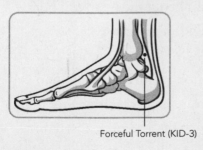

Forceful Torrent (KID-3)

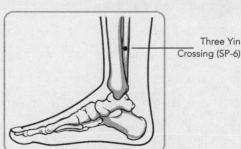

Three Yin Crossing (SP-6)

MENOPAUSE

Repeat on the left foot. This point benefits the urinary system and strengthens the kidneys.

• Find the acupoint Three Yin Crossing (SP-6), four finger-widths above the inner ankle of the right foot. Apply steady pressure with your right thumb until you feel soreness. Hold for 2 minutes. Repeat on the left foot. This point benefits the kidneys and helps strengthen the yin energy.

AVOID

• Nicotine, coffee and alcohol; their use has been shown to worsen menopausal symptoms.

• Stress and emotional upset, which can cause an adrenaline rush that heightens hot flashes and sweats.

MENSTRUAL DISORDERS

MONTHLY MENSTRUAL PERIODS ARE A NORMAL PART of a woman's life. Menstruation is essential for the renewal of the uterine lining in preparation for pregnancy. Major fluctuations in hormone levels precede a menstrual period, and it is normal to feel minor discomfort before and during menstruation. However, many women experience severe symptoms or painful menstruation. Painful menstruation, or dysmenorrhea, is more common in young women in their teens and twenties than in older women, and it can be secondary to an underlying condition such as endometriosis, pelvic inflammatory disease, ovarian cysts, or premenstrual syndrome (PMS). The symptoms of painful menstruation begin days before the onset of menstruation, and can continue throughout the cycle. Symptoms include lower abdominal cramping, a dull ache that often radiates to the lower back, heavy menstrual flow with or without clots, dull headaches, constipation or diarrhea, frequent urination, and mood changes including anxiety or depression. Stress, lack of exercise, and excess caffeine use can also cause menstrual discomfort and PMS. In Western medicine birth control pills or other hormonal agents, diuretics, and antidepressants are often prescribed.

In Chinese medicine, a healthy menstrual cycle relies on several factors, including the condition of the blood, the level of energy, and the proper functioning of the liver and kidneys. For example, if there is heat in the blood or a stagnation of energy resulting from emotional imbalance and stress, the menstrual flow becomes disrupted, causing pain and discomfort. Many women also suffer from a condition in which cold affects the uterus, causing severe menstrual cramps and pain. Stress and intense emotions, especially anger, frustration, and resentment, can easily depress the liver. Over time, the stagnation turns into heat, pushing the blood to flow out heavily with clots and pain.

In one case, a patient of mine would go from being gentle and sweet to rageful and anxious—like Dr. Jekyll and Mr. Hyde—as soon as she hit her ovulation. Two weeks later, when her period would start, she'd return to being her sweet self. Her menstrual pain was unbearable as a result of recurrent endometriosis, which had already been treated with surgery three times. She was referred to me by her gynecologist, and together we created a treatment plan involving diet and nutrition, acupuncture and herbal therapy, exercise, and meditation. After about six months, her symptoms were reduced by about 90 percent. She was quite happy, but the happiest person was her husband, who once remarked that I had saved their marriage.

Following are some recommendations for treating menstrual problems. Be sure to have your gynecologist examine you thoroughly to rule out fibroids, endometriosis, polycystic ovarian syndrome, or other serious disorders.

❋ DIET ❋

• Diet before, during, and after menstruation can have direct bearing on the duration and severity of menstrual symptoms. I recommend a balanced diet rich in green leafy vegetables, whole grains, and moderate to small amounts of organic animal protein. Foods high in essential fatty acids, including cold-water fish, nuts such as almonds and walnuts, and seeds such as sesame and cassia, are helpful. One week prior to the onset of your cycle, I recommend that you incorporate scallions, chives, ginger, fennel, orange peel, spinach, walnuts, hawthorn berries (make tea), raspberries, saffron, tarragon, bay leaf, cinnamon, and black pepper into your diet.

• Alcohol, caffeine, chocolate, and vinegar should be avoided around the time of your menstrual period, as should saturated fats, sugar, raw fruits (except berries), salt, and dairy products. Animal proteins should be eaten in moderation.

❋ HOME REMEDIES ❋

• Make a broth by boiling 3 slices of ginger, 1 chopped green onion, 1 fennel bulb, the dried peel of 1 small orange, and a pinch of black pepper in 3 1/2 cups of water for 10 minutes. Strain, and drink 1 cup 3 times a day beginning 1 week prior to the onset of menstruation.

• Make tea by boiling 1 teaspoon each of hawthorn, cinnamon, and turmeric in 3 1/2 cups of water for 30 minutes. Strain, and drink 3 cups daily. This is a good remedy for abdominal bloating, distention, and pain.

• Take a hot Epsom salt sitz bath daily before the onset of your period. Once your period starts, massage ginger oil into your abdomen and place a heating pad over your abdomen for 30 minutes for pain relief.

❋ DAILY SUPPLEMENTS ❋

• Supplementing with vitamin B complex and vitamin E (800 IU) can help reduce stress and anxiety.

• Taking magnesium (500 milligrams) combined with vitamin B$_6$ (50 milligrams) can help reduce cramps and pain.

• Taking niacin (200 milligrams) combined with rutin (500 milligrams) and vitamin C (1,000 milligrams) is also useful for pain relief.

• Supplementing with evening primrose oil (450 milligrams GLA) can help balance the hormonal system.

• Essential fatty acids in the form of omega-3-rich fish oil (1,000 milligrams EPA; 800 milligrams DHA) and flaxseed oil are natural anti-inflammatories that help reduce menstrual pain and clotting.

———————— ❋ HERBAL THERAPY ❋ ————————

• Herbs can be found in health food or vitamin stores, online, and at the offices of Chinese medicine practitioners. Herbs should be used according to individual needs; consult with a licensed practitioner for a customized formulation. To learn more about the herbs listed here, go to www.ask drmao.com.

• Chamomile tea and valerian tea can help relax the muscles and reduce pain. Chaste tree and black cohosh can also help reduce pain.

• Red raspberry tea helps to strengthen uterine tissue.

• Cramp bark, black cohosh, and Jamaican dogwood can be used to relieve pain and cramping.

• Traditional Chinese herbs used for menstrual difficulties include immature orange peel, nutgrass, silk tree, albizia bark, white peony root, angelica, or dong quai, red clover, motherwort, and bupleurum.

Regular physical activity is very important for promoting the flow of qi in the body. A lack of exercise can increase the severity and duration of symptoms associated with dysmenorrhea. In addition to a regular physical exercise regimen, a good moving meditation can help balance the emotions, reduce stress, strengthen the organs, and regulate menstruation. I recommend the movement section White Crane Twists Its Body to Look Up of the Eight Treasures Qi Gong to my patients for menstrual problems. This exercise helps regulate liver energy, promotes the flow of qi and blood, strengthens the uterine muscles, and helps regulate menstruation. Do this exercise twice daily for best results.

In a quiet, comfortable environment, preferably outdoors, stand with your feet shoulder-width apart, knees slightly bent, spine erect, tailbone tucked in, and head tilted slightly forward. Let your arms hang at your sides, with the shoulders relaxed.

Begin with rhythmic, slow, and relaxed breathing. Inhale deeply but softly, and imagine the breath extending all the way down to the lower abdomen, about two finger-widths below the navel. Exhale gently and softly. Stay in this position for 7 breath cycles, relaxing and calming your mind.

Now, begin the exercise: Inhale, and widen your stance to two shoulder-widths apart. Exhale and bend forward, placing your palms on your knees so that you're bent over at a 90-degree angle.

Inhale, and grasp the back of your left ankle with your right hand while pushing against your left knee with your left hand.

Exhale, and twist your upper torso to the left, twisting your head to look up. You should feel a stretch in your left leg muscles and back.

Inhale, release the grip on your ankle, and return to the forward bend position. Exhale, and place your palms on your knees, remaining bent over. at a 90-degree angle.

Inhale, and grasp the back of your right ankle with your left hand while pushing against your right knee with your right hand.

Exhale, and twist your upper torso to the right, twisting your head to look up. You should feel a stretch in your right leg muscles and back.

Inhale, release the grip on your ankle, and return to the forward bend position. Exhale, and place your palms on your knees, remaining bent over at a 90-degree angle.

Repeat the exercise 3 to 7 times, alternating from one side to the other. Do not overstretch.

Conclude the exercise by returning to the initial standing posture and meditating for 1 minute.

✳ ACUPRESSURE ✳

- Locate the acupoint Valley of Harmony (LI-4), in the web between your thumb and index finger on your right hand. Apply steady pressure with your left thumb until you feel soreness. Hold for 2 minutes. Repeat on the left hand.

- Find the acupoint Great Surge (LIV-3), in the web between the big and second toes on your right foot. Apply steady pressure with your left thumb until you feel soreness. Hold for 2 minutes. Repeat on the left foot.

- Engaging these points helps promote the smooth flow of qi, soothes stagnation, and helps alleviate painful menstruation, cramps, and stress.

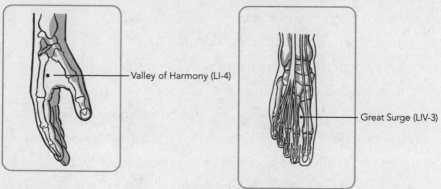

Valley of Harmony (LI-4)

Great Surge (LIV-3)

AVOID

- Coffee, alcohol, and chocolate, as they can aggravate menstrual cramps.

- Food allergies—be observant to determine which foods aggravate menstrual pain and eliminate them from your diet.

- Intrauterine devices (IUDs), which can cause painful menstruation in some women.

- Frequent urinary tract and vaginal infections, which can predispose you to painful menstruation.

- Being overtired—rest and sleep are very important for proper organ function. Get at least eight hours of sleep a night.

MIGRAINES

MIGRAINE HEADACHES ARE DEVASTATING AND DEBILITATING, and they're often confused with other kinds of headaches. Recent studies suggest that, in addition to the common vascular system irregularities, migraines can also be caused by neurological and inflammatory conditions that affect the nerve roots in the neck. Before the onset of a migraine—sometimes up to twenty-four hours before—a large area of neurological activity in the brain is depressed; this causes inflammation, which irritates the cranial nerves. Migraines, unlike ordinary headaches, include symptoms such as nausea, vomiting, auras (light spots), sensitivity to light and sound, numbness, speech difficulty, and pain on one side of the head or in one eye. All of these symptoms are connected to the irritation of the cranial nerves. Migraines can be caused by or accompanied by sinus problems, muscle tension, eyestrain, blood sugar imbalances, or hormonal imbalances, such as premenstrual syndrome (PMS). Migraines tend to last for long periods of time—days or weeks. Researchers believe that there might be a genetic predisposition to migraines.

Migraines respond very well to acupuncture, and many clinical studies have confirmed acupuncture's clinical efficacy for pain management. I had a patient who suffered from intractable migraines for more than fifteen years. He took all the available medication for migraines—including Botox injections—without much relief. I worked with his neurologist to formulate a comprehensive pain management plan consisting of acupuncture and herbal therapies, a hypoallergenic diet, and stress-reduction meditation and stretching exercises. After about four months of treatment, he went from two migraines a week to one or two a month. At this point his neurologist took him off of all medication and the patient continued with the remaining therapies for another two months. That was seven years ago. He now averages one or two migraines a year, and he continues to be off of all medication.

Dietary allergies play a significant role in many people who suffer from migraine headaches. It is important to identify, with the help of an allergist or nutritionist, the foods that may act as triggers for your condition.

Here are some of my favorite home remedies, but always work with your physician to rule out more serious neurological problems.

─────────────── ❊ DIET ❊ ───────────────

• Eat wholesome, organic foods with no preservatives, additives, or artificial flavors or colors. Artificial colors and some preservatives can cause headaches. Add a good variety of fresh fruits, vegetables, whole grains, beans and legumes, fish, and poultry to your diet. Favor fiber-rich foods including leafy green vegetables, parsley, onions, ginger, brown rice, bran, carrots, celery, asparagus, papaya, pineapple, cherries, grapes, prunes, lentils, split peas, mung beans, rosemary, oregano, cilantro, dill, sage, mint, and turmeric. Eat regularly, more frequently, and in smaller quantities. Do not eat while on the run or under stress, and do not eat late at night. Do not eat and lie down immediately afterward.

• Avoid spicy foods, heavy starchy foods, and rich and greasy foods. Alcohol and coffee should be avoided, as should be chocolate, red wine, and dairy products, especially cheese.

___ ❋ HOME REMEDIES ❋ ___

• During an acute episode of migraine headache, place ice packs at your forehead and the base of your neck for 15 to 20 minutes and soak your feet in a hot bath to help lessen the pain. Repeat several times throughout the day.

• Make a tea by boiling 1 tablespoon each of dried chrysanthemum flowers, peppermint, and green tea in 3 1/2 cups of water for 20 minutes. Strain, and drink 3 to 4 cups daily.

• Make fresh carrot and celery juice and drink a 12-ounce glass 3 times a day.

• Drinking a strong cup of coffee can abort the onset of a migraine.

• Apply Tonic Oil (which includes eucalyptus, wintergreen, and menthol) or lavender oil to the temples and forehead and massage gently in a circular motion.

___ ❋ DAILY SUPPLEMENTS ❋ ___

• Supplementing with calcium (1,000 milligrams) and magnesium (100 milligrams) can reduce the intensity and frequency of migraine attacks.

• Vitamin B complex, especially B^6 (50 milligrams) and B^{12} (100 micrograms) can help reduce the symptoms of a migraine.

• Taking niacin (300 milligrams) during an acute attack can dilate and relax the blood vessels in the brain, relieving pain.

─────────── ❋ HERBAL THERAPY ❋ ───────────

• Herbs can be found in health food or vitamin stores, online, and at the offices of Chinese medicine practitioners. Herbs should be used according to individual needs; consult with a licensed practitioner for a customized formulation. To learn more about the herbs listed here, go to www.ask drmao.com.

• Studies show that butterbur (*Petasites hybridus*) extract can provide a 50 percent or more reduction in the frequency of migraines.

• Kudzu (*Pueraria lobata*) can help treat menstrual migraine headaches and cluster headaches.

• White willow bark and turmeric can help reduce the intensity of migraine attacks.

• Traditional Chinese herbs used for migraine headaches include gastrodia, gambir vine, abalone shell, gardenia, skullcap, motherwort, cyathulae, eucommia, loranthus, polygoni, and China root.

─────────── ❋ EXERCISE ❋ ───────────

If you feel a migraine coming on, avoid rigorous exercise, as it may speed up the onset. A gentle 10-minute walk in the fresh air may help relieve stress and reduce the severity of your migraine. Otherwise, a regular regimen of moderate cardiovascular and stretching exercises can help maintain good health and proper circulation.

Daily meditation and tai chi exercises can also help prevent migraines. Here is a simple visualization meditation called White Light Meditation that I've taught to my patients.

Sit or lie down comfortably. Clear your mind, relax your body, and breathe deeply and slowly.

Inhale, and visualize a white light or clear mountain spring water entering your body at the top of your head and flowing down to your abdomen.

Exhale, and visualize the white light or water continuing its downward course from your abdomen to the bottom of your feet, where it drains out.

Repeat this visualization for 10 minutes. Do this meditation as often as necessary. Usually you will experience a quick reduction in symptoms right after completing the exercise.

⁕ ACUPRESSURE ⁕

• Locate the acupoint Wind Pond (GB-20), in the natural indentation at the base of your skull on both sides of your neck. Press and lift up toward the base of your skull with your thumbs and lean your head back. Use the weight of your head against your thumbs for steady pressure on the acupoint. Hold for 5 minutes, breathing deeply and slowly.

• Find the acupoint Greater Yang (Taiyang), in the indentation of the temples. Stimulate the point with the knuckles of your thumbs or the tips of your index fingers. Massage in a circular motion for 5 minutes.

• Find the acupoint Valley of Harmony (LI-4) at the web between your right thumb and index finger. Apply steady pressure with your left thumb until you feel soreness. Hold for 2 minutes. Repeat on the left hand.

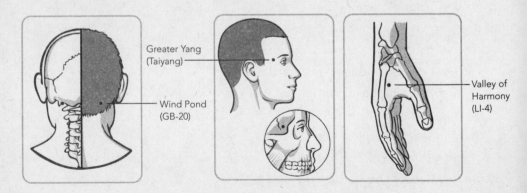

Greater Yang (Taiyang)

Wind Pond (GB-20)

Valley of Harmony (LI-4)

• Make sure that there are no structural imbalances in your spine, neck, or jaw, as these conditions can exacerbate headaches. Structural adjustments may be helpful—consult a chiropractor or osteopath.

AVOID

• Monosodium glutamate (MSG) and aspartame and other artificial sweeteners and preservatives, as they can trigger migraines.

....

• Abrupt alcohol and caffeine withdrawal or missing meals, which can trigger migraines. Contraceptive pills can also cause migraine headaches in some women.

 ## MORNING SICKNESS

IN ABOUT 80 PERCENT OF WOMEN, the elation of being pregnant is soon brought down to earth with sickness—morning sickness—in which nausea, abdominal discomfort, dizziness, lightheadedness, and sometimes vomiting occur throughout the day, not just in the early morning hours. Morning sickness usually goes away by the second trimester of pregnancy, and by itself does not indicate serious illness, but it can have adverse effects on the nutrition of the mother and the fetus, as appetite and nutrient consumption may fall below the required levels.

Acupuncture is probably the most effective non-drug-based therapy for nausea. The National Institutes of Health recognizes acupuncture's efficacy for treating nausea. Many pregnant women—especially those suffering from morning sickness and breach presentation—are referred to acupuncture practitioners by ob-gyn physicians. Often acupuncture, along with dietary changes and the use of mild herbs to settle the stomach, is the only treatment that can help relieve the symptoms. If you are throwing up, you must replenish fluids constantly to avoid dehydration. Make sure your obstetrician properly monitors you during your whole pregnancy.

Below are some remedies for you to try on your own at home.

—————————————— ❊ DIET ❊ ——————————————

• Eat a huge variety of foods and try new foods as often as you like, as appetite can be fickle during pregnancy. Make sure you get adequate protein, including choices such as chicken, turkey, lamb, and eggs, as well as healthful sources of fats, such as nuts and seeds, flaxseed oil, and olive oil. Adequate fiber is important to keep digestion regular, so load up on whole grains such as oats, oat bran, brown rice, millet, quinoa, amaranth, and buckwheat, and fruits such as berries, papaya, bananas, figs, apples, and prunes. Beans and legumes provide excellent whole nutrients and should occupy a large part of a pregnancy diet.

• Try incorporating fresh ginger, with its ability to settle the stomach and relieve nausea, into your diet.

• Don't overeat or skip meals, as both are harmful and can worsen the condition. Eat smaller, more frequent meals and stay away from greasy, fatty foods and heavy meats.

————————— ❊ HOME REMEDIES ❊ —————————

• Make a tea from 3 slices of fresh ginger and a piece of dried tangerine or orange peel by boiling in 3 1/2 cups of water for 20 minutes. Strain, and drink 3 or 4 cups a day.

• Juice 1 medium potato in a juicer or a blender, pass through a strainer, and mix the juice with 1 cup of warm water. Drink on an empty stomach in the morning upon waking. The potato juice will coat your stomach and reduce acid.

• Place some crackers by your bed at night and eat a few upon waking before getting out of bed to soak up excess stomach acid.

• Cook 1 cup each lentils and rice in ample water in a slow cooker overnight and eat it as a hot morning cereal.

─────────── ❋ DAILY SUPPLEMENTS ❋ ───────────

• Taking vitamin B_6 (50 milligrams) can reduce the severity of morning sickness.

• Vitamins K (80 milligrams) and C (1,000 milligrams), when taken together, can help relieve symptoms of nausea.

• Folic acid (2,000 micrograms) is important during pregnancy for prevention of birth defects. It is also an important supplement for digestive health.

• Prenatal vitamins are important to ensure adequate nutrition during pregnancy, especially for those who throw up or have a poor appetite. Try several brands to determine which settles in your stomach the best.

• L-methionine (500 milligrams) can also help in preventing nausea.

─────────── ❋ HERBAL THERAPY ❋ ───────────

• Herbs can be found in health food or vitamin stores, online, and at the offices of Chinese medicine practitioners. Herbs should be used according to individual needs; consult with a licensed practitioner for a customized formulation. To learn more about the herbs listed here, go to www.askdrmao.com.

• Make a tea by boiling 1/2 cup dried chamomile and 3 slices ginger in 3 1/2 cups water for 20 minutes. Strain and drink 3 cups daily, to treat morning sickness. This can help calm the stomach and reduce nausea and vomiting symptoms. Ginger can also be taken in capsule form (500 to 2,000 milligrams).

MORNING SICKNESS

• In Chinese medicine, herbs play an important role in pregnancy care. Those traditionally used for morning sickness include Chinese basil, ginger, giant hyssop, cardamom, bamboo, fermented soybean, and licorice.

❋ EXERCISE ❋

Moderate exercise, ideally walking for 15 minutes in the morning and the evening, is best. Strenuous exercise can exacerbate morning sickness. I also recommend a light sitting meditation to help calm the rebellious qi and stop nausea and vomiting. Do the following meditation once in the morning and once during the day.

Lie down on your back or sit comfortably with your spine erect at the edge of a chair. If you choose to sit, your feet should be flat on the floor, with your legs bent at a 90-degree angle.

Reach up toward the sky with both hands on a deep inhale. As you hold your breath, make tight fists and squeeze, tightening all the muscles in your arms. Slowly exhale, relaxing your arms and bringing your fists down to your chest. Repeat this several times.

Now cross your arms in front of your chest, with your fingers touching just under your collarbone and your wrists crossed at the center of your upper chest.

Lower your chin toward your chest.

Inhale 4 short breaths in a row (without exhaling) through your nose. Fill your lungs completely on the fourth breath. Hold the breath for a few seconds with the chest full and expanded.

Exhale slowly through your mouth.

Repeat this exercise for 2 or 3 minutes, concentrating on your deep and rhythmic breathing.

❋ ACUPRESSURE ❋

• Acupuncture is very effective in treating morning sickness. In severe cases, I've had patients come for treatment every other day to get quick relief. You may use acupressure as often as you need, and you'll see the benefits from regular use.

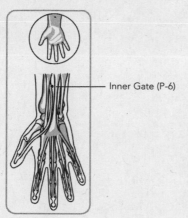

Inner Gate (P-6)

• Find the acupoint Inner Gate (P-6), three finger-widths above the wrist crease, between the two tendons on the inside of the left forearm. Apply moderate pressure with your right thumb. Hold for 3 minutes. Repeat on the right arm. This relieves nausea and vomiting, and reduces anxiety. Do this as often as needed, or you can buy a device that is worn on the wrist to stimulate this acupoint.

AVOID

• Coffee, alcohol and sweets, as they can aggravate morning sickness.

• Being overtired. Rest and sleep are very important, so get at least eight hours of sleep a day.

• Overeating, or going without meals for long periods of time.

MUSCLE PAIN AND SPASM

THE MORE THAN 600 MUSCLES IN YOUR BODY, whether responsible for gross movements like walking or fine, coordinated movements like smiling, are all subject to pain and spasm. Spasm occurs when a muscle contracts but fails to extend back to its original resting position. Spasms are common in adults and often occur at night. Large muscles are more susceptible to spasms, thus they occur more in the legs, abdomen, and sometimes in the back. Muscle cramps and pains occur in early childhood, as well—when they're commonly referred to as growing pains—and they can be very painful. Athletes get muscle cramps when their muscles are required to perform sudden, heavy workloads

MUSCLE PAIN AND SPASM

without proper warm-up. Inactivity, anemia, tobacco use, inflammation, hormonal imbalances, arthritis, arteriosclerosis, dehydration, and hypothyroidism are some of the causes of muscle pain and spasms.

Spasms are caused by an imbalance of the electrolytes calcium, magnesium, and potassium in the muscle tissue. Chronic alcoholics can suffer debilitating muscle spasms as a result of a severe depletion of the body's key electrolytes. Pain and muscle spasms can also be caused by lactic acid or toxin buildup as a result of muscle metabolism, viral infection, or muscle tears from injuries. Most spasms aren't life threatening and often go away without treatment, but they can be treated with muscle relaxants, analgesics, or anti-inflammation drugs. Physical therapists use massage, ultrasound, ice and heat therapy, and exercise for muscle spasms, with pretty good results. If pain and cramping are constant during the day, you should see a physician, as this may be a sign of peripheral circulation problems such as arteriosclerosis.

In Chinese medicine, the liver-gallbladder network is responsible for nourishing the tendons and ligaments of the body. Most muscular disorders are attributed to liver energy stagnation and its inability to clear the body of toxins. Treatment of muscle pain and spasms involves restoring liver energy flow and removing any blockages. It is well documented that muscle pain responds to acupuncture. With several treatments most acute muscle spasms can be relieved quickly. In chronic pain conditions in which there are underlying deficiencies, I incorporate herbal formulations to invigorate the blood, restore electrolyte balance, relax the muscles, and relieve stagnation. I may also use cupping to increase blood flow throughout the muscle, bodywork to stretch and soothe the muscle knots formed by chronic spasms, and moxibustion, which involves heating the acupoint with the herb mugwort. On occasion, postural adjustment will take care of recurring pain. For example, a graphic artist came to me with a shoulder problem that he had suffered with for over two years. A few weeks into his treatment I asked him to show me how he works at his computer. It became obvious to me that he had his mouse pad too high relative to his seat, so I suggested he lower his mouse to below his desktop, allowing his right arm to relax with his elbow bent at a 90-degree angle rather than a 45-degree angle. To his amazement, his shoulder pain vanished a few days after he changed his work position.

❊ DIET ❊

• Favor foods that are particularly good for supporting muscle healing, such as leafy green vegetables rich in minerals, including spinach, collard greens, Swiss chard, mustard greens, dandelion greens, parsley, and cabbage. Fruits with natural anti-inflammatory nutrients like cherries, grapes, papaya, pineapples, and kiwi are a must. Herbs and spices that activate blood flow include cayenne, cinnamon, turmeric, and ginger. Scallions, chives, leeks, and horseradish are also mild analgesics.

• Avoid alcohol, caffeine, sugar, smoking, and stress. Strong emotions like anger and anxiety can block the liver and cause stagnation of its energy, predisposing you to muscle tension and cramps.

❊ HOME REMEDIES ❊

• For acute back injury, apply an ice pack to the painful area for 15 to 20 minutes, 2 to 3 times a day, during the first 24 to 48 hours.

• Take hot Epsom salt baths for 20 minutes a day until the pain is substantially decreased.

• Make a natural anti-inflammatory cocktail by mixing equal parts of unsweetened black cherry juice with dark grape juice. Drink 3 to 6 glasses a day until the pain has eased.

MUSCLE PAIN AND SPASM

• Make a tea from 1 teaspoon each of cinnamon, turmeric, chamomile, and licorice boiled in 4 cups of water for 30 minutes. The tea is good for temporary relief from muscle pain and spasms. Drink 3 or more cups a day.

✳ DAILY SUPPLEMENTS ✳

• Calcium (1,000 milligrams), magnesium (500 milligrams), and potassium (25 milligrams) are essential components for muscle movement, and deficiencies can cause cramps. Proper supplementation can help restore the balance and prevent cramps.

• The enzyme bromelain (450 milligrams), from pineapple, is a natural anti-inflammatory and helps counter muscle and joint pain.

• Vitamin B complex and folate (400 micrograms) are generally diminished with stress and pain, so supplementation can help ease the symptoms.

• Omega-3 fatty acids (1,000 milligrams EPA; 800 milligrams DHA) in fish oil and the antioxidants in vitamin E (800 IU) are helpful for supporting healthy blood circulation and reducing inflammation and pain.

✳ HERBAL THERAPY ✳

• Herbs can be found in health food or vitamin stores, online, and at the offices of Chinese medicine practitioners. Herbs should be used according to individual needs; consult with a licensed practitioner for a customized formulation. To learn more about the herbs listed here, go to www.askdrmao.com.

• Turmeric, white willow bark, and valerian work in conjunction to alleviate inflammation and pain.

• Black haw, horsetail, and Jamaican dogwood are good muscle relaxants, and devil's claw and St.-Johns-wort have anti-inflammatory and analgesic properties.

• Traditional Chinese herbs used for back pain and back health include angelica root, red peony, eucommia, siler, notoginseng, gastrodia, clematis, corydalis, myrrh, frankincense, rehmannia and achyranthes.

✳ EXERCISE ✳

Muscles must be used regularly in order to maintain their vitality and flexibility. Leading a sedentary life is a sure way of predisposing yourself to muscle tension and cramps. Exercise for muscle pain and spasms should focus more on stretching and flexibility and less on strengthening and bulking up. When stretching, never stress the muscle beyond what is comfortable. If it starts to hurt, stop. Always warm up prior to any exercise. Skipping the warm-up is a major cause of muscle strain and sprain. The Eight Treasures Qi Gong exercises help strengthen the tendons and ligaments and increase flexibility without excess stress on the joints. The Fourth Treasure, called the Weeping Willow Shivers in the Morning Breeze, focuses on stretching and relaxing the major muscles of the head, neck, torso, and lower limbs. Practice this sequence twice daily for best results.

In a quiet, comfortable environment, preferably outdoors, stand with your feet shoulder-width apart, knees slightly bent, spine erect, tailbone tucked in, and head tilted slightly forward. Drape your arms at your sides, with your shoulders relaxed.

Begin with rhythmic, slow, and relaxed breathing. Inhale deeply but softly, and imagine your breath extending all the way down to your lower abdomen, about two finger-widths below the navel. Exhale gently and softly. Stay in this position for 7 breath cycles, relaxing and calming your mind.

Now, begin the exercise. You'll be making concentric circular rotations of the major muscles of the head, neck, torso, and lower limbs.

On an inhale, slowly rotate your head one half-circle, then exhale to complete the other half-circle. Do this first clockwise for 3 rotations, then counterclockwise for 3 rotations. Do not strain the muscles.

On an inhale, place your arms above and slightly behind your hips. Begin rotating your hips in a hula-hoop fashion around your pelvis, first in a clockwise direction for 3 rotations, then in a counterclockwise direction for 3 rotations, swaying the body and making the circles as full and as concentric as possible.

Inhale, and draw your feet together with your ankles touching and your knees slightly bent. Bend down and place your palms on top of your knees. Begin making concentric circles with your knees, first clockwise, then counterclockwise. Complete 3 rotations in each direction. Rest your palms against your knees during each brief transitional pause.

Next, make opposing circles with your right and left knees. With your right knee, makes clockwise circles; with your left knee, make counterclockwise circles. Again, repeat for 3 rotations, supporting your knee joints with your hands.

Repeat the previous step with your knees moving in the opposite direction, your right knee making counterclockwise circles, your left knee making clockwise circles.

Return to a standing posture.

Next, raise your right leg off the ground, with your knee slightly bent. Gently shake your leg as though you were shivering. Feel the shiver extend all the way to your foot, relaxing your leg muscles as you shake.

Repeat the shaking with your left leg.

Return to a standing position to conclude the exercise.

❈ ACUPRESSURE ❈

• For muscle cramping of the lower back, gluteal region, and upper thighs, find the acupoint Jumping Circle (GB-30), on the center of the buttocks about midway between the tip of the coccyx and the left hipbone. Position a golf ball on the acupoint and sit on your bed. Press against the ball with your body weight until you feel soreness. Hold for 30 seconds and release. Repeat several times, alternating on the left and right sides. This relaxes muscle spasms, increases joint mobility, and also releases sadness.

. . . .

• For spasms and muscle pain in the lower legs and back, activate the acupoint Yang Spring (GB-34), on the outer part of the lower right leg, just below the bony structure located near the end of the knee crease, about four finger-widths below the kneecap. Apply steady pressure with your right thumb until you feel soreness. Hold for 3 minutes. Repeat on the left leg.

....

• For spasms and muscle pain in the upper extremities, find the acupoint Valley of Harmony (LI-4) in the web between your right thumb and index finger. Apply steady pressure with your left thumb until you feel soreness. Hold for 2 minutes. Repeat on the left hand.

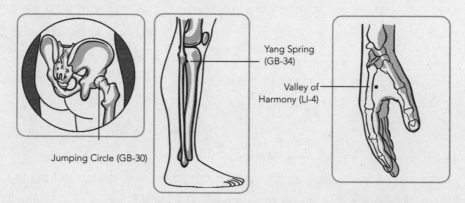

Jumping Circle (GB-30)

Yang Spring (GB-34)

Valley of Harmony (LI-4)

AVOID

• Smoking and excessive use of alcohol. They are irritants, and alcohol depletes the liver energy, leaving tendons and ligaments weak and malnourished.

....

• Certain medications used for weight loss, such as orlistat, as they can reduce levels of fat-soluble essential nutrients because they prevent the absorption of fats in the intestines.

....

• Jumping right back into an exercise program. As you begin an exercise program, be sure to begin gradually and increase over a period of time. Don't assume you can perform at the level you last left off—this is a sure way of triggering a cramp or two.

NAUSEA

NEEDING TO THROW UP PROBABLY RANKS as one of the worst feelings we experience in life. Nausea is not a disease itself but a symptom of many medical conditions, some related to the nervous system and others to the stomach and digestive tract. Nausea is also commonly experienced as a side effect of many drugs, including chemotherapy medications. Morning sickness is a common symptom of pregnancy. Prolonged nausea, if accompanied by vomiting, can cause rapid dehydration, which depletes the body of vital electrolytes and should be addressed immediately. Most cases of nausea are either due to a stomach flu, food poisoning, or motion sickness.

In Chinese medicine, the energies of the body have a specific rhythm and flow. The stomach energy normally flows downward; when it fails to flow in the proper direction and reverses upward, you experience nausea and vomiting. Treating the stomach and digestive tract is key to symptomatic relief, but to resolve the condition the underlying cause must be addressed. Acupuncture is one of the most effective drug-free therapies, and the National Institutes of Health recognizes the efficacy of acupuncture for treating nausea. I've treated many patients for nausea caused by stomach flu, migraine headaches, and the side effects of chemotherapy. Success rests on calming the rebellious energy and harmonizing the stomach with acupuncture and herbal remedies.

Here are some of my favorite home remedies for nausea. If you experience continuous vomiting or unexplained nausea, consult your physician or go to the emergency room immediately.

☀ DIET ☀

• Food plays a key role in digestive system balance. Ginger tops the list of foods to consume for relief of nausea. Stick with clear liquids and avoid heavy and rich foods. Eat wholesome foods containing no preservatives or additives and that have not been sprayed with pesticides. Eat smaller meals more frequently. Favor papayas and pineapples, as they contain bromelain, a digestive enzyme that can help counter indigestion. Eat more yams, potatoes, brown rice, oats, pearl barley, sweet rice, daikon radish, basil, parsley, sage, black sesame seeds, and apples. Drink at least six 8-ounce glasses of room temperature or slightly cool water a day. Sucking on an ice cube can give temporary relief from nausea.

• Do not overeat. Avoid cold or raw foods and spicy foods. Dairy products are hard to digest and should be avoided. Foods high in saturated fats and greasy and fried foods can also distress the stomach and digestive system. Eat unseasoned or mild foods; avoid foods with peppers, onions, and garlic.

❈ HOME REMEDIES ❈

• Make a ginger tea by slicing fresh ginger into 2-inch-long slices and boiling it in 1 cup of water for 5 minutes. Strain, and sip the tea slowly. Drink the tea as often as you need to keep the nausea away. You can sweeten the tea with honey if you find the ginger too spicy.

• Make cinnamon and clove tea by adding 2 cinnamon sticks and 1 teaspoon of ground cloves to 3 cups of water and boiling for 15 minutes. Strain, and drink 3 cups a day. This tea is great in the evenings, as it warms you from the inside and can give you a good night's sleep.

• For morning sickness, have soda crackers ready on your nightstand and eat some upon waking in the morning before getting out of bed to soak up excess stomach acid and help keep nausea to a minimum.

• Slowly sip plain sparkling mineral water or soda water to settle your stomach.

NAUSEA

• Put 5 drops of peppermint oil in a pot of hot water. Place a towel over your head and the pot, and breathe deeply to calm and settle your stomach.

❋ DAILY SUPPLEMENTS ❋

• Vitamin B_6 (50 milligrams) can help alleviate nausea, including morning sickness.

• Vitamin K (200 milligrams) plus vitamin C (1,000 milligrams) can help subdue nausea. (Note that vitamin K can interact with blood-thinning medications—consult your physician.)

• L-methionine (500 milligrams three times a day) can help prevent nausea.

❋ HERBAL THERAPY ❋

• Herbs can be found in health food or vitamin stores, online, and at the offices of Chinese medicine practitioners. Herbs should be used according to individual needs; consult with a licensed practitioner for a customized formulation. To learn more about the herbs listed here, go to www.ask drmao.com.

• Chamomile and ginger are good remedies for morning sickness. As a tea they can help calm the stomach and reduce nausea and vomiting symptoms. Ginger can also be taken in capsule form.

• Traditional Chinese herbs for treating nausea include Chinese basil, ginger, giant hyssop, cardamom, bamboo, fermented soybean, and licorice.

• Make a tea from tarragon and peppermint and sip as a beverage throughout the day.

❋ EXERCISE ❋

The following is a meditation exercise to help treat nausea. You can do it either standing or sitting. If your nausea gets worse, keep your eyes open during the exercise and concentrate on an object in front of you.

Stand or sit with your feet shoulder-width apart, knees bent slightly, spine erect, and arms hanging at your sides. Tilt your head slightly forward. Breathe slowly and deliberately.

Inhale, and gently raise your arms straight up above your head, with your palms facing the ground.

Exhale, and lower your hands as though you were pushing down a large helium-filled balloon.

Repeat the movement 20 times, then place your hands two finger-widths below the navel, with one hand on top of the other, and rub your abdomen in a circular, clockwise motion for 7 rotations.

Vigorously swish around any saliva that has gathered in your mouth. Swallow intently, visualizing the saliva going directly down to your lower abdomen.

※ ACUPRESSURE ※

• Find the acupoint Inner Gate (P-6), three finger-widths above the wrist crease, between the two tendons on the inside of the left forearm. Apply moderate pressure with your right thumb. Hold for 5 minutes. Repeat on the right arm.

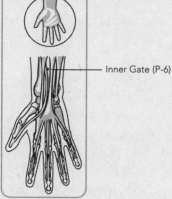

Inner Gate (P-6)

AVOID

• Many prescription and over-the-counter medications that cause nausea, in particular ibuprofen-containing medications such as Advil and Albuterol, and many antibiotics. Check with your doctor.

- Smoking and alcohol, as they irritate the stomach lining and can cause nausea.

- Overeating and lying down immediately after eating, which can cause nausea. Eating rich sauces and heavy foods can also contribute to nausea.

NOSEBLEED

NOSEBLEED, OR EPISTAXIS, AS IT IS KNOWN MEDICALLY, though alarming in appearance, is a relatively benign condition that affects over 45 million Americans. Nosebleeds often appear during the dry and cold autumn and winter months and can be caused by common colds, sinus infections, allergies, excessive use of nasal sprays, environmental irritants, and injuries. Hypertension, drug use, and taking over-the-counter medicines can also cause nosebleeds. The nasal cavities are lined with millions of tiny blood vessels, and they can bleed when injured. Most of the blood is released through the nostrils, but some can escape down the throat, causing an upset stomach. Acute nonstop or chronic nosebleeds require a visit to an ear, nose, and throat specialist for cauterization to stop the bleeding.

In Chinese medicine, bleeding has many origins. Nosebleeds can result from pathogenic heat in the blood, sinus infections, and spleen network weakness that leaves you deficient in bioflavonoids and prone to weakened blood vessels. When aggravated by anger, frustration, and bitterness the liver energy can flare upward and cause nosebleed. This is closely associated with nosebleeds caused by high blood pressure. An unhealthy diet can produce heat in the stomach, which manifests with gum inflammation and nosebleeds. In acute cases, I try to stop the bleeding with topical and oral herbal therapy coupled with acupuncture to lower pressure in the blood vessels. In chronic cases the best approach is to identify and address the underlying condition, whether the culprit is hypertension, allergies, or lifestyle.

Here are some recommendations I give to my patients. Consult with your physician immediately if you feel weak, dizzy, or faint, or if chest pains accompany the nosebleed.

———————————————— ✳ DIET ✳ ————————————————

• A generally healthy and balanced diet with smaller and more frequent meals and ample amounts of complex carbohydrates and wholesome protein sources is a good start. Favor celery, yarrow flower (make tea), bananas, sunflower seeds, honey, soy products, mung beans, bamboo shoots, seaweed, whole grains including buckwheat, and green leafy vegetables such as spinach, broccoli and kale. Dandelion greens, chrysanthemum flowers and cassia seeds (make tea), lotus root, and hawthorn berries (make tea) are also a good addition. Drink at least 8 cups of warm or room temperature water a day.

. . . .

• Avoid overeating and foods that are greasy, deep-fried, barbecued, or spicy. Alcohol and coffee dehydrate and produce dryness; they also induce heat and can cause a rise of yang energy to the head, potentially contributing to nosebleeds.

———————————— ✳ HOME REMEDIES ✳ ————————————

• Soak your feet in a hot foot bath for 20 minutes to guide the heat down and stop the bleeding.

. . . .

• Apply ice packs to the forehead just above the nose and also on the back of the head just inside the back hairline. Apply pressure at the bridge of the nose until the bleeding stops.

NOSEBLEED

• Insert a cotton ball soaked in witch hazel into the nostrils to stop bleeding. Witch hazel acts as an astringent.

———————————— ✳ DAILY SUPPLEMENTS ✳ ————————————

• Supplementing with beta-carotene (800 milligrams) and vitamin A (200 IU) supports the immune system's repair capabilities.

• Vitamin B complex, especially B_6 (50 milligrams), supports vascular health.

• Vitamin C (1,000 milligrams) and K (200 milligrams) can help improve clotting time and prevent excess bleeding.

———————————— ✳ HERBAL THERAPY ✳ ————————————

• Herbs can be found in health food or vitamin stores, online, and at the offices of Chinese medicine practitioners. Herbs should be used according to individual needs; consult with a licensed practitioner for a customized formulation. To learn more about the herbs listed here, go to www.ask drmao.com.

• Yarrow and liverwort tea can help prevent nosebleed.

• For nosebleed associated with colds, respiratory infections, and sinusitis, mulberry, chrysanthemum, imperata, reeds, mouton, gardenia, apricot seeds, platycodon, mint, and licorice are traditionally used.

• For nosebleed due to alcohol abuse, poor diet, or malnutrition, herbs traditionally used include rehmannia, ophiopogonis, anemarrhena, achyranthes, gardenia, and mouton.

• For nosebleed resulting from stress and emotional upset, herbs traditionally used include gentiana, rehmannia, gardenia, biota, cyathulae, alismatis, plantaginis, skullcap, mouton, angelica, and licorice.

During a nosebleed, stop all exercise. Otherwise, a regimen of daily qi gong and tai chi combined with moderate cardiovascular exercise is helpful. Stress can increase episodes of nosebleed, so I teach my patients this stress-release meditation. Follow the simple steps below.

Sit comfortably or lie down on your back. Slow your respiration to deep, abdominal breathing. Say the word "calm" in your mind with every exhalation. You'll be visualizing the relaxation of a body part and releasing tension with every exhalation. Trace the following 3 pathways outlined below.

Start at the top of your head. Inhale, and then exhale and visualize your scalp muscles relaxing. Say "calm" in your mind. Repeat this, saying the word with each body part as you move down through your face, throat, chest, abdomen, thighs, knees, calves, ankles, and feet. When you've relaxed your feet, visualize all the tension in your body leaving through your toes in the form of dark smoke.

Next start at the temple region of your head. This pathway focuses on the sides and upper extremities. Inhale, and then exhale and visualize your temple muscles relaxing. Say the word "calm" in your mind. Repeat this, saying the word with each body part as you move down through your jaw, the sides of your neck, shoulders, upper arms, elbows, forearms, wrists, and hands. Once you've relaxed your hands, visualize all the tension leaving your body through your fingertips in the form of dark smoke.

The final pathway begins on the back of your head. This path relaxes the back of your body. Repeat the breathing-visualization-word routine, as above, as you go from the back of your neck to your upper back, middle back, lower back, back of thighs, calves, and heels. Then focus on the acupoint Bubbling Spring (KID-1), on the soles of your feet, for 1 minute.

Practice this meditation for at least 15 minutes twice a day.

━━━━━━━━ ✳ ACUPRESSURE ✳ ━━━━━━━━

• Find the acupoint Valley of Harmony (LI-4), at the web between your right thumb and index finger. Apply steady pressure with your left thumb until you feel soreness. Hold for 2 minutes. Repeat on the left hand.

NOSEBLEED

• Locate the acupoint Upper Star (DU-23), in the center of the upper forehead, two finger-widths inside the front hairline. Apply steady pressure with your index or middle finger until you feel soreness. Hold for 2 minutes.

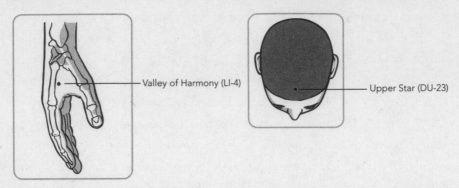

Valley of Harmony (LI-4)

Upper Star (DU-23)

AVOID

• Exposure to dry, dusty and cold conditions by using a warm mist humidifier at home or work. Try to avoid getting a cold or the flu and do not overuse nasal sprays, as they can irritate the nasal passages.

• Stress and overexertion, and keep your blood pressure under control.

OBESITY

FOR THE PAST DECADE THE NUMBER-ONE HEALTH CONCERN in the United States has been the rapidly increasing rate of obesity. Today eight out of ten adults are overweight and some 40 million people are considered obese. Many life-threatening ailments are attributed to obesity, including diabetes, hypertension, heart attack, coronary heart disease, stroke, depression, and the growing problem of infertility. More alarming is pediatric obesity, which has tripled in the last twenty years. Our children are at increasing risk of serious health problems, including insulin resistance, pediatric diabetes, depression, hypertension, developmental problems, and even cancer.

There are physiological and psychological reasons for obesity, but it's often a matter of energy intake versus energy expenditure. We've become extremely sedentary. The quality and quantity of the foods we eat has changed—food now contains tightly packed calories in smaller packages. Our drinks contain high concentrations of sugar, our meats have been treated with hormones and antibiotics, and our streets are littered with fast-food drive-through restaurants serving up heart attacks to go. Our eating habits have also changed. The family dining table has been replaced with individual serving trays positioned comfortably in front of the television, and on-the-go chow downs substitute for lunch and dinner. Breakfast has all but disappeared. All these factors are slowing down our metabolism. It's simple: When you take in too much energy but don't use it up, the body stores it for a rainy day.

Emotions play an important role in obesity as well. We've long known that emotions play a key role in disease. Our hormonal systems react to negative emotional states with the production and release of hormones that help us cope with stressful situations. These hormones are designed to protect the body from harm by shutting down or slowing down bodily functions in order to conserve energy. Thus the stress hormones slow down metabolism and promote the storage of fat. This worked well back when our ancestors were being chased by prey, but now our stressful lifestyle is contributing to the obesity epidemic. A constant state of anxiety and stress creates an imbalance of these hormones in the body, promoting weight gain.

It's not easy to lose weight and keep it off. Many obese people require medical attention and need to be guided in a structured weight loss program. In Chinese medicine, obesity is the accumulation of dampness and phlegm and the result of declining function of the spleen network and metabolic fire of the kidney network due to stress, lack of movement, and poor eating habits. The roles of nutrition, physical activity, and emotions on the body's metabolic functions cannot be over-stated. I work with endocrine and bariatric physicians to design individual weight-loss programs for patients. My treatment program for obesity entails acupuncture and herbal therapies to restore healthy digestion and metabolism and to eliminate dampness and mucus from the body. It also includes Swimming Dragon, a qi gong exercise, and meditation to activate energy flow, besides the diet suggestions below. A study of twenty of our patients on the weight-loss program described above showed an average loss of nineteen over three months.

Here are some simple suggestions that can get you started on your own weight-management program.

───────────────────── ✳ DIET ✳ ─────────────────────

• There are hundreds of fad diet programs out there, ranging from total starvation to high-protein diets promising quick fixes. The problem with dieting is that it deprives the body of food or goes to extremes with a few recommended foods. This is contradictory to our metabolism, and often the results do not last, producing a yo-yo effect and further depressing self-esteem, not to mention metabolic function. We are natural beings requiring a balance of nutrition from all sources.

• I recommend a balanced diet rich in wholesome organic foods, with no preservatives, additives, or artificial colors or flavors. Institute an eating schedule with five small meals each day. Eat sitting down at the table and eat slowly. Do not eat after 7:00 p.m., and do not skip breakfast.

• Diet should consist of a balance of organic sources of lean animal protein, complex carbohydrates, whole grains, legumes, nuts, and fruits and vegetables. Substitute brown rice, bulgur, millet, and buckwheat for white rice and pasta. Favor chlorophyll-rich foods such as broccoli, kale, spinach, asparagus, and dandelion greens. Consume more fruits and nuts, including apples, peaches, cherries, bananas, pomegranates, chestnuts, and pine nuts. Drink at least eight glasses of hot or lukewarm water a day.

• Avoid very spicy foods, as they tend to increase appetite; heavy, starchy foods; simple sugars; and fatty, greasy foods, which cause stagnation. Dairy products, especially cheese, produce dampness and mucus and should be avoided. Sweets of all kinds should be eliminated. Alcohol, soda, and coffee should also be eliminated.

• Do not eat when you are stressed, anxious, or emotional. Practice stress-release meditations or go for a walk. Eating should be a pleasurable event to be savored. Slow down your eating and chew your food well, and you will find that you eat less.

———————— ✳ HOME REMEDIES ✳ ————————

• Replace white sugar with natural alternatives such as stevia or brown rice syrup.

• Drink 2 tablespoons of apple cider vinegar with 1 teaspoon of maple syrup mixed in 12 ounces of warm water every morning on an empty stomach to promote digestion and increase metabolism.

• Instead of reaching for those cookies, create a low-fat trail mix including raw almonds, pumpkin seeds, prunes, and dried apples to eat in between meals to keep your blood sugar even and avoid being famished by lunch or dinner.

• Drink hot water with lemon slices as a beverage throughout the day and before eating to help reduce fluid retention and drain dampness.

• Substitute green or black tea for coffee, as tea contains beneficial polyphenol antioxidants and less caffeine.

---------------------- ✳ DAILY SUPPLEMENTS ✳ ----------------------

• Supplementing with chromium (200 micrograms) can help stabilize blood sugar by increasing cell sensitivity to insulin, which prevents excess blood sugar from being turned into body fat.

• Digestive enzymes such as pancreatin (500 milligrams), lipase, (1,000 IU), and amylase (1,500 IU) taken before each meal can reduce appetite.

• Vitamin B complex and kelp can help reduce water retention.

---------------------- ✳ HERBAL THERAPY ✳ ----------------------

• Herbs can be found in health food or vitamin stores, online, and at the offices of Chinese medicine practitioners. Herbs should be used according to individual needs; consult with a licensed practitioner for a customized formulation. To learn more about the herbs listed here, go to www.askdrmao.com.

• Dandelion greens can be helpful to regulate metabolism and aid in weight reduction, especially if the weight gain is a result of water retention.

• Garcinia cambogia (Malabar tamarind) contains hydroxycitric acid, which has been shown to inhibit fat production and decrease appetite in animals.

• Traditional Chinese herbs for weight management include lotus leaf, green tea, chrysanthemum, Chinese honey locust, atractylodis, astragalus, ginseng, and schizandra fruits. These herbs have metabolic-stimulating properties.

---------------------- ✳ EXERCISE ✳ ----------------------

The number one cause of obesity is inactivity. The human body is designed for physical activity. Our ancestors were hunter-gatherers. They spent most of their natural lives walking long distances to gather food, chase prey, and sometimes be chased as prey. Evolution shaped our metabolic functions for a life on the move, but today we live in opposition to our nature. Most diets fail because we do the opposite of what our bodies are designed for. They aren't designed to subsist on meager foods. They are designed to consume a good amount of energy—and then to burn that energy. Physical activity—not necessarily exercise—is the key to a healthy metabolism. These simple changes can increase activity, helping to speed up metabolism and burn excess calories:

• Take the stairs instead of the escalator or elevator.

• Do your own gardening, or rake your yard once a week.

• Deliberately park far away from your destination.

• Go window shopping at the mall, walking the entire place.

• Get a membership at the local zoo or museums, and take your children there often.

• Step outside during your break at work and take a walk around the building.

The best way to become physically active is to use those evolutionary wonders called legs. Walk as often and for as long as you can. Walk slowly, walk briskly, or just walk. Institute a weekly walkathon or join a local hiking club. You'll be amazed at the beautiful nature you'll find in your neighborhood. Walk for 100 paces after each meal, and start your day or finish your day with a brisk 30-minute walk—this alone can have a wondrous affect on your energy metabolism and will help you get back into shape. Here is a simple qi gong exercise, the Swimming Dragon, that can help speed up your metabolism and reduce your appetite.

This exercise resembles a belly dance—It is a wriggling rhythmic dance of the torso, and it burns energy and promotes fat burning in the abdomen.

OBESITY

In a comfortable, quiet place, stand with your feet together and ankles touching, or as close together as you can get them. Place your hands over your head, with your palms together and fingers pointing up. Be sure to keep your palms together during the entire exercise.

Inhale, and push your waist out to the right side while keeping your head and upper torso straight. Simultaneously move your right elbow to the right, so that it rests at shoulder height.

Exhale, and push your waist out to the left side while keeping your head and upper torso straight. Simultaneously move your left elbow fully to the left, so that it rests at shoulder height.

Repeat this movement several more times. Every time you move your waist to the right, bend your knees a little more, lowering your entire body as you squat. Be sure to keep your upper torso and head straight. As you lower your body, move your hands lower, keeping your palms together and fingers pointing up. When your arms reach your chest, turn your fingers toward the ground and continue the movement.

When your arms reach your knees, you should be squatting. Continue the movements, now rising with each right movement until you reach the standing position. When your arms reach your chest, switch the direction of your fingers so that they're pointing up again.

Throughout this exercise, your hands should make an S-shaped movement and your body should do a rhythmic belly dance. Remember to inhale on the rightward movement and exhale to the left.

Do this exercise during the day on an empty stomach. Begin slowly and increase the speed and vigor, warming up the whole body, but not to the point of perspiration. Practice for 15 to 20 minutes, twice a day, for maximum benefit.

❋ ACUPRESSURE ❋

• Find the acupoint Foot Three Miles (ST-36), four finger-widths below the kneecap on the right leg. Apply moderate pressure with your right thumb until you feel soreness. Hold for 2 minutes. Repeat on the left leg.

• Find the acupoint Abundant Flesh (ST-40), midway between the bottom of the right kneecap and the outer anklebone, two finger-widths to the outside of the shinbone. Apply steady pressure with your right thumb until you feel soreness. Hold for 2 minutes. Repeat on the left leg.

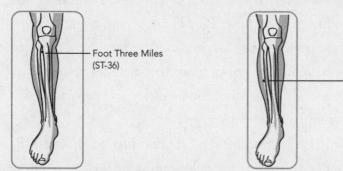

Foot Three Miles
(ST-36)

Abundant Flesh (ST-40)

—————— AVOID ——————

• Sweets and simple sugars, as they pack on the calories and slow down metabolism.

• Alcohol, as it not only increases appetite but also contains a lot of sugar, which ends up deposited as fat.

• Stress and emotional upset, which release stress hormones that can slow down metabolism and promote fat storage.

• Eating after 7 p.m., as it stores most if not all of the energy as fat, especially if you are headed to bed right after eating.

PAINFUL BLADDER SYNDROME

KNOWN AS INTERSTITIAL CYSTITIS (IC) or painful bladder syndrome, this condition is a combination of chronic reoccurring symptoms such as frequent urination with a sense of urgency, sometimes accompanied by burning and pain during urination. About 90 percent of the 1 million Americans diagnosed with IC are women. The most common risk factors include chronic urinary tract infections, and a history of gyne-cological surgeries. IC almost always involves one or more additional chronic conditions such as irritable bowel syndrome, lupus, or allergies. Recent findings show that stress, anxiety, and being overworked often aggravate the condition. Over time, IC can cause permanent damage to the bladder wall, resulting in scarring and ulcerations, which can require surgical intervention. Typical treatment includes oral antihis-tamines, pain and anti-inflammatory medications, and heparin deriv-atives to coat the lining of the bladder.

Like other "irritable" syndromes, painful bladder syndrome is di-rectly linked to an overstressed or overactive immune system. Chinese medicine focuses on identifying lifestyle, diet, environmental, and emotional contributions to the condition. I recall a female patient who suffered from interstitial cystitis for over ten years. After an extensive interview, I could see that her bladder would flare up every time she got emotionally upset—which was just about every other day. Since her urine tests were consistently free of infection, I thought that she might be experiencing spasms of the urethra, the tube that moves urine from the bladder to the vagina. So my approach in her case, as in many oth-ers, was to address her emotional problems while offering acupunc-ture to relieve the spasms and herbal therapy to help support healthy bladder and urethra functions. I also advised her on proper eating habits and stress reduction, and gave her tools such as stress-release meditation to help balance her emotions.

––––––––––––––––––––––––––––––– ❋ DIET ❋ –––––––––––––––––––––––––––––––

• Maintain a diet on the bland side, focusing on vegetables, fruits, whole grains, and fish. Watermelon, pears, carrots, celery, mung beans, adzuki beans, corn, millet, barley, oats, squash, cantaloupe, lotus root, loquats, cranberries, strawberries, grapes, guava, mangoes, and pineapple are good choices.

• Avoid all simple sugars, soft drinks, sweetened juices, fatty meats, and dairy products. Onions, scallions, ginger, black pepper, and other spicy foods can aggravate the condition. Alcohol, spices, chocolate, and caffeine, often contribute to bladder irritation and inflammation. Highly acidic foods, including carbonated beverages, tomatoes, citrus fruits and beverages, and vinegar can aggravate interstitial cystitis. It is important to identify the specific foods that cause irritation and eliminate them from your diet, as these vary from person to person.

❊ HOME REMEDIES ❊

• Drinking 3 cups of unsweetened cranberry juice a day during a flare-up can prevent bacteria from adhering to the walls of the urinary tract. Drink 1 cup a day for prevention.

• Drink freshly squeezed watermelon juice or watermelon seed tea. Boil 1/3 cup watermelon seeds in 3 1/2 cups of water for 30 minutes. Strain. Drink 3 cups daily.

• Drink corn silk tea instead of water during flare-ups. Boil a handful of corn silk in 3 1/2 cups water for 30 minutes. Strain. Drink 3 cups a day.

• A hot sitz bath with Epsom salts can provide temporary relief of pain and discomfort.

❊ DAILY SUPPLEMENTS ❊

• Taking vitamin C (1,000 milligram) and bioflavonoids (2,000 milligrams) is helpful for healthy immune function and is antibacterial.

• Beta-carotene (2,500 milligrams) and zinc (50 milligrams) support healthy immune function and promote healing of mucous membranes.

• Taking probiotics such as acidophilus (3 to 5 billion organisms) can help to maintain healthy immunity in the mucous membranes.

PAINFUL BLADDER SYNDROME

❋ HERBAL THERAPY ❋

• Herbs can be found in health food or vitamin stores, online, and at the offices of Chinese medicine practitioners. Herbs should be used according to individual needs; consult with a licensed practitioner for a customized formulation. To learn more about the herbs listed here, go to www.ask drmao.com.

. . . .

• Buchu, honeybush, uva ursi, thyme and parsley are used for urinary tract conditions. Corn silk and couch grass help soothe the inflammation and ease urination. Horsetail and plantain can help heal the tissue, and goldenseal combined with coneflower is effective in treating chronic infections.

. . . .

• Traditional, Chinese herbs used to support healthy urinary tract function include plantago, akebia, dianthus, water plantain, polyporus, peony, gardenia, and astragalus.

❋ EXERCISE ❋

Tai chi and qi gong can help reduce stress and negative emotions, strengthen immunity, and increase energy. With regular practice, you can harmonize your immune response and reduce the symptoms of interestitial cystitis. The following is a general stress release meditation.

Lie down on your back or sit comfortably with your spine erect at the edge of a chair. If you choose to sit, your feet should be flat on the floor, with your legs bent at a 90-degree angle.

Reach up toward the sky with both hands on a deep inhale. As you hold your breath make tight fists and squeeze, tightening all the muscles in your arms. Slowly exhale, relaxing your arms and bringing your fists down to your chest. Repeat this several times.

Now cross your arms in front of your chest, with your fingers touching just under your collarbone and your wrists crossed at the center of your upper chest.

Lower your chin toward your chest.

Inhale 4 short breaths in a row (without exhaling) through your nose. Fill your lungs completely on the fourth breath. Hold the breath for a few seconds with the chest full and expanded.

Exhale slowly through your mouth.

Repeat this exercise for 2 or 3 minutes, 3 times daily, engaging deep and rhythmic breathing.

※ ACUPRESSURE ※

• Find the acupoint Three Yin Crossing (SP-6), four finger-widths above the inner anklebone, in the depression near the bone on the right leg. Apply steady pressure with your right thumb until you feel soreness. Hold for 3 minutes. Repeat on the left leg.

• Find the acupoint Pure Spring (KID-5), one finger-width below the midpoint of the inner anklebone on the inside of the right foot. This point is tender to the touch. Apply pressure with the tip of your right index finger or thumb until you feel soreness. Hold for 2 minutes. Repeat on the left foot.

• Engaging these points benefits the urinary system and helps modulate the immune system.

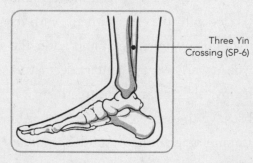

Three Yin Crossing (SP-6)

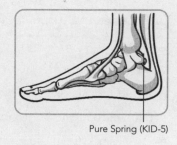

Pure Spring (KID-5)

AVOID

• Alcohol, coffee, and smoking, as they can aggravate the symptoms of interstitial cystitis.

PAINFUL BLADDER SYNDROME

- Stress, anger, and emotional upset, as they can weaken the immune system and produce inflammatory heat in the body.

....

- Being overtired—get plenty of sleep and don't overwork or exhaust yourself, as this weakens the immune system and worsens the condition.

❧ POISON IVY AND POISON OAK ❧

POISONS OAK, POISON IVY, AND POISON SUMAC are species of plants that contain an oily chemical known as urushiol, which is very irritating to the skin and produces a severe allergic reaction in some people. About 15 to 30 percent of the population is immune to urushiol-induced allergies. Those who aren't experience progressively worsening symptoms of itching, redness, and skin oozing accompanied by severe burning pain at the site of contact. It usually takes up to two weeks to resolve the condition, and most of the time it leaves no scars or complications. Itching is the primary concern, since prolonged scratching ulcerates the skin, exposing it to secondary infections.

The skin is the body's largest organ. One of its roles is immune protection, and it acts as an interface with the environment, with its millions of tiny pores through which substances exit and enter the body. In Chinese medicine, poison ivy and related contact dermatitis reactions are classified as toxic fire invading the skin. The treatment approach is to clear the toxin and relieve the symptoms. A neighbor of mine was hiking in the local mountains when he had a sudden sinus allergy attack and started to drain from his nose. He didn't have any tissues with him so he reached for a palm-sized leaf to use to blow his nose. Unfortunately, he used a poison ivy leaf. When I saw him that evening, despite having used antihistamines, he had welts and a rash covering his whole face and hands. He couldn't breathe through his nose because it was swollen shut. The itch was unbearable. I went to my backyard, pulled up a couple of dandelion plants, and put them into a blender with honey and the gel scraped from an aloe leaf. I smeared the poultice all over his face, and I sent him home with dandelions to make into a tea. It wasn't a pretty sight, but next morning his itching and rash were 75 percent better.

Below is a summary of my approach to treating skin allergies and inflammations.

✳ DIET ✳

• Emphasize foods with cooling and cleansing properties, including cucumbers, collard greens, Swiss chard, kale, mustard greens, carrots, celery, broccoli, dandelion greens, mung beans, seaweed, pearl barley, oats, adzuki beans, corn silk, water chestnuts, winter melon, watermelon, brewer's yeast, olives, raspberries, raisins, and grapes. Fish is rich in omega-3 fatty acids, which can nourish the skin. Water is essential for cleansing the body. People who drink at least eight glasses of water a day tend to have better bowel habits and develop fewer allergic reactions.

• Eliminate processed foods, foods containing artificial additives, simple sugars and bleached flour, soft drinks, and spicy, hot, fried, and greasy foods. Avoid dairy products, eggs, shellfish, wheat, tomatoes, eggplant, peanuts, and soy products (such as hydrolyzed soy protein, found in meat substitutes, and protein bars, and powder supplements), which can irritate the skin.

✳ HOME REMEDIES ✳

• Wash the suspected contact area thoroughly with soap and water. It is important to use soap to remove urushiol, as it is an oily substance and water alone will not remove it.

• Crush some dandelion greens and apply to the affected area as a poultice, changing every hour. You can also put the dandelion greens into a blender with 1 cup fresh dandelion greens, 1/2 cup aloe vera gel, and 1 tablespoon honey to make a smoother poultice.

• Apply calamine lotion to the affected area to soothe itching.

• Generously apply aloe vera gel directly from the plant to the affected area to lessen the symptoms of burning, itching, and pain.

• Boil 2 tablespoons licorice root in 2 cups of water, then use the liquid as a compress, changing every 15 minutes for 45 to 60 minutes to soothe the irritation and relieve the symptoms.

• Mash plantain leaves and apply as a poultice, changing every hour to relieve itching. Plantain leaves may be found in Hispanic markets.

❊ DAILY SUPPLEMENTS ❊

• Beta-carotene (1,000 milligrams) and vitamin C (1,000 to 2,000 milligrams) are good anti-inflammatories and can speed up skin healing.

• Vitamin B complex and zinc (50 milligrams) are important for skin tissue renewal.

• Catechin, quercetin, hesperidin, and rutin (up to 300 milligrams daily of each), flavonoids that are found in dark berries, are useful for inflammatory conditions.

❊ HERBAL THERAPY ❊

• Herbs can be found in health food or vitamin stores, online, and at the offices of Chinese medicine practitioners. Herbs should be used according to individual needs; consult with a licensed practitioner for a customized formulation. To learn more about the herbs listed here, go to www.askdrmao.com.

• Jewelweed, aloe vera, marshmallow root, and tea tree oil can treat allergic dermatitis from poison ivy or poison oak.

• Traditional Chinese herbal therapy for allergic skin reactions includes siler, caltrop, schizonepetae, astragalus, licorice, rhubarb, angelica, and skullcap.

❋ EXERCISE ❋

The sweat released through vigorous exercise can irritate the skin. Tai chi and qi gong are perfect exercises for skin problems because they reduce stress, calm the emotions, and promote self-healing. The General Cleansing Qi Gong sequence can help with circulation and promote opening of the pores. Do this sequence indoors and not too vigorously.

Sit comfortably or lie down on your back. Slow your respiration to deep, abdominal breathing. Repeat the word "calm" in your mind with every exhalation. You'll be visualizing the relaxation of a body part and releasing tension with every exhalation. Trace the following 3 pathways outlined below.

Start at the top of your head. Inhale, and then exhale while visualizing your scalp muscles relaxing. Say "calm" in your mind. Repeat this, saying the word with each body part as you move down through your face, throat, chest, abdomen, thighs, knees, calves, ankles, and feet. When you've relaxed your feet, visualize all the tension in your body leaving through your toes in the form of dark smoke.

Start at the temple region of your head. This pathway focuses on the sides and upper extremities. Inhale, and then exhale while visualizing your temple muscles relaxing. Say the word "calm" in your mind. Repeat this, saying the word as you move down through your jaw, the sides of your neck, shoulders, upper arms, elbows, forearms, wrists, and hands. Once you've relaxed your hands, visualize all the tension leaving your body through your fingertips in the form of dark smoke.

The final pathway begins on the back of your head. This pathway relaxes the back of your body. Repeat the breathing-visualization-word routine, as above, as you go from the back of your neck to your upper back, middle back, lower back, back of thighs, calves, and heels. Then focus on the acupoint Bubbling Spring (KID-1), on the soles of your feet, for 1 minute.

Practice this sequence for at least 15 minutes twice a day.

--- ❊ ACUPRESSURE ❊ ---

• Find the acupoint Valley of Harmony (LI-4), at the web between the thumb and index finger of your right hand. Apply steady pressure with your left thumb until you feel soreness. Hold for 2 minutes. Repeat on the left hand.

....

• Locate the acupoint Wind Pond (GB-20), at the natural indentation at the base of your skull on both sides of your neck. Press and lift up toward the base of your skull with your thumbs and lean your head back. Use the weight of your head against your thumbs for a steady pressure on the acupoint for about 5 minutes, breathing deeply and slowly.

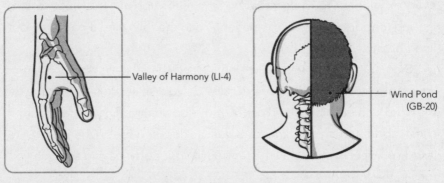

Valley of Harmony (LI-4)

Wind Pond (GB-20)

--- AVOID ---

• Scratching, as it exposes the skin to secondary infections.

....

• Exposure to temperature changes, cold or hot water, and detergents.

....

• Constipation, and make sure to keep your skin clean.

....

• Alcohol, smoking, and caffeine. They are irritants and can worsen allergies.

PSORIASIS

PSORIASIS IS A COMMON SKIN CONDITION that affects more than 6 million Americans, possibly the result of several factors, including heredity, lifestyle, and diet. It is a symptom of a faulty skin cell regeneration mechanism. Normal skin cells take up to a month to mature, but in patients with psoriasis this process is shortened to 5 to 7 days, producing excessive skin cells that cause the skin to thicken in raised red areas with silvery scales. Psoriasis commonly appears on the elbows, knees, groin, and scalp. Lesions that ooze and ulcerate may appear, causing pain. Flaking and itching are common, and about 10 percent of chronic psoriasis patients develop arthritis as well. Stress, obesity, exposure to environmental toxins, skin infections, alcohol use, and certain drugs can worsen the condition. Western medicine relies on steroidal creams, tar cream with UV light treatment, antibiotics, and immunosuppressants for relief.

In Chinese medicine, diseases of the skin have a direct link to the lung–large intestine network, which also governs the immune system. When the lungs are weak and attacked by pathogenic wind or microbes, the skin doesn't receive proper nourishment. Heat toxins in the blood can also manifest as skin disease. Psoriasis is best treated when the underlying conditions are addressed either by dispersing the wind or clearing the heat and toxins from the skin.

I've worked with dermatologists on some very stubborn cases of psoriasis. One case involved a man who had severe psoriasis for six years—the thick patches of his skin wouldn't clear up with steroids

PSORIASIS

and tar and UV light treatments. After a cleansing and detoxification program, I put him on a vegetarian diet with no animal products at all. I administered a full course of acupuncture and herbal therapy to cleanse his body of heat and toxins and to harmonize his immune system to lower inflammatory reaction. After about five months, his skin cleared up by about 95 percent. With proper dietary and lifestyle adjustments and regular treatments, many of my patients have experienced relief from their symptoms.

Here is a summary of my approach.

❊ DIET ❊

• What you eat eventually ends up in your skin. People often eat without a second thought as to the content of their food. Many of our foods today contain chemical and artificial ingredients that can cause allergic reactions and irritate the immune system. Keep a diary of your meals, be more attentive to what you eat and your physical and emotional reactions, and soon you will discover whether you have allergic reactions to foods that contribute to your psoriasis. Avoiding these foods can significantly reduce flare-ups.

• Eat a wholesome diet with foods that nourish the skin. Favor broccoli, dandelion greens, mung beans, lentils, split peas, chickpeas, black beans, lima beans, pinto beans, seaweed, pearl barley, oats, adzuki beans, water chestnuts, winter squash, winter melon, watermelon, carrots, brewer's yeast, olives, raspberries, papaya, pineapple, cherries, peaches, apples, pears, raisins, and grapes. Water is essential for cleansing the body. People who drink at least 80 ounces of water a day tend to have better bowel habits and develop fewer allergic reactions.

• Eliminate processed foods, foods containing artificial additives, bleached white flour, sugars, soft drinks, and spicy, deep-fried, and greasy foods. Stay off all animal foods, including meat, fish, poultry, dairy products, eggs, and shellfish, as well as highly allergenic foods such as wheat, corn, tomatoes, eggplant, peanuts, caffeinated beverages, alcohol, citrus fruits, and some soy products.

✳ HOME REMEDIES ✳

• Soak in a sulfur bath or hot spring for 20 minutes regularly to help the skin heal, or if that isn't possible, soak in a warm Epsom salt bath for 20 minutes nightly until skin improves.

• Peel and slice 15 water chestnuts and place in a nonmetallic pot with 1 cup of rice vinegar. Slowly simmer for 20 minutes to allow the chestnuts to absorb the vinegar. Remove from the heat and let cool, drain the excess vinegar, and mash the chestnuts into a paste. Seal in a jar to store. Apply this solution with a loofah sponge and lightly scrub to thin out the thick patches of skin once a day.

• Boil 1 cup each of pearl barley and mung beans with 8 cups of water and drink 3 cups of the water every day. You should also eat the solids.

• Detoxify—some people benefit from a one-week cleansing diet based on our Tao of Wellness Cleansing and Detoxification Program, which includes fresh vegetables juice and broths, herbal therapy, body brushing, Tui Na lymphatic massage, acupuncture, cupping, far infrared sauna, and mind-body exercises. Go to www.taoofwellness.com for more information on the detoxification program.

✳ DAILY SUPPLEMENTS ✳

• Gamma-linolenic acid (GLA; 450 milligrams) taken daily can help regulate inflammatory response. Evening primrose oil and borage oil are good sources of GLA. Omega-3 fatty acids (1,000 milligrams EPA; 800 milligrams DHA) from fish and flaxseeds are also helpful.

- Vitamins B$_{12}$ (200 micrograms), folate (400 micrograms), vitamin E (800 IU), zinc (50 milligrams), selenium (100 micrograms), and quercetin (500 milligrams) taken before meals help treat psoriasis.

- Taking probiotics (3 to 5 billion organisms) can help remove toxic substances and regulate immune response.

─────────────── ❋ HERBAL THERAPY ❋ ───────────────

- Herbs can be found in health food or vitamin stores, online, and at the offices of Chinese medicine practitioners. Herbs should be used according to individual needs; consult with a licensed practitioner for a customized formulation. To learn more about the herbs listed here, go to www.ask drmao.com.

- Burdock, red clover, licorice, chamomile, and calendula can help support skin health.

- Milk thistle stops the breakdown of substances that contribute to psoriasis and protects the liver. Other herbs helpful for treating psoriasis include yellow dock and sarsaparilla.

- Our Exquisite Skin Chinese herbal formula helps support healthy skin function and reduce itching. It contains siler, caltrop, schizonepetae, astragalus, peony, dong quai, Fo-Ti, rhubarb, licorice, and other Chinese herbs.

- For topical relief from itching, mix 10 drops of Tonic Oil (containing wintergreen, eucalyptus, menthol, and other herbs) with fresh aloe vera gel and apply liberally and frequently.

─────────────── ❋ EXERCISE ❋ ───────────────

Stress and anxiety can make psoriasis worse and possibly trigger outbreaks. I recommend that you include stress-reduction exercises in your regular workout routine. Tai chi and qi gong are great for reducing stress and calming the emotions. The General Cleansing Qi Gong exercise that follows can help with circulation and promote the opening of the pores. Do this exercise indoors and not too vigorously.

Sit comfortably or lie down on your back. Slow your respiration to deep, abdominal breathing. Say the word "calm" in your mind with every exhalation. You'll be visualizing the relaxation of a body part and releasing tension with every exhalation. Trace the following 3 pathways outlined below.

Start at the top of your head. Inhale, and then exhale and visualize your scalp muscles relaxing. Say "calm" in your mind. Repeat this, saying the word with each body part as you move down through your face, throat, chest, abdomen, thighs, knees, calves, ankles, and feet. When you've relaxed your feet, visualize all the tension in your body leaving through your toes in the form of dark smoke.

Next, start at the temple region of your head. This pathway focuses on the sides and upper extremities. Inhale, and then exhale while visualizing your temple muscles relaxing. Say the word "calm" in your mind. Repeat this, saying the word with each body part as you move down through your jaw, the sides of your neck, shoulders, upper arms, elbows, forearms, wrists, and hands. Once you've relaxed your hands, visualize all the tension leaving your body through your fingertips in the form of dark smoke.

The final pathway begins at the back of your head. This pathway relaxes the back of your body. Repeat the breathing-visualization-word routine, as above, as you go from the back of your neck to your upper back, middle back, lower back, back of thighs, calves, and heels. Then focus on the acupoint Bubbling Spring (KID-1), on the soles of your feet, for 1 minute.

Practice this exercise for at least 15 minutes twice a day.

─────────── ❋ ACUPRESSURE ❋ ───────────

• Locate the acupoint Wind Pond (GB-20), in the natural indentation at the base of your skull on either side of your neck. Press and lift up toward the base of your skull with your thumbs and lean your head back. Use the weight of your head against your thumbs for a steady pressure. Hold for 5 minutes, breathing deeply and slowly.

. . . .

• Find the acupoint Valley of Harmony (LI-4), in the web between your right thumb and index finger. Apply steady pressure with your left thumb until you feel soreness. Hold for 2 minutes. Repeat on the left hand.

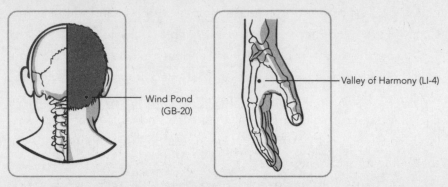

Wind Pond (GB-20)

Valley of Harmony (LI-4)

 RINGING IN THE EAR

THE CONDITION OF UNWELCOME NOISES IN YOUR EARS—which are often described as buzzing, roaring, ringing, whistling, or hissing sounds—is called tinnitus, which is the Latin word for ringing. Though not considered a serious or fatal condition, tinnitus does affect quality of life for many people. One in twenty Americans experiences prolonged tinnitus, and its occurrence increases with age. Tinnitus is almost always associated with hearing loss, and although the exact mechanism that produces the sounds is not well known, the sounds aren't imaginary. The sounds may be intermittent, continuous, or pulsing. Tinnitus can interfere with normal activities and, because it usually is worse in the evenings, it tends to disturb sleep. There are many causes for tinnitus, including a degenerative auditory nerve, ear infections, neurological problems, and Ménière's disease. Many prescription medications and chemotherapy can also cause tinnitus.

In Chinese medicine, the kidney-bladder network governs hearing and the ears. Tinnitus, then, is often associated with progressive kidney weakness brought on by overstrain, lack of sleep, and excessive sexual activity. Negative emotions are also often associated with tinnitus. Anger, frustration, resentment, and hatred block the liver energy, which over time produces fire rising up to the head, which disrupts hearing.

Diet plays a role as well. Overconsumption of cold and raw foods and dairy products promotes the formation of mucus, causing congestion and preventing proper nourishment of the ears. Digital audio player and cell phone use have contributed to the increased rate of hearing problems. I had a patient in his fifties who suddenly lost 50 percent of his hearing in one ear and lived with a terrible ringing in both of his ears for several years. He saw many hearing specialists, and all advised him to get a hearing aid. Unconvinced or perhaps unwilling to acknowledge his problems, he came to see me as a last resort. He was a typical type-A personality. He worked sixty hours a week and was constantly traveling by plane for work. He also suffered from chronic sinus allergies. I focused on strengthening his kidney network, which was weakened from the wear and tear of his life, and regulating his emotions to ease stress, while at the same time clearing away mucus blockage. In doing so, I removed the root causes of the condition and allowed his body to heal itself. By using acupuncture and herbal therapy and advising him on appropriate diet and lifestyle—I insisted that he not travel for three months—his hearing has improved and the tinnitus is hardly noticeable. His audiologist is quite happy with the results—and so is he.

—————————— ❊ DIET ❊ ——————————

• A healthy and balanced diet with smaller and more frequent meals including ample amounts of complex carbohydrates and wholesome proteins is a good start. Adding more warming foods, such as organic chicken and lamb, can help strengthen the kidney yang energy. Scallions, sesame seeds, fish, baked tofu, soybeans, walnuts, eggs, lentils, black beans, lotus seeds, ginger, and cinnamon bark are also helpful.

• Avoid cold and raw foods and icy beverages, as the coldness may constrict the eustachian tubes, causing poor drainage from the inner ears. Maintain a diet low in saturated fats and eliminate fried and greasy foods. Avoid processed meats and dairy products, as they have a tendency to increase mucus production. Protein deposits similar to those in milk have been found in the inner ears of patients with partial hearing loss.

—————————— ❊ HOME REMEDIES ❊ ——————————

• Simple ear irrigation can remove excess wax buildup, which may be a cause of tinnitus. Earwax kits are available at some local pharmacies. You may also want to visit your ENT specialist if the problem becomes severe.

• Make a tea by boiling 1 heaping tablespoon each of dried oregano, cilantro, rosemary, sage, and cinnamon and 3 slices of fresh ginger in 4 cups of water for 15 minutes. Seal the pot to prevent steam from escaping as it boils. Drink 3 cups a day for at least 3 weeks.

- Heat 2 tablespoons of salt and place in a cotton pouch, seal it, and use as a heat compress by placing it over the ear for 10 minutes a day.

❋ DAILY SUPPLEMENTS ❋

- Melatonin (1 to 3 milligrams) taken daily can lessen symptoms of tinnitus.

- Zinc (50 milligrams) and manganese (5 milligrams) taken daily can help diminish tinnitus.

- Vitamin B complex supplements, including B_{12} (200 micrograms) can relieve tinnitus resulting from noise damage.·

❋ HERBAL THERAPY ❋

- Herbs can be found in health food or vitamin stores, online, and at the offices of Chinese medicine practitioners. Herbs should be used according to individual needs; consult with a licensed practitioner for a customized formulation. To learn more about the herbs listed here, go to www.ask drmao.com.

- Cordiceps taken 3 times daily has been shown in clinical studies to reduce tinnitus.

- Ginkgo biloba can help stabilize hearing loss and ringing by increasing capillary blood circulation.

- Traditional Chinese herbs for supporting healthy hearing function include rehmannia, wild yam, schizandra, Asian cornelian, and magnetite.

❋ EXERCISE ❋

Exercise is important for stimulating blood circulation, reducing cholesterol, and preventing the premature decline of vital energy. I recommend a regular regimen of daily qi gong and tai chi combined with moderate cardiovascular exercise. I use qi gong exercises with my patients to help maintain good hearing and reduce degeneration. The Liver Cleansing Qi Gong is very useful, as are the Immortal Beating the Heavenly Drum and Immortal Sounding the Heavenly Bell exercises, which can be found in the hearing loss section (page 317). Do these exercises daily for optimum results.

For the Liver Cleansing Qi Gong, stand with your feet shoulder-width apart in front of a tree. Inhale, and raise your right leg. Exhale, and place your right foot on the ground in front of you between your body and the tree.

Inhale, and raise both arms from the sides until they come together over your head. Exhale, and lower your hands in front of your face. Visualize green light running down your face as your hands move down to your chest.

Inhale, and move your hands to the right rib cage over your liver. Exhale, and move your arms down your right abdomen and right leg, as if pushing down and out with your hands. Visualize a green light moving the toxins out of the liver and down the liver meridian on the inside of your right leg and out of the big toe.

The tree is a receptacle of liver energy and is capable of regenerating itself, much like its ability to absorb toxic carbon dioxide and produce oxygen.

❊ ACUPRESSURE ❊

• Find the acupoint Outer Gate (SJ-5), two thumb-widths above the outer wrist crease of the right hand, between the two tendons. Apply pressure with your left thumb until you feel soreness. Hold for 2 minutes.

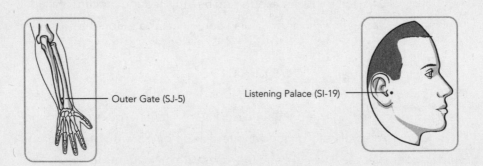

Outer Gate (SJ-5)

Listening Palace (SI-19)

• Locate the acupoint Listening Palace (SI-19), directly in front of the right ear canal, in the depression formed when the mouth is slightly open. Apply steady pressure with your index or middle finger until you feel soreness. Hold for 2 minutes. Repeat on the left side.

AVOID

• Certain antibiotics, including aminoglycosides, gentamicin, and tobramicin, which can cause hearing loss. Consult your physician.

• Aspirin, as it can cause tinnitus.

• Some diuretics, such as furosemide (Lasix), in high doses and some antihypertensive drugs, such as the combination bisoprolol and hydrochlorothiazide (Ziac), which can cause hearing loss. Consult your physician.

• Exposure to loud noise, and turn down ambient noises.

• Alcohol use and smoking, which speed up hearing decline and promote plaque buildup, preventing proper nourishment of the ears.

ROSACEA

ROSACEA, OR ACNE ROSACEA, IS A CHRONIC ACNE CONDITION. It affects the forehead, nose, cheeks, and sometimes the chin, and it occurs mainly in people with light skin and of northwestern European descent. The exact cause of rosacea is unknown, though genetics are thought to play a role. Diet and lifestyle are key contributors as well. Recent research suggests that parasitic mites, known as demodex mites, are more abundant in people with rosacea. (Demodex mites are also thought to cause some severe cases of acne.) In severe cases, untreated rosacea may be disfiguring to the face. Many well-documented triggers have been identified, including extreme weather and temperature exposure, excessive sunlight or sunburn, alcohol, caffeine, spicy foods, and certain medications. Topical steroid use can also trigger an outbreak. Western medicine offers a variety of palliative treatments, including antibiotics, creams, and light therapy involving broad spectrum pulsed-light therapy.

In Chinese medicine, flushing of the face has many causes, and several organ networks may be involved. The skin is governed by the lung network, so heat in the lungs will affect the quality of the skin. Too much alcohol or rich and spicy foods creates excess heat in the stomach network, which can end up on the face as rosacea. Emotion also shows itself in the face. Stress and anxiety can flare up the fire energy of the heart, which governs the spirit, causing rosacea. My treatment for rosacea focuses on soothing and calming the spirit, clearing heat, and removing any circulation blockages through acupuncture, herbal therapy, and lifestyle and dietary changes.

Here are some of my recommendations.

✳ DIET ✳

• Foods play a major role in triggering rosacea. Your diet should be on the bland side, with a healthy mix of whole grains, green leafy vegetables, and fresh fruits. Identifying and avoiding triggers can dramatically reduce your symptoms. Incorporate more prunes, guava, pearl barley, water chestnuts, lotus seeds (cook like beans), lotus leaves, mulberries, goji berries, cucumbers, beets, beet tops, dandelion greens, squash, and mung beans into your diet. Omega-3 fatty acids, found in cold-water fish, can help nourish the skin. Water is essential for cleansing the body, so drink at least 60 ounces a day.

• Eliminate processed foods, foods containing artificial additives, simple sugar and bleached flour, soft drinks, and spicy, fried, and oily foods. Animal proteins should be avoided. Excessive sun exposure should also be avoided. Alcohol, especially red wine, and aged cheeses, are notorious for triggering the condition.

❊ HOME REMEDIES ❊

• Shave the skin of one fresh cucumber, put it in a blender, and puree with 1 egg white. Apply with cotton ball to the affected area and leave on for 30 minutes, then wash with cold water. Repeat daily.

• Make chamomile tea and soak the affected area using a clean soft gauze, changing the application every 15 minutes. Repeat twice a day.

• Take 1 tablespoon flaxseed oil or fish oil daily; you can use it in a salad as a dressing.

❊ DAILY SUPPLEMENTS ❊

• Taking vitamin B complex and pancreatic and digestive enzymes can help reduce rosacea.

• Topical application of vitamin A (5,000 IU), often used for acne, can help with the inflammation of rosacea.

• Taking betaine hydrochloride (300 milligrams) at mealtimes aids stomach acid production and may be helpful, as some people with rosacea do not produce sufficient stomach acid.

❊ HERBAL THERAPY ❊

• Herbs can be found in health food or vitamin stores, online, and at the offices of Chinese medicine practitioners. Herbs should be used according to individual needs; consult with a licensed practitioner for a customized formulation. To learn more about the herbs listed here, go to www.ask drmao.com.

• Burdock, yellow dock, red clover, and cleavers are used to relieve symptoms of rosacea.

ROSACEA

• Chinese medicine herbal prescriptions for rosacea include the herbs pagoda tree flower, skullcap, coptidis, cape jasmine fruit, rehmannia, peony, and cardamom.

• Our Exquisite Skin Chinese herbal formula helps support healthy skin function and reduce itching. It contains siler, caltrop, schizonepetae, astragalus, peony, dong quai, Fo-Ti, rhubarb, and licorice.

────────────── ✳ EXERCISE ✳ ──────────────

Stress and anxiety can trigger and worsen rosacea. Tai chi and qi gong are great for reducing stress and calming the emotions, and they are also physically beneficial. A qi gong meditation called Heart Nourishing Qi Gong helps calm anxiety, reduce stress, promote healthy circulation, and relieve symptoms.

Inhale, and from the sides of your body, gently raise your arms to your head with your palms facing up. When you reach your head, turn your palms so that they face the top of the head at the acupoint Hundred Meeting (DU-20).

Exhale, imagining that you are exhaling through the centers of your palm (at the Labor Palace acupoint) into the top of your head.

Inhale, and then exhale, gently bringing your arms down with your palms facing down. At about head level, start exhaling out of the middle of your palms. Visualize bringing the energy down through your lower abdomen. End by turning your palms so that they face your abdomen.

At this point, your arms should be curved and relaxed at about waist level. Hold this posture, gently breathe, and meditate.

Inhale, and bring the energy up from your perineum to the top of your upper back just below the cervical vertebrae (the vertebrae in your neck).

Exhale, imagining you are exhaling down the inside of your left arm, out of the Labor Palace point, and into your lower abdomen.

Inhale from the middle of your palms and bring the energy up your left arm, to the center of your chest.

Exhale, and visualize the energy moving down and around your lower abdomen, starting down your right side and finishing up around your left side.

Inhale, and bring the energy up from your perineum to the top of your upper back just below the cervical vertebrae.

Exhale down your right arm, out of the middle of your palms and into the lower abdomen.

Inhale from the middle of your palms and bring the energy up your right arm to the center of your chest.

Exhale, and visualize the energy moving down and around your lower abdomen, starting down your left side and finishing up around your right side.

Inhale from the center of your left sole, bringing the energy up your left leg, to your thigh, and then your hip.

Exhale, and visualize the energy moving around your abdomen, starting up your lower left side, to the top of the abdomen, down your right side and ending up around the left side of your lower abdomen.

Inhale from the center of your right sole, bringing the energy up your right leg, to your thigh, and up to your hip.

Exhale, and visualize the energy moving around your lower abdomen, starting from your right side, to the top, down your left side, and ending up the right side of your lower abdomen.

Inhale, and visualize the energy at the the top of the head moving down to the center of your chest.

Exhale, and visualize the energy moving around your lower abdomen, starting up the top, moving down your left side, and ending up at the right side of your lower abdomen.

Begin to return the qi to your body.

Inhale, bringing your hands to your sides. Then with your palms facing toward your back, gather the energy around you (making a circle), bringing your arms in front of you, with your palms facing your lower abdomen.

Exhale, visualizing the gathered energy entering your lower abdomen and swirling around the navel.

Quickly inhale, and slowly raise your hands with your palms facing down and level with your lower abdomen.

Exhale, and bring the energy back to your lower abdomen.

Repeat this exercise twice a day. In evening, do this exercise before 7 p.m.

✻ ACUPRESSURE ✻

• Find the acupoint Inner Gate (P-6), three finger-widths above the wrist crease, between the two tendons on the inside of the left forearm. Apply moderate pressure with your right thumb. Hold for 3 minutes. Repeat on the right arm.

• Find the acupoint Foot Three Miles (ST-36), four finger-widths below the kneecap on the right leg. Apply moderate pressure with your right thumb until you feel soreness. Hold for 5 minutes. Repeat on the left leg.

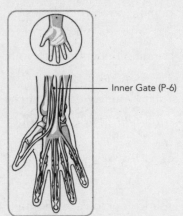

Inner Gate (P-6)

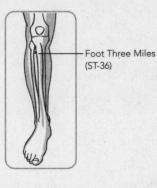

Foot Three Miles (ST-36)

AVOID

• Exposure to temperature changes, cold or hot water, and detergents.

• Exposure to sunlight UVA rays, which can trigger an outbreak.

• Excessive use of cosmetics, creams, and abrasive skin cleansers.

- Alcohol, smoking, and caffeine, which are irritants and generate heat that contributes to flare-ups.

- Stress, anxiety, and emotional upset, which can initiate flare-ups.

 ## SCIATICA

THE LARGEST NERVE BUNDLE IN YOUR BODY can become the largest pain in the rear. The sciatic nerve originates from the lowest part of your spine and serves the lower body. When the nerve gets irritated, inflamed, or compressed, unbearable pain shoots down your buttocks, to the back of your legs, and down to your feet. You may also experience numbness in the leg or feet, difficulty walking or standing, or even bladder problems and fever. Anything from prolonged sitting on hard surfaces to carrying a large wallet can cause sciatica. Herniated disks, muscular pressure, and spinal stenosis (narrowing of the space in the spinal column through which the nerve extends) are possible causes as well. Sciatica mostly affects people ages twenty-five to forty-five, most often the result of sudden twisting movements or the improper lifting of heavy objects. The easiest preventives for sciatica are proper posture, good physical fitness, taking special care when lifting or moving heavy objects, and a healthy lifestyle in general.

There is a condition in Chinese medicine known as painful obstruction syndrome, which describes a situation in which the energy meridians and blood vessels become compressed, blocking the flow of energy and blood and causing severe pain. Sciatica is one such painful obstruction syndrome, often caused by dampness in addition to energy and blood constriction. In Chinese medicine, there are further differentiations of dampness-related painful obstruction, such as dampness and cold, dampness and wind, and dampness and heat classifications. See the section on arthritis (pages 195–202) for recommendations for each of these. I've treated many acute and chronic sciatica conditions using acupuncture and herbal therapy with good results. Acupuncture is effective for all kinds of pain, but particularly for sciatica. My approach is to unblock the stagnation, promoting the flow of energy and blood. I also advise my patients on exercises to strengthen the core muscles.

Here are some of my recommendations.

✳ DIET ✳

• A healthy, well-balanced diet rich in complex carbohydrates, whole grains, fresh vegetables, and organic animal protein is important for a healthy body. I recommend foods high in potassium, including bananas, potatoes, oranges, spirulina, and chlorella, as well as dark green leafy vegetables, and saltwater fish such as flounder, salmon, and sardines. Soybeans, kidney beans, black beans, garlic, onions, kale, grapes, mulberries, anise seeds, cinnamon, almonds, walnuts, and prunes are also beneficial.

• Avoid alcohol and smoking, as they can irritate the sciatic nerve. Sugar, especially processed bleached sugar, should be eliminated. Irritating foods such as spicy, greasy, or fried foods, as well as dairy and other foods that create dampness, should also be avoided.

✳ HOME REMEDIES ✳

• Chamomile tea is a muscle relaxant, and can help alleviate the pain of sciatica. Steep chamomile tea bags in boiling water for 5 minutes. Drink 3 cups daily.

• Prepare a shallow bath with lukewarm water (about body temperature), add 1 cup Epsom salts, 2 tablespoons eucalyptus oil, and a few drops of lavender and chamomile oils. Sit in the bath for 20 minutes to relax your body, then take a lukewarm shower. Take a bath twice daily until the pain is substantially relieved.

❋ DAILY SUPPLEMENTS ❋

• Taking vitamin B complex can speed up healing in sciatica conditions.

• Taking calcium (2,000 milligrams) and magnesium (1,000 milligrams) helps relieve muscle spasms and reduce pressure on the nerves.

• The enzyme bromelain (800 milligrams) is an natural anti-inflammatory and helps alleviate back pain.

• MSM (2,000 milligrams) is also useful for general pain relief.

❋ HERBAL THERAPY ❋

• Herbs can be found in health food or vitamin stores, online, and at the offices of Chinese medicine practitioners. Herbs should be used according to individual needs; consult with a licensed practitioner for a customized formulation. To learn more about the herbs listed here, go to www.ask drmao.com.

• Evening primrose oil, horsetail, and chamomile are good Western herbs used to treat sciatica.

• White willow bark, valerian, and passionflower work as relaxants and are natural pain relievers.

• Chinese herbal formulations for sciatica includes the herbs gentiana root, cnidium, peach kernel, safflower, licorice, notopterygium root, myrrh, angelica, dong quai, pteropus, nutgrass, achyranthes, and other Chinese herbs.

SCIATICA

✳ EXERCISE ✳

There is a definite advantage to exercising regularly, as exercise tones and strengthens your muscles and helps maintain healthy joints. Exercise can also help prevent sciatica. During sciatica flare-ups, pain may preclude you from exercising and bed rest can help reduce the irritation of the nerve. In addition to cardiovascular exercise such as swimming or walking for 30 minutes a day, yoga, tai chi, and qi gong can help strengthen the body without causing too much stress.

I recommend Dao In Qi Gong, which is gentle on the body and provides great benefits. The sequence Stretching the Well helps the sciatic nerve. Practice this regularly to attain relief and prevent flare-ups.

Sit with your right leg as when cross-legged and your left leg turned out to the left so your left heel is touching your left buttock. Hold your left ankle with your left hand and hold your right heel with your right hand.

Inhale, and turn your head to the right, twist your torso to the right, and lean to the right, still holding on to your heel.

Exhale, and twist your head and upper body to the left, lowering your body and bringing your right shoulder to your right knee, still holding your ankle.

Inhale, lift yourself up, and twist to the left, looking behind you.

Exhale, and return to the beginning posture.

Repeat the steps above for a total of 3 times on this side.

Then switch sides: Sit with your left leg as when cross-legged and your right leg turned out to the right so your right heel is touching your right buttock. Hold your right ankle with your right hand and hold your left heel with your left hand.

Inhale, and turn your head to the left, twist your torso to the left, and lean to the left, still holding your heel.

Exhale, and twist your head and upper body to the right, and lowering your body and bringing your left shoulder to your left knee, still holding your ankle.

Inhale, lift yourself up, and twist to the right, looking behind you.

Exhale, and return to the beginning posture.

Repeat the steps above for a total of 3 times on this side.

❋ ACUPRESSURE ❋

• Find the acupoint Jumping Circle (GB-30), on the center of the buttocks about midway between the tip of the coccyx and the right hipbone. Apply heavy pressure with your right thumb or index finger until you feel soreness. Hold for 30 seconds and release. Repeat several times, alternating the right and left sides.

. . . .

• Find the acupoint Yang Spring (GB-34), on the outer part of the lower right leg, just below the bony structure located near the end of the knee crease about four finger-widths below the kneecap. Apply steady pressure with your right thumb until you feel soreness. Hold for 3 minutes. Repeat on the left leg.

. . . .

• Engaging the combination of these points is excellent for relaxing and strengthening the tendons and treating sciatica.

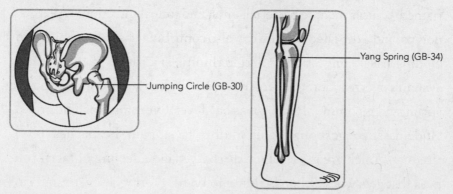

Jumping Circle (GB-30)

Yang Spring (GB-34)

AVOID

• Smoking and excessive use of alcohol, as they can deplete the body of vital nutrients needed for bone health. Nicotine especially irritates the sciatic nerve.

. . . .

SCIATICA

- The insomnia drug Ambien, which has been linked to sciatica in some people. Consult your physician for alternatives.

- Stress, worry, and tension, as these emotions irritate the nervous system and predispose you to sciatica.

- Poor posture—always sit with your back erect with support in the lumbar area. Do not sit for prolonged periods on hard surfaces. If you carry a wallet, take it out of your rear pocket when sitting. Take frequent breaks at work and stretch your lower back and buttocks.

SINUS PROBLEMS

SINUS PROBLEMS CAN INCLUDE A SLEW OF CONDITIONS related to the nasal passageway and the cavities beyond it. Acute or chronic sinus infections or sinusitis, affect some 37 million people in the United States. In a sinus infection, the mucous linings of the sinuses are inflamed. Causes include bacterial, viral, and fungal infections. Allergies, polyps, and a deviated septum can also contribute to sinus problems including nasal congestion. Allergic rhinitis is a result of the immune system's overreaction to allergens in the air; it often occurs during the spring and is commonly known as hay fever. Symptoms of sinusitis include nasal congestion, postnasal drip, facial pain, headaches, fever, tiredness, thick green or yellow discharge, and a feeling of facial fullness that gets worse when bending forward. During a severe sinus infection some people get toothaches. In chronic cases, the sense of smell can be diminished.

In Chinese medicine, the nose and sinuses are directly linked to the lung–large intestine network and the spleen-pancreas-stomach network. Invasion by pathogens or foreign particles causes clogging of the lung network and leads to nasal congestion and heat signs that include inflammation or infection. The digestive system is involved in providing proper nourishment and supporting the immune system. A weak digestive system can produce dampness that further congests the upper respiratory tract with mucus. In my clinical experience, strengthening the digestive system is fundamental to long-term relief of all sinus problems. Only with strong digestive function can there be a healthy immune system. I use acupuncture for immediate symptomatic relief and herbal therapy to clear the pathogens. I also recommend special breathing exercises, and I educate patients about an appropriate diet. Here are some of my favorite remedies.

❊ DIET ❊

• A wholesome, balanced diet with a high concentration of fiber and complex carbohydrates can help improve and maintain good respiratory health. Incorporate lots of whole grains, including quinoa, amaranth, and brown rice rather than wheat, rye, and barley, which are typically high-allergy grains. Favor papaya, cranberries, pears, pineapples, wild cherries, mangoes, and citrus fruits such as grapefruit and limes, cauliflower, and green vegetables such as artichokes, Brussels sprouts, broccoli, kale, and spinach. Herbs and spices such as ginger, scallions, basil, garlic, oregano, cayenne pepper, white pepper, horseradish, and turmeric also help to fight inflammation and help open passageways. Drink 8 glasses of warm or hot water a day.

• Foods that produce mucus and dampness, including dairy products, cold and raw foods, wine, greasy foods, and simple sugars, should be avoided. Soft drinks and some store-bought juices have a high content of corn syrup, which also produces dampness and mucus.

❊ HOME REMEDIES ❊

• Add a few drops of oil of wintergreen or menthol to a vaporizer. Inhale the vapor through your nose until the passageways clear. If you don't own a vaporizer, simply drop the oil into a pot of boiling water and inhale the steam with a towel covering your head and the pot, being careful not to burn yourself with the steam vapor.

....

• Make a tea by boiling 2 ounces magnolia flowers, 1 teaspoon chopped basil, 2 slices of ginger, and 1 chopped scallion in 3 1/2 cups of water for 20 minutes. Strain, and drink 1 cup 3 times a day for 1 week, or until the condition clears up.

....

• Mix 1 pressed garlic clove with 1 teaspoon olive oil and soak 2 clean cotton balls with the mixture. Wash your nostrils with warm salt water, then place the cotton balls in your nostrils. Leave in for 20 minutes; repeat 3 times a day until the symptoms clear up.

....

• Irrigate your nasal passageways with a solution of 1 teaspoon sea salt and 1 drop each of oregano oil and wintergreen oil in a cup of warm water. Fill a small squeeze bottle with the solution, and squirt it into one nostril at a time, and blow out through the nose. Alternate nostrils until you use up the solution. Repeat daily.

─────────────── ✳ DAILY SUPPLEMENTS ✳ ───────────────

• Supplementing with vitamins A (200 IU) and C (1,000 milligrams) can help ward off infections and regulate immune response. Zinc (50 milligrams) also helps supports a healthy immune system and prevents infections.

....

• Taking bromelain (500 milligrams) and quercetin (400 milligrams) can reduce histamine release, the body's natural allergic response.

....

• Gamma-linolenic acid (GLA; 450 milligrams) contains omega-6 fatty acids, which regulate inflammatory response.

─────────────── ✳ HERBAL THERAPY ✳ ───────────────

• Herbs can be found in health food or vitamin stores, online, and at the offices of Chinese medicine practitioners. Herbs should be used according

to individual needs; consult with a licensed practitioner for a customized formulation. To learn more about the herbs listed here, go to www.ask drmao.com.

• Ginger and licorice root are used to reduce inflammation and fight off allergies.

• Elderberry and astragalus are immune moderators and are useful in fighting upper respiratory infections and allergies.

• Magnolia flowers, mint, angelica, platycodon, dandelion, xanthium fruit, perilla seeds, and siler root all have anti-allergic properties and help reduce nasal inflammation and congestion.

• Traditional Chinese herbs used to strengthen the digestive system and support a healthy immune system include ligustrum, atractylodis, oryza, Cherokee rosehip, mulberry, honeysuckle, self-heal spike, Fo-Ti and eclipta.

❋ EXERCISE ❋

Exercise strengthens the body against infections and illnesses, and it helps balance immune function. Daily 30-minute cardiovascular exercise such as brisk walks (2 to 3 miles per hour) or aerobic workouts can help improve circulation and strengthen the body. I also recommend two Dao In Qi Gong exercises, Immortal Pressing the Sun and Moon Corners, and Immortal Massaging the Nose, simple yet effective exercises for relieving sinus congestion.

For Immortal Pressing the Sun and Moon Corners, sit at the tip of a sturdy chair with your back erect, spine stretched, and your head tilted slightly forward.

Inhaling, press your forehead just inside the temples with your palms.

Exhale, and release.

Repeat for a total of 3 times.

For Immortal Massaging the Nose, sit at the tip of a sturdy chair with your back erect, spine stretched, and your head tilted slightly forward.

Cross your middle and index fingers by placing the tips of your middle fingers on top of the fingernails of your index fingers.

Rub the sides of your nose 36 times in a circular motion, warming your fingers first if they're cold. You can apply a small amount of peppermint or spearmint essential oils to the area to enhance the massage.

❋ ACUPRESSURE ❋

• Find the acupoint Valley of Harmony (LI-4), at the web between your right thumb and index finger. Apply steady pressure with your left thumb until you feel soreness. Hold for 2 minutes. Repeat on the left hand.

• Locate the acupoint Welcome Fragrance (LI-20), on either side of the nostrils, next to the nose flap. Using the fingertips or the nails of your index fingers, gently press and dig in until you feel soreness. Hold the pressure for 2 minutes. Repeat as needed to clear nasal congestion.

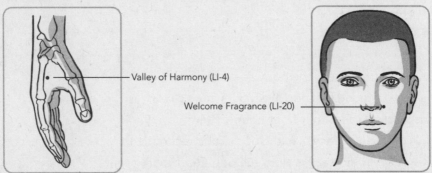

Valley of Harmony (LI-4)

Welcome Fragrance (LI-20)

AVOID

• Extreme temperature and weather fluctuations, as any sudden changes will worsen the condition. Air conditioners and heaters are particularly bad offenders.

• Exposure to environmental triggers, including dusty, dirty, and polluted air, which aggravate the nasal passages.

- Stress, and get plenty of sleep. Sinus congestion is often worse with lack of sleep and rest.

- Alcohol and smoking, both of which are irritating to the respiratory tract and make inflammation worse.

SNORING

MORE THAN 40 MILLION AMERICANS SNORE AT NIGHT. In itself, snoring is not a serious condition, but it can affect your quality of sleep and can be very disturbing to your loved ones. Snoring affects more men than women. There are severe types of snoring that are associated with sleep disorders such as sleep apnea, a condition in which a person may stop breathing for as long as ninety seconds. Symptoms of snoring include the wheezing, gurgling, and snorting noises made by the soft palate as air is forced through the oral and nasal cavity at high speeds. The vibration of the soft palate produces these sounds. Obesity plays a major role in snoring. Losing just 5 percent of body weight can reduce snoring dramatically and help improve quality of sleep. Asthma is one the most common medical conditions that can cause snoring. Smoking, alcohol use, and poor diet can also instigate snoring. Western medicine offers a variety of mechanical and surgical solutions to the problem. One treatment involves radio frequency tissue ablation—a surgical technique for cutting away the flap of skin at the uvula in the back of the throat. When left untreated, people who snore are at higher risk for high blood pressure, heart disease, and stroke.

In Chinese medicine, snoring is considered energy stagnation. The most common underlying cause of the stagnation is a buildup of dampness and phlegm. Dampness in the body is the direct result of improper

SNORING

diet, which weakens spleen and digestive functions and impairs the body's ability to transform and transport vital nutrients. Residue then lingers in the body and forms dampness, impairing cellular function, congealing into phlegm, and obstructing flow.

Excess dampness and mucus also translate into obesity. I had a patient who came in for a chronic sinus condition and a weight problem. It took three to four months of acupuncture to clear his nasal passageways and herbal therapy to eliminate mucus and mobilize the metabolic fire. I recently saw his wife, who thanked me for getting rid of her husband's snoring problem. By taking care of his sinus condition and helping him lose weight, the acupuncture also helped his snoring disappear. It is imperative to establish good dietary and lifestyle habits to prevent a buildup of dampness and energy blockage. Here are some simple recommendations I give to my patients.

—————————————— ✳ DIET ✳ ——————————————

• A wholesome, seasonally balanced diet rich in soluble fiber and complex carbohydrates can help maintain good respiratory health and vitality of defensive qi. Incorporate more whole grains (including quinoa, brown rice, and millet), cabbage, beets, beet tops, carrots, and yams, into your diet. Papaya, cranberries, pears, pineapple, wild cherries, mangoes, and citrus fruits, such as grapefruit and limes, are also helpful. Green leafy vegetables including spinach, broccoli, and kale provide essential nutrients for healthy immunity. Ginger, onions, basil, garlic, bamboo shoots, black mushrooms, dandelion greens, and chrysanthemum flowers also help fight inflammation.

....

• Drink 80 ounces of hot or warm water a day—that's ten 8-ounce glasses. Water intake is essential for proper lymphatic drainage. All vegetables need to be thoroughly washed in running water to remove any pesticide and chemical residues.

....

• Foods that produce mucus and dampness, including dairy products, cold and raw foods, greasy foods, white sugar, and bleached flour, should be avoided. Wheat, chocolate, shellfish, potatoes, tomatoes, and eggplant may overstimulate the immune response and should be eaten in moderation. Soft drinks and some packaged fruit juices have a high content of corn syrup and produce dampness and mucus.

────────────── ❋ HOME REMEDIES ❋ ──────────────

• Practice good sleeping habits. Clear your airways and nasal passages before going to bed. Sleep on your right side rather than on your back to reduce, if not eliminate, snoring. Pillows should not be too thick to avoid kinking your neck and obstructing the airways.

• Gargle with warm salt water before going to bed to shrink the tissues, moisten the oral cavity, and prevent dryness.

• Drink green tea and chamomile tea—they contain natural antihistamines and can help reduce mucus production and balance the immune system.

────────────── ❋ DAILY SUPPLEMENTS ❋ ──────────────

• Chromium (200 micrograms) and essential fatty acids found in fish and flaxseed oils (1,000 milligrams EPA; 800 milligrams DHA) can help with inflammatory conditions and reduce tissue swelling. Chromium is also good for reducing blood sugar, a form of dampness.

• Probiotics (3 to 5 billion organisms), with their beneficial organisms for intestinal flora are essential for protecting against allergic reactions.

• Bromelain (450 milligrams) and the antioxidant quercetin (500 milligrams) can work to modulate histamine release, which causes allergic response.

────────────── ❋ HERBAL THERAPY ❋ ──────────────

• Herbs can be found in health food or vitamin stores, online, and at the offices of Chinese medicine practitioners. Herbs should be used according

SNORING

to individual needs; consult with a licensed practitioner for a customized formulation. To learn more about the herbs listed here, go to www.ask drmao.com.

. . . .

• Drink ginger and peppermint tea at night before bedtime to reduce swelling and keep the sinus passageways open.

. . . .

• Unripe orange, tangerine, and lemon peels are good for digestion and reduce dampness and mucus.

. . . .

• Our family formula Allergy Tamer is made up of herbs including magnolia flowers, xanthium, mint, dandelion, Chinese basil, siler root, schizandra, and other herbs that support healthy immune function and relieve allergic reactions.

❋ EXERCISE ❋

Physical activity helps maintain good digestion, helps you lose weight and maintain a healthy body weight, and also helps reduce stress, anxiety, and strong emotions. A daily fitness program consisting of 30-minute walks and qi gong or tai chi is very beneficial for a healthy digestive system and can help treat snoring.

The following two Dao In Qi Gong exercises, Immortal Pressing the Sun and Moon Corners and Immortal Massaging the Nose are simple yet effective exercises for relieving sinus congestion and alleviating snoring.

For Immortal Pressing the Sun and Moon Corners, sit at the tip of a sturdy chair with your back erect, spine stretched, and your head tilted slightly forward.

Inhaling, press your forehead just inside the temples with your palms. Exhale, and release.

Repeat for a total of 3 times. Practice 3 or 4 times a day.

For Immortal Massaging the Nose, sit at the tip of a sturdy chair with your back erect, spine stretched, and your head tilted slightly forward.

Cross your middle and index fingers by placing the tips of your middle fingers on top of the fingernails of your index fingers.

Rub the sides of your nose 36 times in a circular motion, warming your fingers first if they're cold. You can apply a small amount of peppermint or spearmint essential oils to the area to enhance the massage.

✳ ACUPRESSURE ✳

• Find the acupoint Valley of Harmony (LI-4), at the web between your right thumb and index finger. Apply steady pressure with your left thumb until you feel soreness. Hold for 2 minutes. Repeat on the left hand.

• Locate the acupoint Welcome Fragrance (LI-20), on either side of the nostrils, next to the nose flap. Using the fingertips or the nails of your index fingers, gently press and dig in until you feel soreness. Hold the pressure for 2 minutes. Repeat every hour during periods of congestion.

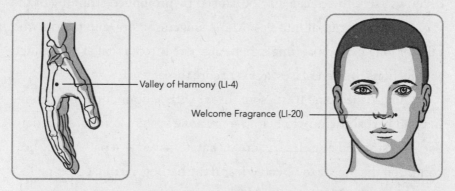

Valley of Harmony (LI-4)

Welcome Fragrance (LI-20)

AVOID

• Evening snacks, decrease alcohol consumption, and stop smoking.

• Using antihistamines and sleeping medications, as well as muscle relaxants, as they can loosen the musculature and cause the obstruction of the airways that causes snoring. Consult your physician for alternatives.

SORE THROAT

SORE THROAT, MEDICALLY KNOWN AS PHARYNGITIS, occurs when the tonsils in the pharynx acquire a viral or bacterial infection, creating inflammation and irritation. A sore throat often accompanies or precedes the common cold and flu. Some of the better-known culprits include the adenovirus, mononucleosis, the Epstein-Barr virus, and streptococcus. A sore throat can also be caused by prolonged straining of the vocal cords and throat muscles. Many singers, actors, and people who talk for long periods of time experience sore throats that aren't related to infections. In some cases, a severe sore throat can cause loss of voice.

Chinese medicine treats sore throat with acupuncture for pain relief and herbal therapy to help the immune system combat infections and heal strained muscles. A sore throat is viewed as a pathogenic heat condition that needs to be cooled, and the pathogens must be expelled. I see many noninfectious cases of sore throat that result from postnasal drip or acid reflux, both of which can be addressed with Chinese medicine. I use topical herbal sprays and solutions of herbs for gargling that soothe the throat muscles and relieve swelling and inflammation, helping patients to quickly recover from the symptoms. Here I offer some advice for sore throat relief. If a sore throat doesn't clear up within three days and is accompanied by fever, you should see your physician immediately. In rare cases, a potentially dangerous infection of diphtheria can cause sore throat and should be addressed immediately by a physician.

─────────────── ❋ DIET ❋ ───────────────

• Adding more cooling dandelion greens, chrysanthemum flowers, mint, scallions, cabbage, cilantro, burdock root, apples, pears, bitter melon, and rose hips to your diet can help ward off infections and relieve sore throat. Drink plenty of warm or room temperature water, at least eight glasses a day.

• Pear juice is soothing to the throat, as are cucumber juice and honey.

• Avoid foods that are greasy, deep-fried, barbecued, and spicy, as they can irritate the throat. Shellfish should be avoided as well.

─────────────── ❋ HOME REMEDIES ❋ ───────────────

• Slowly swallow 1 tablespoon of honey to coat the throat. Repeat 3 to 6 times a day until the sore throat is gone. The honey works as a natural antibiotic.

• As a throat cleanser, make a solution of 1 part 3 percent hydrogen peroxide and 3 parts warm water, and gargle in the back of your throat for 1 minute twice a day. Do not swallow the solution. This will help disinfect the throat and kill any bacteria or viral infection. A less potent but still effective gargle can be made with sea salt and warm water.

• Cut thin slices of ripe lemons. Add a pinch of salt and eat whole with the peel. This acts as an astringent and kills bacteria.

• Mix 1 tablespoon horseradish, 1 tablespoon honey, and 1 teaspoon ground cloves in a glass of warm water and stir well. Sip slowly to soothe the throat and inhibit the development of microbes.

SORE THROAT

✳ DAILY SUPPLEMENTS ✳

• Taking vitamin C (1,000 milligrams) 3 times a day can help fight infections.

• Vitamin A (200 IU) or beta-carotene (1,000 milligrams) taken twice a day helps to strengthen immunity.

• Zinc (50 milligrams) lozenges taken every 2 hours at the onset of a colds can reduce duration.

✳ HERBAL THERAPY ✳

• Herbs can be found in health food or vitamin stores, online, and at the offices of Chinese medicine practitioners. Herbs should be used according to individual needs; consult with a licensed practitioner for a customized formulation. To learn more about the herbs listed here, go to www.ask drmao.com.

• Andrographis (king of bitters) 3 times daily can reduce symptoms of colds quickly and inhibit microbe formation.

• Drink chamomile, echinacea and goldenseal tea to support immune function and reduce the frequency and shorten the duration of sore throats.

• Boil 1 teaspoon dried honeysuckle, 1 teaspoon mint leaves, and 1 teaspoon licorice root in 12 ounces of water for 15 minutes, and add 1 teaspoon honey. Strain, and drink as a tea 3 times a day to relieve a sore throat. This is a good remedy for children.

• Traditional Chinese herbs for relieving sore throat and fighting infections include fructus arctii, mulberry leaves, rehmannia, licorice, forsythia, honeysuckle, prunella, and andrographis.

✳ EXERCISE ✳

Exercise is important for stimulating blood circulation, maintaining a healthy immune system, and preventing colds. I recommend a regimen of daily qi gong and tai chi combined with moderate cardiovascular exercise.

The following is an ancient Taoist vocal qi gong exercise called the Six Healing Sounds meditation. When practiced twice a day it can help relieve sore throat, build strong vocal cords, harmonize the organs, and strengthen the body.

Sit comfortably at the tip of a sturdy chair with your spine erect, your arms placed on your legs, and your head tilted slightly forward.

Begin breathing slowly and rhythmically, inhaling deeply and gently and exhaling slowly through the mouth for 1 minute.

Now begin the practice. You'll be making 6 different sounds, all soft and quiet, barely audible. You'll repeat each sound 6 times, for a total of 36 vocalizations.

The first sound is for the liver: a prolonged "shh" (as if quieting a baby). Utter the sound softly and gently on an exhale 6 times.

The second sound is for the heart: a prolonged "ho" (as in "hi ho"). Utter the sound softly and gently on an exhale 6 times.

The third sound is for the spleen and stomach: a prolonged "hoo" (as in "who"). Utter the sound softly and gently on an exhale 6 times.

The fourth sound is for the lungs: a prolonged "sss" (as in "hiss" without the "hi"). Utter the sound softly and gently on an exhale 6 times.

The fifth sound is for the kidneys: a prolonged "foo" (as in "food" without the "d"). Utter the sound softly and gently on an exhale 6 times.

The sixth and final sound is for the gallbladder: a prolonged "shii" (as in "she"). Utter the sound softly and gently on an exhale 6 times.

Conclude the practice with 1 minute of relaxed, rhythmic breathing.

✳ ACUPRESSURE ✳

• Find the acupoint Valley of Harmony (LI-4), at the web between your right thumb and index finger. Apply steady pressure with your left thumb until you feel soreness. Hold for 2 minutes. Repeat on the left hand.

SORE THROAT

• Locate the acupoint Fish Belly (LU-10), in the fleshy part of your right palm just beneath your thumb. Apply steady pressure with your left thumb until you feel soreness. Hold for 2 minutes. Repeat on the left hand.

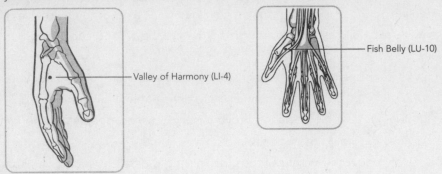

Valley of Harmony (LI-4)

Fish Belly (LU-10)

AVOID

• Exposure to dry, dusty, and cold conditions. Use a humidifier in dry climates.

• Alcohol, overeating, eating spicy foods, and smoking, all of which produce heat and can irritate the throat.

• Stress and overexertion, and get plenty of rest and sleep.

• Using old toothbrushes; change them often, or soak them in hydrogen peroxide every other day, as bacteria may collect on the brush.

SUNBURN

THERE IS A FINE LINE BETWEEN A SUNTAN AND A SUNBURN. The skin is very sensitive to ultraviolet rays, and sensitive skin can get a sunburn in less than five minutes of exposure to direct sunlight. Most people think that they can avoid sunburn by staying in the shade, but ultraviolet rays can penetrate the shade. Prolonged and repeated sunburns can cause aging of the skin, loss of skin elasticity, and skin cancer.

Symptoms of acute sunburn include itching, blisters, pain, redness, and swelling accompanied by chills, headache, fever, and nausea. Severe sunburn is treated like a first-degree burn and requires the care of a dermatologist.

In Chinese medicine, sunburn is considered a summer heat invasion. The condition resembles the common cold with the additional symptoms of a rash. As the heat from the sun enters the body, it gets trapped in the energy meridians and skin. This trapped heat is often combined with dampness, causing the typical symptoms. I approach sunburn by providing immediate relief with topical herbal therapy along with acupuncture to release the trapped heat from the skin and to soothe the symptoms of burning and pain. I then follow up with oral herbal therapy and dietary advice. The key, of course, is to take precautions to prevent sunburn in the first place.

Here are some good home remedies and recommendations for caring for sunburn.

✳ DIET ✳

• During acute sunburn, overeating is not recommended. Fluids are important to rehydrate the body and skin. Cooling foods including watermelon, cucumber, cantaloupe, honeydew, celery, broccoli, bok choy, lentils, mushrooms, squash, zucchini, pears, peaches, prunes, pineapple, and apples are useful for removing the trapped heat and cooling the body. Drink a glass of water hourly.

• Avoid greasy, barbecued, spicy, and deep-fried foods, as they may worsen the condition. Dairy products in general should be avoided, as they promote the formation of dampness in the body. The exception is yogurt, as the acidophilus in yogurt is helpful for immune function in the healing process. Alcohol and coffee dehydrate the body and produce heat, so they should be avoided.

• Drink a mixture of 12 ounces each of pineapple and black cherry juice to help reduce inflammation and heat. Drink 3 cups daily.

• Apply a thin layer of plain yogurt to the burn area to cool and soothe the irritation.

• Aloe vera gel applied topically is a tried-and-true remedy for skin burns.

• To prevent sunburn, limit exposure to sun, especially between 10 a.m. and 3 p.m.

• Use a UVA sunscreen with an SPF factor of 30 to 50.

• Wear a long-sleeved shirt, long pants, and a wide-brimmed hat.

───────────── ❊ DAILY SUPPLEMENTS ❊ ─────────────

• Taking beta-carotene (1,000 milligrams) or other carotenoids (500 milligrams) can prevent severe sun sensitivity.

• Taking fish oils containing omega-3 fatty acids (1,000 milligrams EPA; 800 milligrams DHA) lessen the symptoms of sunburn.

• Vitamins B_3 (100 milligrams), C (1,000 milligrams), and E (800 IU) can be taken as a protective measure to prevent sunburn.

• Taking vitamin D (600 IU) supplements helps protect the skin from UVB lights.

───────────── ❊ HERBAL THERAPY ❊ ─────────────

• Herbs can be found in health food or vitamin stores, online, and at the offices of Chinese medicine practitioners. Herbs should be used according to individual needs; consult with a licensed practitioner for a customized formulation. To learn more about the herbs listed here, go to www.ask drmao.com.

· Green tea and calendula can inhibit cell damage from sunburn. They can be taken internally as a tea or topically as a wash.

· Crush some dandelion greens and apply to the affected area as a poultice, changing every hour. You also can put 1 cup of dandelion greens in a blender and blend with 1/2 cup aloe vera gel and 1 tablespoon honey to make a smoother poultice. Repeat 4 to 6 times a day for maximum relief.

· Traditional Chinese remedies used to treat summer heat syndrome include mung beans, lotus leaf, sweet wormwood, momordica fruit, fermented soy, eupatorium, and elsholtzia.

❋ EXERCISE ❋

Don't exercise strenuously during a summer heat wave or when you have a bad sunburn. Calm, rest, and relaxation will help with your recovery. I recommend the following general stress-release meditation to calm and relax you while your body heals.

Lie down on your back or sit comfortably with your spine erect at the edge of a chair. If you choose to sit, your feet should be flat on the floor, with your legs bent at a 90-degree angle.

Reach up toward the sky with both hands on a deep inhale. As you hold your breath make tight fists and squeeze, tightening all the muscles in your arms. Slowly exhale, relaxing your arms and bringing your fists down to your chest. Repeat this several times.

Next, cross your arms in front of your chest, with your fingers touching just under your collarbone and your wrists crossed at the center of your upper chest.

Lower your chin toward your chest, and inhale 4 short breaths in a row through your nose (without exhaling). Fill your lungs completely on the

SUNBURN

fourth breath and hold the breath for a few seconds with the chest full and expanded.

Exhale slowly through your mouth.

Repeat this exercise for 2 or 3 minutes, concentrating on deep and rhythmic breathing.

❋ ACUPRESSURE ❋

• Find the acupoint Valley of Harmony (LI-4), at the web between your thumb and index finger. Apply steady pressure with your left thumb until you feel soreness. Hold for 2 minutes. Repeat on the left hand.

• Locate the acupoint Wind Pond (GB-20), is in the natural indentation at the base of your skull on either side of your neck. Press and lift up toward the base of your skull with your thumbs and lean your head back. Use the weight of your head against your thumbs for steady pressure on the acupoint. Hold for 5 minutes, breathing deeply and slowly.

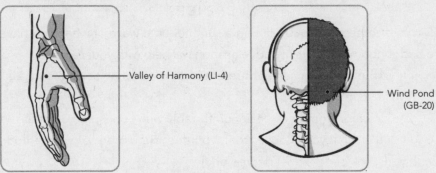

Valley of Harmony (LI-4)

Wind Pond (GB-20)

AVOID

• Strenuous activities and outdoor exposure. Rest in a cool but not cold environment.

• Further exposure to the sun or heat, as this may worsen the condition.

• Sun exposure if you're taking certain drugs that make your skin more susceptible to sunburn, such as tetracycline, thiazide diuretics, anti-anxiety medications such as alprazolam, and NSAIDs such as piroxicam.

TENDINITIS

YOUR SKELETAL STRUCTURE IS HELD IN PLACE by thousands of fibers that form tendons. The tendons attach the muscles to the bones and play a key role in all movements. Tendons and ligaments—which connect one bone to another—can become irritated and inflamed as a result of overuse, repetitive stress, and injury, causing a condition known as tendinitis. Acute tendinitis may develop into a chronic condition if left untreated. The most commonly affected joints include the shoulder (rotator cuff tendinitis), the elbow (tennis elbow or golfer's elbow), the wrist and thumb, the knee, and the ankles (Achilles tendinitis). Metabolic disorders such as diabetes can cause calcified tendinitis, which occurs when calcium deposits build up in a joint. Symptoms of tendinitis include joint pain that gets worse with movement, swelling accompanied by warmth and redness, tenderness of the limb, and crackling sounds when moving the affected joint. Typical treatment involves anti-inflammatory and pain medication along with physical therapy and rest. In unresponsive cases, an orthopedic physician will most likely recommend cortisone injections to reduce inflammation.

Known as painful obstruction syndrome, tendinitis in Chinese medicine represents blockage of energy and blood flow accompanied by dampness and heat in the affected joint and meridian system. The liver-gallbladder network is responsible for nourishing the tendons and joints of the body, so if this network is weakened as a result of emotional stress or toxic overload, the tendons become malnourished and prone to injury and damage. Tendons have much less blood supply than muscles, so tendon injuries are slower to heal than muscle injuries. I've found that tendinitis pain responds very well to acupuncture, as acupuncture can pinpoint where restored blood and energy flow are needed for healing a specific body part. With the addition of herbal therapy, I've treated many acute and chronic tendinitis conditions with excellent results. I also work with orthopedists, physical therapists, and other specialists to devise a treatment plan for complete recovery. My approach is to unblock the stagnation, promote the flow of energy and blood, strengthen the liver, and nourish the tendons and ligaments. I also advise my patients on appropriate exercises and lifestyle changes to prevent relapse of the condition.

Here are some of my recommendations.

 DIET

• Eat a healthy, well-balanced diet rich in vegetables and fruits, whole grains, and organic animal protein sources. The connective tissue structure also requires calcium and other minerals. Foods high in calcium and vitamin D (needed to enhance calcium absorption) include broccoli, chestnuts, clams, dark green vegetables, flounder, salmon, sardines, shrimp, mussels, and soybeans. Kidney beans, black beans, garlic, onions, kale, tempeh, pineapple, grapes, mulberries, anise seeds, cinnamon, cloves, almonds, walnuts, and prunes are also beneficial for the bones.

• Avoid carbonated soft drinks, alcohol, and smoking. Yeast, sugars, especially processed, bleached sugar, should be eliminated as well. Salt in small quantities can help strengthen the bones but should be used in moderation.

• For acute tendon or ligament injury, apply an ice pack to the painful area for 15 to 20 minutes 2 to 3 times a day in the first 24 to 48 hours.

• Take hot Epsom salt baths for 20 minutes a day until the pain is substantially decreased.

• Make a natural anti-inflammatory cocktail by mixing equal parts of unsweetened black cherry juice with dark grape juice. Drink 3 to 6 glasses a day until the pain has eased.

• Make a tea with 2 slices of ginger, 1/3 cup chopped parsnip, and 1 teaspoon of cinnamon in 3 1/2 cups of water. Simmer for 15 minutes. Strain, and drink 3 cups a day for 1 month or until condition improves.

• For pain and swelling, crush taro root to make a poultice, and apply to the affected joint, changing every 4 hours.

※ DAILY SUPPLEMENTS ※

• The enzyme bromelain (450 milligrams), from pineapple, is a natural anti-inflammatory and helps with muscle and joint pain.

• B complex vitamins and folate are generally diminished with stress and pain, so supplementation can help with the symptoms.

• Glucosamine (1,000 milligrams), chondroitin sulfate (400 milligrams), and MSM (1,000 milligrams) taken together can help support healthy bones and joints.

• Omega-3 fatty acids (1,000 milligrams EPA; 800 milligrams DHA) from fish or flaxseed oil are also naturally anti-inflammatory.

TENDINITIS

• Herbs can be found in health food or vitamin stores, online, and at the offices of Chinese medicine practitioners. Herbs should be used according to individual needs; consult with a licensed practitioner for a customized formulation. To learn more about the herbs listed here, go to www.ask drmao.com.

• A substance in turmeric known as curcumin reduces inflammation.

• White willow bark, licorice, and comfrey are traditionally used for tendinitis and other injuries.

• Traditional Chinese herbs used for tendinitis include angelica root, red peony, eucommia, siler, notoginseng, gastrodia, clematis, corydalis, myrrh, frankincense, rehmannia, and achyranthes.

———— ✳ EXERCISE ✳ ————

There is a definite advantage to exercising regularly. Exercise tones muscles and strengthens joints, and can help prevent tendinitis. Pay special attention to strenuous, repetitive, or jarring movements—especially in active sports—to prevent injury. Never stress the joints beyond their designed flexibility range. And always warm up prior to exercise. Most acute tendinitis cases are caused by not properly warming up before playing strenuous sports. Tai chi and qi gong can help strengthen the body without causing too much stress. The warm-up section of the Eight Treasures Qi Gong helps strengthen the joints and increase flexibility. Practice it twice a day for best results.

In a quiet, comfortable environment, preferably outdoors, stand with your feet shoulder-width apart, knees slightly bent, spine erect, tailbone tucked in, and head tilted slightly forward. Place your arms palms down on your lower abdomen just below the navel, one hand overlapping the other.

Begin with rhythmic, slow, and relaxed breathing. Inhale deeply but softly, and imagine the breath extending all the way down to the lower abdomen, about two finger-widths below the navel. Exhale gently and softly. Stay in this position for 7 breath cycles, relaxing and calming your mind.

Make your right hand into a loose fist and begin tapping your lower abdomen with mild to moderate strength in a rhythmic fashion. Proceed to the middle and upper abdomen, then the chest.

Start tapping under the armpit of the left arm, then the inner part of the arm and down to the palm. Then tap the outer part of the arm back up to the shoulder. Tap the shoulder muscle seven times.

Repeat the same movement with the left hand.

Begin tapping the lower back on both sides with both hands made into loose fists. Move the tapping down the backs of the legs to the outside of the ankles.

Start tapping on the insides of the ankles, working your way up the inside of the calves and thighs.

Finally, return to standing position, again tapping your lower abdomen. End by placing your palms on your lower abdomen, left hand on top of the right. Make clockwise circles, rubbing the lower abdomen 36 times.

✳ ACUPRESSURE ✳

• Find the acupoint Jumping Circle (GB-30), on the center of the buttocks about midway between the tip of the coccyx and the right hipbone. Apply heavy pressure with your thumb or index finger until you feel soreness. Hold for 30 seconds and release. Repeat several times, alternating the left and right sides.

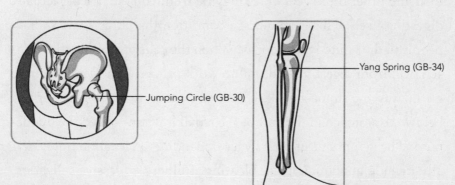

Jumping Circle (GB-30)

Yang Spring (GB-34)

• Find the acupoint Yang Spring (GB-34), on the outer part of the lower right leg, just below the bony structure located near the end of the knee crease, about four finger-widths below the kneecap. Apply steady pressure with your right thumb until you feel soreness. Hold for 3 minutes. Repeat on the left leg.

AVOID

• Smoking, and excessive use of alcohol, as they are irritants, and alcohol especially depletes the liver energy, leaving tendons weak and malnourished.

• Certain medications used for weight loss, such as Xenical (orlistat), as well as minoxidil, which can cause tendinitis. Talk to your doctor about alternatives.

• Repetitive tasks at work or repetitive sports activities. Be mindful of your physical activities and posture and make sure you warm up before exercising.

ULCERS

THAT GNAWING PAIN IN THE STOMACH that sometimes gets better with food and other times gets worse may be from your stomach's actually digesting itself! This is an ulcer, a condition that affects five million people in the United States today. When the cells protecting the stomach wall from digestive acids fail to work properly, the acids begin to burn away the stomach wall. Ulcers can occur in the stomach or just below the stomach in the part of the small intestine called the duodenum. The symptoms of ulcers vary depending on location but generally include abdominal pain, bloating, fullness, excessive salivation, nausea, vomiting, loss of appetite, and weight loss. You can tell where the ulcer is located based on the pattern of pain—if the ulcer is in the duodenum, the pain gets better after eating but worse an hour later; if it's in the stomach, the pain gets worse when eating. In severe cases there may be vomiting of blood or passing of a tarlike black stool, which is a result of bleeding from the duodenum. A major cause of ulcers is bacterial infection. The bacteria *Helicobacter pylori* erode the stomach lining, reducing the protective mucous membrane and stimulating the production of excessive stomach acid. Prolonged use of aspirin and other nonsteroidal anti-inflammatory drugs has also been linked with ulcers, as have smoking, alcohol use, and stress. Antibiotics and acid blocker medications are commonly prescribed for ulcers.

Chinese medicine recognizes that pathogens, diet, and stress play key roles in the development of digestive disorders. Ulcers in particular are viewed as a disharmony between the stomach and liver networks. I see many more conditions of gastroesophageal reflux disorder (GERD)—a precursor condition—than ulcers. The treatment for both conditions focuses on harmonizing the stomach and liver systems, healing the lining of the digestive tract, supporting the functions of digestion, and easing pain and discomfort.

I once had a patient with stomach pain and other symptoms of an ulcer, including a black, tarlike stool. Her gastroenterologist had confirmed the diagnosis with an endoscopy. After three separate courses of antibiotics she was still experiencing pain and an occasional dark bowel movement, and her GI specialist referred her to me. I put her on a treatment program of acupuncture and herbal therapies, and I changed her diet and taught her stress-reduction techniques. Within six weeks, her symptoms disappeared and have not returned.

Here are some of my favorite remedies for ulcers. If you are experiencing severe, doubling-over pain that spreads across the entire abdomen, vom-

ULCERS

iting with blood, or black, tarlike stools for more than three days, you should consult your physician immediately.

❋ DIET ❋

• The single most important thing you can do to help treat ulcers is to improve your diet. Eating in smaller amounts and more frequently, as well as eating a good breakfast, are essential. According to Chinese medicine, the energy of the stomach network is at it peak between 7:00 and 9:00 a.m., so skipping breakfast robs the stomach of its vital energy source. A high-fiber diet rich in whole grains, legumes, fruits, and vegetables is helpful. Favor alkalinizing foods such as potatoes, cabbage, figs, papaya, kale, spinach, mustard greens, Swiss chard, winter squashes, zucchini, carrots, sweet potatoes, yams, lentils, split peas, and persimmons.

• Do not overeat, skip meals, or eat late at night. Deep-fried and greasy foods stimulate acid and bile production, and should be avoided. Spicy foods, acidic foods, and alcohol are irritants to the stomach lining. Sugar and salt can also act to increase stomach acid and should be minimized. Each person reacts to certain foods differently—there may be particular foods that aggravate ulcers for you, so be watchful of these foods and keep a diary to eliminate foods that are particularly uncomfortable for you. Tomatoes, eggplant, citrus fruits, pineapple, vinegar, and chilies tend to be prime offenders.

❋ HOME REMEDIES ❋

• Cabbage contains several anti-ulcer compounds, so including cabbage in your diet can speed up the healing of ulcers. Try this simple cabbage soup recipe: Combine 2 cups shredded cabbage, 1 cup chopped celery, 1 cup diced potatoes, 1/2 cup okra, 1/2 cup diced onions with 6 cups water and bring to a boil over high heat, then simmer for 30 minutes, or until the vegetables are tender. Season with a pinch of ginger, cumin, and oregano and garnish with cilantro. Eat the cabbage soup 3 to 4 times a week for 1 month, or until the condition improves.

• Make a healing shake with 1 chopped banana, 1/3 cup chopped raw potato, 1/2 cup blueberries, a pinch each of ground cinnamon, cloves, and ginger, and 1 tablespoon honey. Blend in a blender with 1 cup rice milk and 1/2 cup low-fat plain yogurt. Drink with breakfast every morning for 1 month.

• Eat 1 tablespoon of honey on an empty stomach several times throughout the day, keeping the honey in your mouth and allowing it to slowly move down your esophagus. Honey is nature's antibiotic and has been found to inhibit *Helicobacter pylori*.

✳ DAILY SUPPLEMENTS ✳

• Supplementing with zinc (50 milligrams), vitamin A (200 IU), and selenium (100 micrograms) can help heal ulcers.

• Taking flavonoid supplements (500 milligrams) can help with the absorption of vitamin C (1,000 milligrams) and support the healing process.

• Quercetin (500 milligrams) taken 3 times a day can help to suppress ulcer formation and also has anticancer properties.

✳ HERBAL THERAPY ✳

• Herbs can be found in health food or vitamin stores, online, and at the offices of Chinese medicine practitioners. Herbs should be used according to individual needs; consult with a licensed practitioner for a customized formulation. To learn more about the herbs listed here, go to www.ask drmao.com.

• A specialized licorice preparation called deglycyrrhized licorice (DGL) taken in chewable form before meals and at bedtime can help relieve ulcer symptoms and help with healing.

ULCERS

• Make a tea by boiling 2 tablespoons dried marigold flowers in 3 1/2 cups of water for 15 minutes. Strain, and drink 1 cup 3 times a day for 2 weeks or until the condition improves. Marigold has traditionally been used to heal ulcers.

....

• Reishi mushrooms in capsule or tablet form can help the immune system fight inflammation in the stomach.

....

• Traditional Chinese herbs such as sepia, skullcap, bamboo, and coptidis have antibacterial and acid-neutralizing properties.

✳ EXERCISE ✳

Walking is the best exercise for moving the food along the digestive tract and improving digestion and absorption. The energetic meridians of the digestive organs run along the large muscles of the legs, so walking stimulates energy flow within the channels and promotes digestion. Take an easy 10-minute walk after each meal and massage your abdomen as you walk, making circles around your navel with your palms. This helps move your food through your digestive tract without prolonged accumulation.

A simple walking exercise called Merry-Go-Around Circle Walk is quite helpful for people who can't exercise vigorously because of a health condition or other prohibiting circumstances.

In a quiet outdoor setting—a park or yard—find a tree with at least 5 feet of clear space around the trunk in all directions. If you were to draw a circle around the tree, its diameter would be around 10 to 12 feet, though larger or smaller circles are fine as well. Perform the exercise for 15 minutes twice a day.

For the first half of the exercise walk clockwise around the tree. For the second half, walk counterclockwise.

With each completed circle change the position of your arms by slightly raising or lowering your hands in front or on the sides of your trunk.

• Find the acupoint Valley of Harmony (LI-4), at the web between your right thumb and index finger. Apply steady pressure with your left thumb until you feel soreness. Hold for 2 minutes. Repeat on the left hand. This is good for reducing heat and inflammation and opening energy blockages in the GI tract.

• Find the acupoint Inner Gate (P-6), three finger-widths above the wrist crease, between the two tendons on the inside of the left forearm. Apply moderate pressure with your right thumb. Hold for 5 minutes. Repeat on the right arm. This settles the stomach, helps reduce acidity, and calms anxiety.

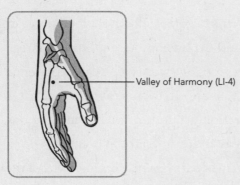

Valley of Harmony (LI-4)

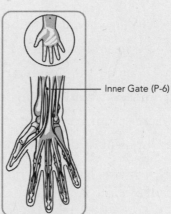

Inner Gate (P-6)

AVOID

• Coffee, alcohol, and smoking; they all can cause or worsen ulcers.

• Excessive use of nonsteroidal anti-inflammatory drugs such as aspirin, which can injure the stomach lining, potentially leading to ulcers. Talk to your doctor about alternatives if you are taking this type of medication.

• Stress, anxiety, and emotional upset before eating and while you're eating, as this can worse the condition.

ULCERS

VARICOSE VEINS AND SPIDER VEINS

THOSE UNSIGHTLY AND SOMETIMES PAINFUL VEINS that resemble twisted ropes are called varicose veins. A milder form of this condition is known as telangiectasia, or spider veins. Varicose veins are the result of faulty operation of the valves within the veins, which normally help the blood move from the arms and legs back up to the heart. I liken the action of these valves to locks on the Panama Canal—each lock prevents the backflow of seawater, which allows the ship to move from the lower elevation of the Pacific to the higher elevation of the Atlantic Ocean.

When the valves within the veins become defective, blood pools in these areas, enlarging the veins and producing bulging, ropelike features on the skin. With varying degrees of severity, one can experience pain, heavy sensations in the legs that are often worse at night and after exercise, ankle swelling, discoloration around the veins, and the development of dry, itchy, thin areas that can lead to eczema (venous eczema). In the worst cases, the skin is permanently discolored as a result of waste products building up in the legs. More common in women than in men, varicose veins can result from hereditary predisposition, pregnancy, obesity, menopause, aging, prolonged standing, or the prolonged straining that often accompanies chronic constipation.

In Chinese medicine, varicose result from weakness of the muscles and connective tissues, which are governed by the spleen network or the digestive system. With chronic weakness comes the pooling of blood and energy, leading to varicose veins or spider veins. My treatments focus on strengthening the spleen network, supporting healthy digestive function, toning the muscles, and activating the movement of blood and energy. I use acupuncture, acupressure, and massage to stimulate blood circulation, and I target local varicose veins with topical and oral herbal therapy to help reduce swelling and discoloration. I also recommend specific lower-leg exercises to keep the muscles and veins strong.

Here are some of my favorite remedies for varicose veins and spider veins. If you experience severe pain, bleeding, or lumps around the varicose veins you should see a vascular specialist immediately.

❄ DIET ❄

• A high-fiber diet helps prevent constipation, which can build up pressure and aggravate varicose veins. Concentrate your meals around whole grains, legumes, fruits, and vegetables. Citrus fruits (with the rind), apricots, blueberries, blackberries, cherries, rose hips, buckwheat, and millet all contain rutin, a bioflavonoid routinely used to treat varicose veins. Garlic, onions, ginger, and cayenne pepper contain compounds that strengthen the tissues and walls of the veins. Eat plenty of fish, as they are rich in omega-3 fatty acids and can help strengthen the veins and reduce plaque and inflammation.

• Do not overeat. Cut out red meat entirely and restrict fats, refined sugars, and simple carbohydrates. Avoid foods containing preservatives and artificial coloring and flavoring. Salt, alcohol, cheese, and ice cream should be avoided as well.

❄ HOME REMEDIES ❄

• Boil 1 cup of hawthorn berries in 4 cups of water for 20 minutes. Strain, and drink 3 cups a day for 1 month, or until the condition improves. Hawthorn berry can help to tone the cardiovascular system.

• Make tea from 2 tablespoons each of yarrow, horse chestnut, ginger, and prickly ash bark by boiling them in a pot of about 3 1/2 cups of water. Strain, and drink 1 cup 3 times a day for 1 month, or until the condition improves.

• Massaging witch hazel cream twice a day into the affected area can reduce the formation of spider and varicose veins.

• Apply a rag saturated with warmed apple cider vinegar to the varicose veins for 20 minutes twice a day. Follow this treatment with an 8-ounce glass of warm water mixed with apple cider vinegar and 1 teaspoon honey.

❈ DAILY SUPPLEMENTS ❈

• Taking zinc supplements (50 milligrams) can help retain vitamin E (800 IU) in the bloodstream and strengthen the veins.

• Vitamin E supplements (800 IU) can be a preventive against varicose veins.

• Taking vitamin A (400 IU) can help ease varicose ulcerations and speed up healing.

• Taking vitamin C (3,000 milligrams) daily can help strengthen vein walls and prevent dilation.

• Bioflavonoids (800 milligrams) contain properties beneficial for vascular health.

❈ HERBAL THERAPY ❈

• Herbs can be found in health food or vitamin stores, online, and at the offices of Chinese medicine practitioners. Herbs should be used according to individual needs; consult with a licensed practitioner for a customized formulation. To learn more about the herbs listed here, go to www.ask drmao.com.

• Horse chestnut (*Semen Aesculus hippocastanum*) taken daily can be helpful in reducing varicose veins.

• Butcher's broom (*Ruscus aculeatus*) is traditionally used to strengthen loose and bulging veins.

....

• Traditional Chinese herbs used for varicose and spider veins and to support healthy vascular function include angelica, safflower, peach seed, peony, motherwort, cinnamon, ligusticum, cyathulae root, hare's ear root, balloon flower root, bitter orange, and licorice.

❉ EXERCISE ❉

Use gravity to reduce the pressure on the veins in your legs. Lie flat on the floor and rest your legs on a chair or straight up against a wall for 5 minutes twice a day to help drain blood from swollen veins. Daily exercise is one of the most effective treatments for strengthening your muscles and vasculature, and swimming is by far the best exercise, as it doesn't put weight on your legs. If you don't have access to a pool, use a recumbent stationary bike. Swim or bike for at least 30 minutes a day. Daily stretching exercises upon waking also help.

The following Dao In Qi Gong exercise, Immortal Straightening the Leg, can help strengthen the muscles and promote blood circulation in the legs. Do this exercise for 10 minutes twice a day.

Lie on your back with your legs straight, feet apart, and arms straight and resting naturally alongside your body with your palms up.

Inhale, and bend your left knee, folding your left leg up to your chest.

Clasp your leg with your hands; interlace and lock your fingers. Your body should be relaxed with your head on the floor.

Exhale, and make a circle with your foot at your ankle. Do 5 clockwise circles, then 5 counterclockwise circles.

Inhale, and straighten your knee so your leg is straight up, perpendicular to the floor.

Exhale, and gently and slowly lower your straight leg to the floor, returning to the beginning posture.

Repeat the sequence with your right leg.

• Find the acupoint Foot Three Miles (ST-36), four finger-widths below the kneecap on the right leg. Apply moderate pressure with your right thumb until you feel soreness. Hold for 5 minutes. Repeat on the left leg.

• Find the acupoint Three Yin Crossing (SP-6), four finger-widths above the inner right anklebone, in the depression near the bone. Apply steady pressure with your right thumb until you feel soreness. Hold for 3 minutes. Repeat on the left leg.

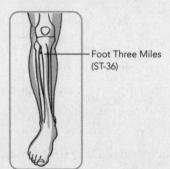

Foot Three Miles (ST-36)

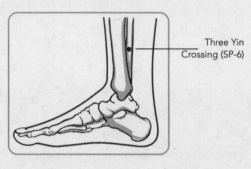

Three Yin Crossing (SP-6)

———————— AVOID ————————

• Smoking and alcohol, which are irritants and damage the walls of the blood vessels.

• Prolonged standing or straining. If your job requires you to stand for long periods of time, do the above exercise every hour and stretch your legs at least twice during the day.

WARTS

A COMMON SKIN CONDITION CAUSED by the human papillomavirus (HPV), warts come in a variety of sizes and shapes, and they can occur on the extremities, the face, the genital region, and the soles of the feet. Genital warts are contagious, whereas flat and common warts are not. Mostly harmless and painless, common warts are more of an aesthetic challenge to most people. Those with compromised immune systems, such as people with HIV/AIDS, autoimmune conditions, and those debilitated as a result of severe illnesses, alcohol abuse, and smoking are at an increased risk of getting warts. Hygiene also plays a role—unclean communal baths, showers, and pools are breeding grounds for the HPV virus. Conventional medical treatment involves topical applications of salicylic and lactic acids or surgical removal.

In Chinese medicine, warts are seen as an invasion by a dampness toxin and as a stasis of energy and blood. An underlying weakness in the immune system allows the invasion of pathogens. The best approach is to boost immune function by activating the lung and spleen networks, unblock the stagnation, and expel the pathogenic accumulation. I work with dermatologists to treat children with recurring warts—mainly on their hands and feet—with good success in preventing recurrence. The immunity of children is often inadequately developed, so strengthening immune function is paramount in the prevention and treatment of skin warts. I administer both oral and topical herbal therapy, and dietary and hygiene measures are often part of the treatment. Here are some recommendations I give to my patients.

❊ DIET ❊

• A well-balanced, organic diet is important for maintaining a well-functioning immune system and for nourishing the skin. In many cases of warts (especially flat warts) there is an identified nutritional deficiency of vital substances. Your diet should be based on whole grains, fresh vegetables, nuts and seeds, and organic sources of animal protein. Essential fatty acids obtained from cold-water fish, seeds, and nuts are also important.
• Alcohol consumption increases your risk of getting warts. Caffeine and refined, processed foods, simple sugars, and soft drinks should be eliminated. Dairy and saturated fats and animal fats should be minimized.

• Apply fresh milky juice from a calendula plant (purchased from a plant nursery) directly on the wart 3 or 4 times a day.

• Aloe vera gel applied directly from the plant to the wart can help remove warts.

• Cut a small square patch from a fresh banana peel. Place it face down on the wart and secure it in place with a bandage or medical tape. Leave it on overnight, changing it every day for 2 to 3 weeks, until the wart is gone.

• Before bed, apply a thin layer of castor oil or olive oil to the affected area, then place slices of garlic on top of the wart and secure it with medical tape or a bandage. Change daily for 2 to 3 weeks, or until the wart is gone.

• Make an immunity broth by cooking 1/2 cup each of broccoli, cauliflower, Brussels sprouts, cabbage, asparagus, and shiitake mushrooms in 6 to 8 cups water and simmer for 1 hour. Add miso to taste. Eat 1 bowl every day until the wart subsides.

━━━━━━━━ ✻ DAILY SUPPLEMENTS ✻ ━━━━━━━━

• Supplementing with vitamin C (1,000 milligrams), beta-carotene (800 milligrams), vitamin E (800 IU), and zinc (50 milligrams) can help support immune function and facilitate healing. Vitamin E in oil form may be used as topical antiviral.

• Vitamin B complex helps with stress and depression, which can weaken your immune system. Selenium (200 micrograms) also supports the immune function.

• Folic acid (800 micrograms) is recommended for treating genital warts.

• Taking L-lysine (1,000 milligrams), garlic (800 milligrams), and bee propolis (450 milligrams) can reduce viral activity.

• Traditional Chinese herbs for warts include brucia seed, tribulus, drynaria, smoked plum, perilla leaf, coix seeds, isatis, angelica, peony, cardamon, apricot seeds, and cork tree bark.

....

• Other herbs that are antiviral and detoxify include sephora, smilacis, gentian, magnetite, honeysuckle, phellodendri, and safflower.

────────── ❋ EXERCISE ❋ ──────────

The General Cleansing Qi Gong is a meditation practice designed to cleanse the body of toxins and strengthen the immune system. It helps with circulation, promotes movement of qi and blood, and cleanses the skin and channels of pathogens.

Sit comfortably or lie down on your back. Slow your respiration to deep, abdominal breathing. Say the word "calm" in your mind with every exhalation. You'll be visualizing the relaxation of a body part and releasing tension with every exhalation. Trace the following 3 pathways outlined below.

Start at the top of your head. Inhale, and then exhale and visualize your scalp muscles relaxing. Say "calm" in your mind. Repeat this, saying the word with each body part as you move down through your face, throat, chest, abdomen, thighs, knees, calves, ankles, and feet. When you've relaxed your feet, visualize all the tension in your body leaving through your toes in the form of dark smoke.

Next, start at the temple region of your head. This pathway focuses on the sides and upper extremities. Inhale, and then exhale and visualize your temple muscles relaxing. Say the word "calm" in your mind. Repeat this, saying the word with each body part as you move down through your jaw, the sides of your neck, shoulders, upper arms, elbows, forearms, wrists, and hands. Once you've relaxed your hands, visualize all the tension leaving your body through your fingertips in the form of dark smoke.

The final pathway begins at the back of your head. This pathway relaxes the back of your body. Repeat the breathing-visualization-word rou-

WARTS

tine, as above, as you go from the back of your neck to your upper back, middle back, lower back, back of thighs, calves, and heels. Then focus on the acupoint Bubbling Spring (KID-1), on the soles of your feet, for 1 minute.

Practice this exercise for at least 15 minutes twice a day.

❋ ACUPRESSURE ❋

• Locate the acupoint Winding Gulch (LI-11), in the depression at the outer part of the right elbow crease, between the elbow tendon and the bone. The point is best located when the arm is bent at 90 degrees with the palm facing the abdomen. Apply steady pressure with your left thumb until you feel soreness. Hold for 3 minutes. Repeat on the left arm.

• Find the acupoint Foot Three Miles (ST-36), four finger-widths below the kneecap on the right leg. Apply moderate pressure with your right thumb until you feel soreness. Hold for 5 minutes. Repeat on the left leg.

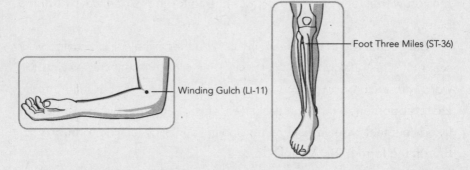

Foot Three Miles (ST-36)

Winding Gulch (LI-11)

AVOID

• Using public facilities, and practice healthy hygiene. Wash your hands regularly.

• Alcohol and smoking, as they drastically increase your chances of developing warts.

• Stress and avoid emotional extremes.

THE CANDIDA YEAST ORGANISM is a normal part of the intestinal flora—the microorganisms that live in the digestive tract. The balance of the intestinal flora can be disturbed by the use of antibiotics, birth control pills, immunosuppressant drugs, hormones, poor diet, excess stress, alcohol consumption, and other factors. In cases of extreme imbalance, candida flourishes. Initially its overgrowth is limited to the intestines, but it can invade other parts of the body, the most common of which is the vaginal tract. When left untreated, yeast overgrowth produces alcohol and other toxic by-products that put stress on the body. Over 75 percent of women suffer a vaginal yeast infection at least once. The humid, moist, and warm environment of the vagina is very hospitable to yeast. The most common symptom of a yeast infection is a creamy, curdlike discharge accompanied by vaginal itching and burning, painful urination, and pain during intercourse. The condition often gets worse after receiving antibiotic treatments. Conventional medicine typically treats yeast infections with topical or oral antifungal medications.

Chinese medicine classifies candida as an accumulation of dampness and heat toxin in the body. Often a result of a weakened spleen-pancreas-stomach network, digestion is impaired, leading to a buildup of dampness, which tends to permeate the lower parts of the body. The sticky, congealing nature of dampness combined with emotional stress blocks the free flow of energy, generating heat and toxins. The dampness and heat toxin discharge through the vaginal opening, giving rise to the symptoms of candida infection. The relationship between the digestive system and yeast is the key to long-term relief from recurrent yeast infections; this is the case for most of the patients I see for yeast infections. Yeast infections can also result from a weakened immune system, as in chronic fatigue syndrome. My approach to treatment starts with a diet free of ingredients that fuel the growth of yeast, such as refined carbohydrates. I use acupuncture and herbal therapies to support healthy immune function and to inhibit fungal activity and expel dampness and heat toxins.

Below are recommendations I give to my patients.

❊ DIET ❊

• The most important line of defense against candida imbalance, which is almost always the cause of vaginal yeast infections, is proper diet. The diet should be low in carbohydrates—all breads, including wheat and rye breads—should be eliminated, as well as dairy products, cheeses of all kinds, alcohol, sugar, pastries, candy, vinegar, and all pickled foods. Cold and raw foods cause digestive dampness and therefore should be avoided. Leftovers should be frozen, not refrigerated, since mold has a great opportunity to grow overnight.

• Eat more leafy green vegetables, including spinach, collard greens, Swiss chard, mustard greens, dandelion greens, beet tops, carrot tops, as well as barley, garlic, mung beans, citrus fruits, kohlrabi, cabbage, artichokes, and shiitake mushrooms. Fish and nuts should replace red meat and animal fats. Walnut, sesame, flaxseed, olive, and virgin coconut oils are most desirable. Eat little or no fruits, as their sugars fuel the growth of yeast.

❊ HOME REMEDIES ❊

• Make a tea by boiling 1 cup of fresh dandelion in 3 1/2 cups of water for 30 minutes. Strain, and drink 3 cups a day.

• Eat 2 steamed artichokes a day for 1 week, or until the condition clears up. Artichokes have natural antifungal properties.

• Juice 1 bunch beet tops, 1 bunch carrot tops, and 1 large daikon radish. Drink 2 to 3 glasses a day for 1 week, or until the condition subsides.

─────────── ❋ DAILY SUPPLEMENTS ❋ ───────────

• Vitamins C (1,000 milligrams) and E (800 IU) and selenium (200 micrograms) act as anti-inflammatory agents and help support immune function.

....

• Omega-6 (450 milligrams GLA) and omega-3 (1,000 milligrams EPA; 800 milligrams DHA) essential fatty acids are useful as natural anti-inflammatories.

....

• Probiotics such as acidophilus (3 to 5 billion organisms) are commonly used supplements to control candida overgrowth.

....

• Taking enteric-coated garlic pills (900 milligrams) can inhibit the growth of candida.

....

• Taking caprylic acid (500 milligrams) work as an effective antifungal.

....

• Make sure all vitamins and supplements that you take are yeast free.

─────────── ❋ HERBAL THERAPY ❋ ───────────

• Herbs can be found in health food or vitamin stores, online, and at the offices of Chinese medicine practitioners. Herbs should be used according to individual needs; consult with a licensed practitioner for a customized formulation. To learn more about the herbs listed here, go to www.askdrmao.com.

....

• Chinese herbs that have specific and general antifungal properties include pagoda tree fruit, chaulmoogra seeds, erythrina bark, aloe vera, and genkwa flower.

....

• Traditional Chinese herbs used to treat yeast infections include gentian root, skullcap, gardenia, akebia, plantain, alisma, bupleurum, rehmannia, angelica, and licorice.

....

• Herbs to strengthen the spleen-pancreas-stomach network and digestive function include hawthorn, astragalus, codonopsis, atractylodis, tangerine, cardamom, and dioscorea.

❈ EXERCISE ❈

In addition to a regular exercise regimen, I recommend the General Cleansing Qi Gong, which helps with circulation, cleanses the body of toxins, and enhances immune function.

Sit comfortably or lie down on your back. Slow your respiration to deep, abdominal breathing. Say the word "calm" in your mind with every exhalation. You'll be visualizing the relaxation of a body part and releasing tension with every exhalation. Trace the following 3 pathways outlined below.

Start at the top of your head. Inhale, and then exhale and visualize your scalp muscles relaxing. Say "calm" in your mind. Repeat this, saying the word with each body part as you move down through your face, throat, chest, abdomen, thighs, knees, calves, ankles, and feet. When you've relaxed your feet, visualize all the tension in your body leaving through your toes in the form of dark smoke.

Next, start at the temple region of your head. This pathway focuses on the sides and upper extremities. Inhale, and then exhale and visualize your temple muscles relaxing. Say the word "calm" in your mind. Repeat this, saying the word with each body part as you move down through your jaw, the sides of your neck, shoulders, upper arms, elbows, forearms, wrists, and hands. Once you've relaxed your hands, visualize all the tension leaving your body through your fingertips in the form of dark smoke.

The final pathway begins at the back of your head. This path relaxes the back of your body. Repeat the breathing-visualization-word routine, as above, as you go from the back of your neck to your upper back, middle back, lower back, back of thighs, calves, and heels. Then focus on the acupoint Bubbling Spring (KID-1), on the soles of your feet, for 1 minute.

Practice this exercise for at least 15 minutes twice a day.

❊ ACUPRESSURE ❊

• Find the acupoint Foot Three Miles (ST-36), four finger-widths below the kneecap on the right leg. Apply moderate pressure with your right thumb until you feel soreness. Hold for 2 minutes. Repeat on the left leg.

• Find the acupoint Abundant Flesh (ST-40), midway between the bottom of the right kneecap and outer anklebone, two finger-widths to the outside of the shinbone. Apply steady pressure with your right thumb until you feel soreness. Hold for 2 minutes. Repeat on the left leg.

• Engaging these points can strengthen digestive function and enhance immunity to prevent candida buildup.

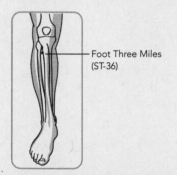

Foot Three Miles
(ST-36)

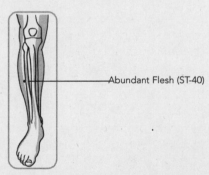

Abundant Flesh (ST-40)

AVOID

• Improper hygiene, to prevent vaginal yeast infections.

• Douches, vaginal deodorants, and long bubble baths taken often, which can change the pH balance of the vaginal canal in favor of yeast overgrowth.

• Broad-spectrum antibiotics, which radically alter balance and can cause yeast overgrowth. Consult your physician.

• Alcohol use and overeating sweets, which also contribute to yeast buildup.

. . . .

IN ANCIENT CHINA, parents were respected and revered by their children. Traditionally, when someone is your teacher, even for just a day, you pay respect and reverence to him or her as you would to a parent. I owe my knowledge of healing to my father, Hua-Ching Ni, who was my first teacher of Chinese medicine. According to tradition, this makes him my father many times over. It was my father whose healing brought me back to life from a near-death coma when I was a child, whose inspiration encouraged me to enter the medical profession, and whose extensive writing forms the philosophical foundation upon which this book is based. I am fortunate to be his son and student, and I am forever indebted to him.

I am appreciative to my many patients over the years, who taught me how to listen and be compassionate, and who gave me the chance to show them how to activate their innate self-healing powers.

I am grateful to Aram Akopyan, a business partner and former student of outstanding aptitude—and now a licensed practitioner of Chinese medicine—whose research and compilations contributed enormously to the second part of this book.

Special thanks to my editor, Jeff Galas, for his conviction about the value of my work and his patience and editorial expertise; to Megan Newman, Avery's publisher; to Leda Scheintaub, my copy editor; and to all the folks at Avery/Penguin whose collective efforts brought this book to fruition.

My deep gratitude to Laurie Dolphin, my unwavering collaborator and partner, for her complete dedication to my writing endeavors. Her thoughtful design graces the pages of this book and has made it infinitely more accessible. Special thanks to her assistant, Allison Meierding, the project manager extraordinaire, and to Patty Wu, who did an amazing job on the illustrations of acupuncture points.

I am thankful to Stuart Shapiro, who has believed in my abilities since the early days of my professional career. Stuart is a maverick strategist whose insights in the publishing world compare with his extraordinary work in the political world.

Special recognition goes to Cathy McNease for helping me bring Chinese nutrition remedies to Western readers more than twenty years ago as the coauthor of my first book on self-healing, *The Tao of Nutrition*.

I could not ask for a better partner in our medical practice than my brother Dr. Daoshing Ni and his wife, Sumyee, who share the same vision for wellness medicine. Both have been there with me each and every step from the beginning of the Tao of Wellness Center to the founding of Yo San University. Thank you for being there for me.

I could not have completed this book in a timely fashion without the patience and loving support of my wife, Emm, and my children, Yu-Shien Michelle, Yu-Shing Natasha, and Yu-Kai Nicolas. They have been the recipients of many of the self-healing remedies described in this book. Thank you for making my life fulfilling.

Finally, I thank my mother, who not only nurtured me from birth to adulthood with her maternal love, a powerful medicine, but is still to this day a constant source of wonderful home healing remedies. Thank you for making me eat and drink all those strange-tasting but effective natural preparations. I am a testament to the power of self-healing.

. . . .

ASK DR. MAO

The official website for *Secrets of Self Healing* and Dr. Mao's other books. It is a natural health search engine that contains thousands of searchable health questions and answers as well as articles on health, wellness, and longevity. You may also look up herbs and purchase Dr. Mao's herbal products here.
www.askdrmao.com
info@askdrmao.com

ACUPUNCTURE.COM

The oldest, most comprehensive, and most informative website for acupuncture, acupressure, Chinese herbal medicine, nutrition, Tui Na bodywork, tai chi, qi gong, and related healing practices. This excellent resource for self-healing for both consumers and practitioners offers access to an acupoints database and hundreds of publications and herbal products, and a directory of licensed practitioners throughout the United States.
www.acupuncture.com
info@acupuncture.com

ARTHRITIS ALTERNATIVE

This is an excellent resource for people suffering from arthritis, with a wealth of educational information on various types of arthritis and natural healing options including diet, herbs, and supplements.
www.arthritis-alternative.com
info@arthritis-alternative.com

CHI HEALTH INSTITUTE (CHI)

The Chi Health Institute is a nonprofit association that is dedicated to promoting health and self-healing through the mind-body movement arts. The Institute offers public courses as well as professional-level education and certification programs for tai chi, qi gong, and meditation from the Ni family tradition. It also maintains a directory of certified CHI instructors around the world.
www.chihealth.org
info@chihealth.org

GNC

GNC is the nation's largest retailer of nutritional supplements, with more than 5,000 retail locations throughout the United States. For store locations, go to the website.
www.gnc.com

HEALING PEOPLE NETWORK

A comprehensive website on complementary and alternative medicine (CAM) for consumers and practitioners. In-depth coverage of subjects such as acupuncture, aromatherapy, ayurveda, bodywork, Chinese medicine, cancer-risk reduction, environmental toxicology, fitness training, herbalism, homeopathy, naturopathy, nutrition and lifestyle, pet health, and other natural-healing modalities. The site also provides a referral network of CAM practitioners throughout the United States and access to more than 1,000 professional-grade supplement products.

www.healingpeople.com
contact@healingpeople.com

HERB RESEARCH FOUNDATION

Provides useful information on well-researched therapeutic herbs and publishes a magazine, *HerbalGram*.
4140 15th St.
Boulder, CO 80304
www.herbs.org

INTEGRAL LIVING INSTITUTE

The Integral Living Institute is a nonprofit educational organization that offers distance-learning courses and certification programs in Chinese Nutrition and Dietary Therapy. Students learn at home through DVDs and workbooks the theories and practice of Chinese Nutrition in the three-module course at their own pace. Future programs planned include Chinese herbal therapy and acupressure. Great for people interested in natural self-healing for themselves as well as for those looking to become a natural-health educator or consultant.

www.Integralliving.net
tot@traditionsoftao.com

TAO OF WELLNESS

The medical and wellness centers in Southern California founded by Dr. Mao with his brother Dr. Daoshing Ni. They both practice here, along with a team of associates. The center focuses on delivering exceptional treatments in acupuncture and Chinese medicine. Besides its general medicine practice, Tao of Wellness is renowned for its work in fertility, women's health, longevity, immune health, and oncology support.
1131 Wilshire Blvd., Suite 300
Santa Monica, CA 90401
www.taoofwellness.com
contact@taoofwellness.com

VITAMIN SHOPPE
A retail chain of more than 300 stores nationwide, it offers a large selection of vitamin and herbal supplements in stores and online. For store locations, consult the website.
www.vitaminshoppe.com

WHOLE FOODS MARKET
Founded in 1980 as one small store in Austin, Texas, Whole Foods Market is now the world's leading retailer of natural and organic foods, with close to 200 stores in North America and the United Kingdom. These stores are a good place for healthy, mostly organic food, herbs, dietary supplements, and household supplies.
www.wholefoods.com

WILD OATS MARKET
Founded in 1987 as Crystal Market, this was the only vegetarian natural food store in Boulder, Colorado. Wild Oats is now the second-largest retailer of natural and organic foods, with more than 100 stores in North America. These stores are a good source for healthy, natural, and organic food, herbs, supplements, and household supplies.
www.wildoats.com

WORLD RESEARCH FOUNDATION
WRF established a unique international nonprofit health information network to help people stay informed about all available treatments around the world. This is one of the few organizations that provide health information on both allopathic and alternative medicine techniques.
www.wrf.org
info@wrf.org

YO SAN UNIVERSITY
An accredited graduate school of traditional Chinese medicine founded by Dr. Mao and his family. Its rigorous academic, clinical, and spiritual development programs train students for the professional practice of acupuncture and Eastern medicine, and carry on the authentic medical tradition.
13315 W. Washington Blvd., Suite 200
Los Angeles, CA 90066
www.yosan.edu
admissions@yosan.edu

REFERENCES

Balch, P.A. *Prescription for Nutritional Healing*. 4th ed. New York: Avery, 2006.

Beers, M.H., and R. Berkow, eds. *The Merck Manual of Diagnosis and Therapy.* 17th ed. Whitehouse Station, NJ: Merck Research, 1999.

Benskey, D., and R. Barolet. *Chinese Herbal Medicine Formulas and Strategies.* Seattle: Eastland, 2000.

Blumenthal, M., ed. *The Complete German Commission E Monographs: Therapeutic Guide to Herbal Medicines*. Boston, MA: Integrative Medicine, 1998.

Bunney, S., ed. *The Illustrated Encyclopedia of Herbs: Their Medicinal and Culinary Uses.* New York: Dorset, 1984.

Cameron, M. *Lifetime Encyclopedia of Natural Remedies*. Paramus, NJ: Prentice Hall, 1993.

Chen, J., and T. Chen. *Chinese Medical Herbology and Pharmacology.* Los Angeles: Art of Medicine Press, 2005.

Cline, D., H. W. Hofstetter, and J. R. Griffin. *Dictionary of Visual Science*. 4th ed. Boston, MA: Butterworth-Heinemann, 1997.

Crook, W. G. *The Yeast Connection: A Medical Breakthrough*. Jackson, TN: Professional Books, 1986.

Cummings, S., and D. Ullman. *Everybody's Guide to Homeopathic Medicines*. 3rd ed. New York: Putnam, 1997.

Dambro, M.R. *Griffith's 5 Minute Clinical Consult*. Baltimore, MD: Lippincott Williams & Wilkins, 1999.

Dunkell, S. *Goodbye Insomnia, Hello Sleep*. New York: Carol, 1994.

Fauci, A.S., E. Braunwald, K. J. Isselbacher, et al., eds. *Harrison's Principles of Internal Medicine*. 14th ed. New York: McGraw-Hill, 1998.

Gibney, M. J., H. H. Vorster, and J. K. Frans. *Introduction to Human Nutrition*. London: Blackwell Science, 2002.

Goodman-Gilman, A., T. Rall, A. Nies, and T. Palmer. *The Pharmacological Basis of Therapeutics*. 8th ed. New York: Pergamon, 1990.

Gruenwald, J., T. Brendler, C. Jaenicke, et al., eds. *PDR for Herbal Medicines*. Montvale, NJ: Medical Economics, 1998.

Jonas, W. B., and J. Jacobs. *Healing with Homeopathy: The Doctors' Guide.* New York: Warner, 1996.

Kaatz, D. *Characters of Wisdom: Taoist Tales of the Acupuncture Points.* London: Petite Bergerie, 2005.

Koopman, W. J., ed. *Arthritis and Allied Conditions.* 13th ed. Baltimore, MD: Williams & Wilkins, 1997.

Maciocia, G. *The Practice of Chinese Medicine.* Edinburgh: Churchill Livingstone, 2000.

Maclean, Will, and Jeff Littleton. *Clinical Handbook of Internal Medicine.* Sydney: Sydney University Press, 2003.

Martin, J. M., and Z. P. Rona. *The Complete Candida Yeast Guidebook.* Rocklin, CA: Prima, 1996.

Middleton, E. ed. *Allergy: Principles and Practice.* 5th ed. St. Louis, MO: Mosby-Year Book, 1998.

Morrison, R. *Desktop Companion to Physical Pathology.* Nevada City, NV: Hahnemann, 1998.

————.*Desktop Guide to Keynotes and Confirmatory Symptoms.* Albany, CA: Hahnemann Clinic, 1993.

Mowrey, D. *The Scientific Validation of Herbal Medicine.* New Canaan, CT: Keats, 1986.

Murray, M.T., and J. E. Pizzorno. *Encyclopedia of Natural Medicine.* 2nd ed. Rocklin, CA: Prima, 2001.

Newall, C. et al. *Herbal Medicines: A Guide for Health-Care Professionals.* London: Pharmaceutical Press, 1996.

Ni, D. *Crane Style Qi Gong Video.* Los Angeles: Seven Star, 2004.

Ni, H. *Attune Your Body with Dao In.* Los Angeles: Seven Star, 1989.

————. *Power of Natural Healing.* Los Angeles: Seven Star, 1995.

————. *Tao, the Subtle Universal Law.* Los Angeles: Seven Star, 1979.

Ni, M. *Chinese Herbology Made Easy.* Los Angeles: Seven Star, 1986.

————. *Dr. Mao's Harmony Tai Chi.* San Francisco: Chronicle, 2006.

————. *The Eight Treasures: Energy Enhancement Exercises.* Los Angeles: Seven Star, 1996.

————. *Secrets of Longevity: Hundreds of Ways to Live to be 100.* San Francisco: Chronicle, 2006.

————. *Self-Healing Qi Gong Video*. Los Angeles: Seven Star, 1995.

————. *The Yellow Emperor's Classic of Medicine*. Boston: Shambhala, 1995.

Ni, M., and C. McNease. *The Tao of Nutrition*. Los Angeles: Seven Star, 1987.

Oschman, J. L. *Energy Medicine: The Scientific Basis*. Edinburgh: Churchill Livingstone, 2002.

Snider, R.K., ed. *Essentials of Musculoskeletal Care*. Rosemont, IL: American Academy of Orthopaedic Surgeons, 1997.

Time-Life Books, eds. *The Medical Advisor*. Alexandria, VA: Time-Life, 1996.

Trattler, R. *Better Health Through Natural Healing*. Victoria, Australia: Hinkler, 2001.

Werbach, M.R. *Nutritional Influences on Illness*. New Canaan, CT: Keats, 1987.

Williams, R.H., and P. R. Larsen, eds. *Williams Textbook of Endocrinology*. Amsterdam: Elsevier, 2003.

Wisneski, L. A., and Lucy Anderson. *The Scientific Basis of Integrative Medicine*. Boca Raton, FL: CRC, 2005.

REFERENCES FOR SPECIFIC CONDITIONS

ACNE

Amer, M., et al. 1982. Serum zinc in acne vulgaris. *Int. J. Dermat.* 21:481.

Bassett, I.B., D. L. Pannowitz, and R. S. Barnetson. 1990. A comparative study of tea-tree oil versus benzoylperoxide in the treatment of acne. *Med. J. Aust.* 153(8): 455–58.

Michaelsson, G., L. Johlin, and K. Ljunghall. 1977. A double-blind study of the effect of zinc and oxytetracycline in acne vulgaris. *Br. J. Dermatol. 97(5):561–66*.

Ni, M. *Self Healing Qi Gong Video*. Los Angeles: Seven Star, 1992.

Ni, M., and C. McNease. *The Tao of Nutrition*. Los Angeles: Seven Star, 1987.

ALLERGIES

Eby, G. A. 1997. Zinc ion availability—the determinant of efficacy in zinc lozenge treatment of common colds. *J. Antimicrob. Chemother.*

Ni, H. *Attune Your Body with Dao In*. Los Angeles: Seven Star, 1989.

Ni, M., and C. McNease. *The Tao of Nutrition*. Los Angeles: Seven Star, 1987.

Ogasawara, H., and E. Middleton, Jr. 1985. Effect of selected flavonoids on histamine release (HR) and hydrogen peroxide (H_2O_2) generation by human leukocytes. *J. Allergy Clin. Immunol.* 75:184.

Yoshimoto, T., et al. 1983. Flavonoids: Potent inhibitors of arachidonate 5-lipoxygenase. *Biochem. Biophys. Res. Commun.* 116:612–618.

ARTERIAL PLAQUE

Benskey, D., and R. Barolet. *Chinese Herbal Medicine.* Seattle: Eastland, 1990.

Chen, J.K., and T. Chen. *Chinese Medical Herbology and Pharmacology.* Los Angeles: Art of Medicine Press, 2005.

Glagov, S., E. Weisenberg, C. K. Zarins, R. Stankunavicius, and G. J. Kolettis. 1987. Compensatory enlargement of human atherosclerotic coronary arteries. *N. Engl. J. Med.* 316:131—137.

Ni, M. *The Eight Treasures: Energy Enhancement Exercises.* Los Angeles: Seven Star, 1996.

Ni, M. and C. McNease. *The Tao of Nutrition.* Los Angeles: Seven Star, 1987.

ARTHRITIS

Altman, R. D., and C. J. Lozada. 1998. Practice guidelines in the management of osteoarthritis. *Osteoarthritis and Cartilage* 6(Suppl A):22–24.

D'Ambrosio, E., B. Casa, and G. Bompani, et al. 1981. Glucosamine sulphate: a controlled clinical investigation in arthrosis. *Pharmatherapeutica* 2(8):504–8.

Eberhardt, R., T. Zwingers, and R. Hofmann. 1995. DMSO in patients with active gonarthrosis. A double-blind placebo controlled phases III study. *Fortschr. Med.* 113:446–50.

Elkayam, O., J. Ophir, and S. Brener, et al. 2000. Immediate and delayed effects of treatment at the Dead Sea in patients with psoriatic arthritis. *Rheumatol. Int.* 19(3):77–82.

Ernst, E., and S. Chrubasik. 2000. Phyto—anti-inflammatories. A systematic review of randomized, placebo-controlled, double-blind trials. *Rheum. Dis. Clin. North Am.* 26(1):13–27.

Felson, D.T., Y. Zhang, and J. M. Anthony, et al. 1992. Weight loss reduces the risk for symptomatic knee osteoarthritis in women: The Framingham Study. *Ann. Intern. Med.* 116:535–39.

Felson, D.T., Y. Zhang, and M. T. HanNan, et al. 1997. Risk factors for incident radiographic knee osteoarthritis in the elderly: The Framingham Study. *Arthritis Rheum.* 40:728–33.

Giordano, N., P. Nardi, and M. Senesi, et al. 1996. The efficacy and safety of glucosamine sulfate in the treatment of gonarthritis. *Clin. Ter.* 147:99–105.

McAlindon, T.E., P. Jacques, and Y. Zhang. 1996. Do antioxidant micronutrients protect against the development and progression of knee osteoarthritis? *Arthritis Rheum.* 39(4):648–56.

Morrison, R. *Desktop Companion to Physical Pathology.* Nevada City, NV: Hahnemann, 1998.

Müller-Fassbender, H. 1987. Double-blind clinical trial of s-adenosylmethionine versus ibuprofen in the treatment of osteoarthritis. *Am. J. Med.* 83(suppl 5A):81–83.

Ni, M. *Dr. Mao's Harmony Tai Chi.* San Francisco: Chronicle, 2006.

———. *The Eight Treasures: Energy Enhancement Exercises.* Los Angeles: Seven Star, 1996.

Ni, M., and C. McNease. *The Tao of Nutrition.* Los Angeles: Seven Star, 1987.

Tapadinhas, M.J., I. C. Rivera, and A. A. Bignamini. 1982. Oral glucosamine sulphate in the management of arthrosis: report on a multi-centre open investigation in Portugal. *Pharmtherapeutica.* 3:157–68.

ASTHMA

Bielory, L., and R. Gandhi. 1994. Asthma and vitamin C. *Ann. Allergy* 73(2):89–96.

Dry, J., and D. Vincent. 1991. Effects of a fish oil diet on asthma: results of a one-year double-blind study. *Int. Arch. Allergy Immunol.* 95:156–57.

Gupta, I., V. Gupta, and A. Parihar, et al. 1998. Effects of Boswellia serrata gum resin in patients with bronchial asthma: results of a double-blind, placebo-controlled, 6-week clinical study. *Eur. J. Med. Res.* 3(11):511–14.

Monteleone, C.A., and A. R. Sherman. 1997. Nutrition and asthma. *Arch. Intern. Med.* 157:23–24.

Ni, M. *The Eight Treasures: Energy Enhancement Exercises.* Los Angeles: Seven Star, 1996.

Ni, M., and C. McNease. *The Tao of Nutrition.* Los Angeles: Seven Star, 1987.

Shivpuri, D.N., et al. 1969. A crossover double-blind study on Tylophora indica in the treatment of asthma and allergic rhinitis. *J. Allergy* 43:145–50.

Shivpuri, D.N., S. C. Singhal, and D. Parkash. 1972. Treatment of asthma with an alcoholic extract of Tylophora indica: a crossover, double-blind study. *Ann. Allergy* 30:407–12.

Sur, S., M. Camara, and A. Buchmeier, et al. 1993. Double-blind trial of pyridoxine (vitamin B_6) in the treatment of steroid-dependent asthma. *Ann. Allergy* 70:147–52.

Wright, J. 1989. Vitamin B_{12}: Powerful protection against asthma. *Int. Clin. Nutr. Rev.* 9(4):185–88.

BAD BREATH

Fitchie, J.G., R. W. Comer, P. J. Hanes, and G. W. Reeves. 1989. The reduction of phenytoin-induced gingival overgrowth in a severely disabled patient: a case report. *Compendium* 10(6):314.

Francetti, L., E. Maggiore, and A. Marchesi, et al. 1991. Oral hygiene in subjects treated with diphenylhydantoin: effects of a professional program. [in Italian] *Prev. Assist. Dent.* 17(30):40–43.

Ni, M. *The Eight Treasures: Energy Enhancement Exercises.* Los Angeles: Seven Star, 1996.

Ni, M., and C. McNease. *The Tao of Nutrition.* Los Angeles: Seven Star, 1987.

Pack, A. R. C. 1984. Folate mouthwash: effects on established gingivitis in periodontal patients. *J. Clin. Periodontol.* 11:619–28.

Pack, A. R. C., and M. E. Thomson. 1980. Effects of topical and systemic folic acid supplementation on gingivitis in pregnancy. *J. Clin. Periodontal.* 7:402–14.

Steinberg, S.C., and A. D. Steinberg. 1982. Phenytoin-induced gingival overgrowth control in severely retarded children. *J. Periodontol.* 53(7):429–33.

Vogel, R. I., R. A. Fink, O. Frank, and H. Baker. 1978. The effect of topical application of folic acid on gingival health. *J. Oral Med.* 33(1):20–22.

Vogel, R.I., R. A. Fink, and L. C. Schneider, et al. 1976. The effect of folic acid on gingival health. *J. Periodontol.* 47:667–68.

BONE LOSS

Alekel, D.L., A. St. Germain, C. T. Peterson, K. B. Hanson, J. W. Stewart, and T. Toda. 2000. Isoflavone-rich soy protein isolate attenuates bone loss in the lumbar spine of perimenopausal women. *Am. J. Clin. Nutr.* 72:844–52.

Blanch J., and A. Pros. 1999. Calcium as a treatment of osteoporosis. *Drugs Today.* 35:631–39.

Blumenthal, M., A. Goldberg, and J. Brinkmann, eds. *Herbal Medicine: Expanded Commission E Monographs.* Newton, MA: Integrative Medicine Communications, 2000: 201–04.

Carlisle, E.M. 1976. In vivo requirement for silicon in articular cartilage and connective tissue formation in the chick. *J. Nutr.* 106(4):478–84.

Chiechi, L.M. 1999. Dietary phytoestrogens in the prevention of long-term post-menopausal diseases. *Int. J. Gynaecol. Obstet.* 67(1):39–40.

Gillespie, W. J., A. Avenell, D. A. Henry, D. L. O'Connell, and J. Robertson. Vitamin D and vitamin D analogues for preventing fractures associated with involutional and post-menopausal osteoporosis (*Cochrane Review*). In *The Cochrane Library,* Issue 1. Oxford: Wiley, 2001.

Kiel, D. P., et al. 1990. Caffeine and the risk of hip fracture: the Framingham study. *Am. J. Epidemiol.* 132(4):675–84.

Melhus, H., K. Michaelsson, and A. Kindmark, et al. 1998. Excessive dietary intake of vitamin A is associated with reduced bone mineral density and increased risk for hip fracture. *Ann Intern Med.* 129:770–78.

Ni, M. *The Eight Treasures: Energy Enhancement Exercises.* Los Angeles: Seven Star, 1996.

Ni, M., and C. McNease. *The Tao of Nutrition.* Los Angeles: Seven Star, 1987.

Tucker, K. L., M. T. Hannan, H. Chen, L. A. Cupples, P. W. F. Wilson, and D. P. Kiel. 1999. Potassium, magnesium and fruit and vegetable intakes are associated with greater bone mineral density in elderly men and women. *Am. J. Clin. Nutr.* 69:727–36.

BRONCHITIS

Balch, P. A. *Prescription for Nutritional Healing.* 4th ed. New York: Avery, 2006.

Benskey, D., and R. Barolet. *Chinese Herbal Medicine Formulas and Strategies.* Seattle: Eastland, 2000.

Ni, M. *The Eight Treasures: Energy Enhancement Exercises.* Los Angeles: Seven Star, 1996.

Ni, M., and C. McNease. *The Tao of Nutrition.* Los Angeles: Seven Star, 1987.

CANDIDA

Crook, W.G. *The Yeast Connection: A Medical Breakthrough.* Jackson, TN, Professional Books, 1983, 1984, 1986.

Martin, J. M., and Z. P. Rona. *The Complete Candida Yeast Guidebook.* Rocklin, CA: Prima, 1996.

Ni, M. *Self Healing Qi Gong Video.* Los Angeles: Seven Star, 1992.

Ni, M., and C. McNease. *The Tao of Nutrition.* Los Angeles: Seven Star, 1987.

Williams, L.R., et al. 1989. The composition and bactericidal activity of oil of Melaleuca alternifolia (tea tree oil). *Int. J. Aromather.* 1(3):15.

CARPAL TUNNEL SYNDROME

Banner R., and E. W. Hudson. 2001. Case report: acupuncture for carpal tunnel syndrome. *Can. Fam. Physician* 47:547–49.

Bartram, T. *Encyclopedia of Herbal Medicine.* Dorset, England: Grace, 1995, 369–370.

Ellis, J. M. 1987. Treatment of carpal tunnel syndrome with vitamin B$_6$. *South. Med. J.* 80(7):882–84.

Ellis, J. M., et al. 1997. Survey and new data on treatment with pyridoxine of patients having a clinical syndrome including the carpal tunnel and other defects. *Res. Commun. Chem. Pathol. Pharmacol.* 17(1):165–77.

Ellis, J.M., et al. 1976. Vitamin B$_6$ deficiency in patients with a clinical syndrome including the carpal tunnel defect. Biochemical and clinical response to therapy with pyridoxine. *Res. Commun. Chem. Pathol. Pharmacol.* 13(4):743–57.

Heller, A., and T. Koch. 2000. Immunonutrition with omega-3-fatty acids. Are new anti-inflammatory strategies in sight? *Zentralbl. Chir.* 125(2):123–36.

Koopman, W.J., ed. *Arthritis and Allied Conditions.* 13th ed. Baltimore:Williams & Wilkins, 1997.

Morrison, R. *Desktop Guide to Keynotes and Confirmatory Symptoms.* Albany, CA: Hahnemann Clinic, 1993,174, 27–29, 36–38.

Ni, M. *The Eight Treasures: Energy Enhancement Exercises.* Los Angeles: Seven Star, 1996.

Ni, M., and C. McNease. *The Tao of Nutrition.* Los Angeles: Seven Star, 1987.

Raederstorff, D., et al. 1996. Anti-inflammatory properties of docosahexaenoic and eicosapentaenoic acids in phorbol-ester-induced mouse ear inflammation. *Int. Arch. Allergy. Immunol.* 111(3):284–90.

CHRONIC FATIGUE SYNDROME

Cleare, A. J., V. O'Keane, and J. P. Miell. 2004. Levels of DHEA and DHEAS and responses to CRH stimulation and hydrocortisone treatment in chronic fatigue syndrome. *Psychoneuroendocrinology* 29.6:724–32.

Forsyth, L.M., H. G. Preuss, A. L. MacDowell, L. Chiazze, Jr., G. D. Birkmayer, and J. A. Bellanti. 1999. Therapeutic effects of oral NADH on the symptoms of patients with chronic fatigue syndrome. *Ann. Allergy Asthma. Immunol.* 82.2:185–191.

Hartz, A.J., S. Bentler, R. Noyes, J. Hoehns, C. Logemann, S. Sinift, Y. Butani, W. Wang, K. Brake, M. Ernst, and H. Kautzman. 2004. Randomized controlled trial of Siberian ginseng for chronic fatigue. *Psychol. Med.* 34.1:51–61.

Ni, M. *Self-Healing Qi Gong Video*. Los Angeles: Seven Star, 1992.

Ni, M., and C. McNease. *The Tao of Nutrition*. Los Angeles: Seven Star, 1987.

Warren, G., M. McKendrick, and M. Peet. 1999. The role of essential fatty acids in chronic fatigue syndrome. A case-controlled study of red-cell membrane essential fatty acids (EFA) and a placebo-controlled treatment study with high dose of EFA. *Acta. Neurol. Scand.* 99.2:112–16.

COLD AND FLUS

Braunig, B., et al. 1992. Echinacea purpura root for strengthening the immune response in flu-like infections. *Z. Phytother.* 13:7–13.

Caceres, J., et al. 1997. Prevention of common colds with Andrographis paniculata dried extract: A pilot double blind trial. *Phytomedicine* 4(2):101–04.

Eby, G. A. 1997. Zinc ion availability—the determinant of efficacy in zinc lozenge treatment of common colds. *Antimicrob. Chemother.* 40(4):483–93.

Hemila, H. 1992. Vitamin C and the common cold. *Br. J. Nutr.* 67(1):3–16.

Ni, H. *Attune Your Body with Dao In*. Los Angeles: Seven Star, 1989.

Ni, M., and C. McNease. *The Tao of Nutrition*. Los Angeles: Seven Star, 1987.

COLD HANDS AND FEET

DiGiacomo, R.A., J. M. Kremer, and D. M. Shah. 1989. Fish-oil dietary supplementation in patients with Raynaud's phenomenon: a double blind, controlled, prospective study. *Am. J. Med.* 86:158–64.

Johnson, J. A., PhD. *Chinese Medical Qigong Therapy*. Palm Desert, CA: International Institute of Medical Qi Gong, 2000.

Ni, M. *The Eight Treasures: Energy Enhancement Exercises*. Los Angeles: Seven Star, 1996.

Ni, M., and C. McNease. *The Tao of Nutrition*. Los Angeles: Seven Star, 1987.

Pitchford, Paul. *Healing with Whole Foods*. 3rd ed. Berkeley, CA: North Atlantic Books, 2002.

Ringer, T. V., et al. 1989. Fish oil blunts the pain response to cold pressure testing in normal males (Abstract). *J. Am. Coll. Nutr.* 8(5):435.

Sunderland, G. T., J. J. F. Belch, and R. D. Sturrock, et al. 1988. A double blind randomized placebo-controlled trial of Hexopal in primary Raynaud's disease. *Clin. Rheumatol.* 7(1):46–49.

CONSTIPATION

Chang, H. M. 1986. Pharmacology and applications of Chinese materia medica. World Scientific I: 620–24.

Ni, H. *Attune Your Body with Dao In.* Los Angeles: Seven Star, 1989.

Ni, M. *The Eight Treasures: Energy Enhancement Exercises.* Los Angeles: Seven Star, 1996.

Ni, M., and C. McNease. *The Tao of Nutrition.* Los Angeles: Seven Star, 1987.

COUGH

Barolet, B. *Chinese Herbal Medicine Formulas and Strategies.* Seattle: Eastland, 2000.

Ni, M. *The Eight Treasures: Energy Enhancement Exercises.* Los Angeles: Seven Star, 1996.

Ni, M., and C. McNease. *The Tao of Nutrition.* Los Angeles: Seven Star, 1987.

DANDRUFF

Balch, P. A. *Prescription for Nutritional Healing.* 4th ed. New York: Avery, 2006.

Ni, M. *Self Healing Qi Gong Video.* Los Angeles: Seven Star, 1992.

Ni, M., and C. McNease. *The Tao of Nutrition.* Los Angeles: Seven Star, 1987.

DIABETES

Casassus, P., A. Fontbonne, and N. Thibult, et al. 1992. Upper-body fat distribution: a hyperinsulinemia-independent predictor of coronary heart disease mortality. *Arterioscler. Thromb.* 1387–92.

Isida, K., A. Mizuno, T. Murakami, and K. Shima. 1996. Obesity is necessary but not sufficient for the development of diabetes mellitus. *Metabolism* 45:1288–95.

Karter, A. J., E. J. Mayer-Davis, J. V. Selby, et al. 1996. Insulin sensitivity and abdominal obesity in African-American, Hispanic, and non-Hispanic white men and women. *Diabetes* 45:1547–55.

Natural Medicines Comprehensive Database. Coenzyme Q-10. Natural Medicines Comprehensive Database website. Accessed May 17, 2005.

Ni, H. *Power of Natural Healing.* Los Angeles: Seven Star, 1995.

Ni, M., and C. McNease. *The Tao of Nutrition*. Los Angeles: Seven Star, 1987.

Yeh, G. Y., D. M. Eisenberg, and T. J. Kaptchuk, et al. Systematic review of herbs and dietary supplements for glycemic control in diabetes. *Diabetes Care* 26(4): 1277–94.

DIARRHEA

de Roos, N.M., and M. B. Katan. 2000. Effects of probiotic bacteria on diarrhea, lipid metabolism, and carcinogenesis: a review of papers published between 1988 and 1998. *Am. J. Clin. Nutr.* 71(2):405–11.

Kasper, D.L., E. Braunwald, A. K. Fauci, S. L. Hauser, D. L. Longo, and J. L. Jameson. *Harrison's Principles of Internal Medicine*. New York: McGraw-Hill, 2005.

Longstreth, G.L., W. G. Thompson, W. D. Chey, L. A. Houghton, F. Mearin, and R. C. Spiller. 2006. Functional bowel disorders. *Gastroenterology* 130:1480–91.

Ni, H. *Attune Your Body with Dao In*. Los Angeles: Seven Star, 1989.

Ni, M. *Self Healing Qi Gong Video*. Los Angeles: Seven Star, 1992.

Ni, M., and C. McNease. *The Tao of Nutrition*. Los Angeles: Seven Star, 1987.

DIZZINESS

Cameron, M. *Lifetime Encyclopedia of Natural Remedies*. Paramus, NJ: Prentice Hall, 1993.

Chen, J. K. *Chinese Medical Herbology and Pharmacology*. Los Angeles: Art of Medicine Press, 2003.

Ni, M. *Self Healing Qi Gong Video*. Los Angeles: Seven Star, 1992.

Ni, M., and C. McNease. *The Tao of Nutrition*. Los Angeles: Seven Star, 1987.

Yardley, L. *Vertigo and Dizziness*. New York: Routledge, 1994.

ECZEMA

Aertgeerts, P., M. Albring, and F. Klaschka, et al. 1985. Comparison of Kamillosan cream (2 g ethanolic extract from chamomile flowers in 100 g cream) versus steroid (0.25% hydrocortisone, 0.75% fluocortin butyl ester) and non-steroid (5% bufexamac) external agents in the maintenance therapy of eczema [translated from German]. *Z. Hautkr.* 60:270–77.

Anderson, C., M. Lis-Balchin, and M. Kifk-Smith. 2000. Evaluation of massage with essential oils in childhood atopic eczema. *Phyother Res.* 14(6):452–56.

Andreassi, M., P. Forleo, A. Di Lorio, S. Masci, G. Abate, and P. Amerio. 1997. Efficacy of gamma-linolenic acid in the treatment of patients with atopic dermatitis. *J. Int. Med. Res.* 25(5):266–74.

Biagi, P.L., et al. 1994. The effect of gamma-linolenic acid on clinical status, red cell fatty acid composition and membrane microviscosity in infants with atopic dermatitis. *Drugs Exp. Clin. Res.* 20(2):77–84.

Billmann-Eberwein, C., F. Rippke, T. Ruzicka, and J. Krutmann. 2002. Modulation of atopy patch test reactions by topical treatment of human skin with a fatty acid-rich emollient. *Skin Pharmacol. Appl. Skin Physiol.* 15(2):100–04.

Borrek, S., A. Hildebrandt, and J. Forster. 1997. Gamma-linolenic-acid-rich borage seed oil capsules in children with atopic dermatitis. A placebo-controlled double-blind study [Article in German]. *Klin Padiatr.* 209(3):100–04.

Calder, P.C., and E. A. Miles. 2000. Fatty acids and atopic disease. *Pediatr Allergy Immunol.* 11 Suppl 13:29–36.

Kanny, G. 2005. Atopic dermatitis in children and food allergy: combination or causality? Should avoidance diets be initiated? *Ann. Dermatol. Venereol.* 132 Spec. No. 1:1S90-103.

Macnair, Trisha. Complementary treatment for eczema. BBC Health. bbc.co.uk.

Ni, M. *Self Healing Qi Gong Video.* Los Angeles: Seven Star, 1992.

Ni, M., and C. McNease. *The Tao of Nutrition.* Los Angeles: Seven Star, 1987.

Whitaker, D.K., et al. 1996. Evening primrose oil (Epogam) in the treatment of chronic hand dermatitis: disappointing therapeutic results. *Dermatology* 193:115–20.

FLATULENCE

Ganiats, T.G., W. A. Norcross, A. L. Halverson, P. A. Burford, and L. A. Palinkas. 1994. Does Beano prevent gas? A double-blind crossover study of oral alpha-galactosidase to treat dietary oligosaccharide intolerance. *J. Fam. Pract.* 39(5):44–45.

Murray, Michael, N.D., and Joseph Pizzorno, N.D. *Encyclopedia of Natural Medicine.* Roseville, CA: Prima, 1998.

Ni, H. *Attune Your Body with Dao In.* Los Angeles: Seven Star, 1989.

Ni, M. *Self Healing Qi Gong Video.* Los Angeles: Seven Star, 1992.

Ni, M., and C. McNease. *The Tao of Nutrition.* Los Angeles: Seven Star, 1987.

FLOATERS

Cline, D., H. W. Hofstetter, and J. R. Griffin. *Dictionary of Visual Science.* 4th ed. Boston: Butterworth-Heinemann, 1997.

Ni, H. *Attune Your Body with Dao In.* Los Angeles: Seven Star, 1989.

Roth, M., P. Trittibach, F. Koerner, and G. Sarra. 2005. Pars plana vitrectomy for idiopathic vitreous floaters. *Klin. Monatsbl. Augenheilkd.* 222(9):728–32.

GOUT

Ferri, F.F. *Ferri's Clinical Advisor: Instant Diagnosis and Treatment.* St. Louis, MO: Mosby-Year Book, 1999.

Larson, D.E., ed. *Mayo Clinic Family Health Book.* 2nd ed. New York: Morrow, 1996.

Murray, M.T., and J. E. Pizzorno. *Encyclopedia of Natural Medicine.* 2nd ed. Rocklin, CA: Prima, 1998.

Ni, H. *Attune Your Body with Dao In.* Los Angeles: Seven Star, 1989.

Ni, M., and C. McNease. *The Tao of Nutrition.* Los Angeles: Seven Star, 1987.

Rose, B. *The Family Health Guide to Homeopathy.* Berkeley, CA: Celestial Arts, 1992.

Theodosakis, J., B. Adderly, and B. Fox. *The Arthritis Cure.* New York: St. Martin's, 1997.

Tierney, L.M., Jr., S. J. McPhee, and M. A. Papadakis, eds. *Current Medical Diagnosis and Treatment.* Norwalk, CT: Appleton & Lange, 1994.

Werbach, M.R. *Nutritional Influences on Illness.* New Canaan, CT: Keats, 1987.

GUM DISEASE

Fitchie, J.G., R. W. Comer, P. J. Hanes, and G. W. Reeves. 1989. The reduction of phenytoin-induced gingival overgrowth in a severely disabled patient: a case report. *Compendium* 10(6):314.

Francetti, L., E. Maggiore, and A. Marchesi, et al. 1991. Oral hygiene in subjects treated with diphenylhydantoin: effects of a professional program. [in Italian] *Prev. Assist. Dent.* 17(30):40–43.

Ni, M. *The Eight Treasures: Energy Enhancement Exercises.* Los Angeles: Seven Star, 1996.

Ni, M., and C. McNease. *The Tao of Nutrition.* Los Angeles: Seven Star, 1987.

Pack, A.R.C. 1984. Folate mouthwash: effects on established gingivitis in periodontal patients. *J. Clin. Periodontol.* 11:619–28.

Pack, A.R.C., and M. E. Thomson. 1980. Effects of topical and systemic folic acid supplementation on gingivitis in pregnancy. *J. Clin. Periodontol.* 7:402–14.

Steinberg, S.C., and A. D. Steinberg. 1982. Phenytoin-induced gingival overgrowth control in severely retarded children. *J. Periodontol.* 53(7):429–33.

Vogel, R.I., R. A. Fink, O. Frank, and H. Baker. 1978. The effect of topical application of folic acid on gingival health. *J. Oral. Med.* 33(1):20–22.

Vogel, R.I., R. A. Fink, and L. C. Schneider, et al. 1976. The effect of folic acid on gingival health. *J. Periodontol.* 47:667–68.

HAIR LOSS

Balch, P. A. *Prescription for Nutritional Healing.* 4th ed. New York: Avery, 2006.

Ni, H. *Attune Your Body with Dao In.* Los Angeles: Seven Star, 1989.

Ni, M., and C. McNease. *The Tao of Nutrition.* Los Angeles: Seven Star, 1987.

Rebora, A. 2004. Pathogenesis of androgenetic alopecia. *J. Am. Acad. Dermatol.* 50(5):777–79.

HEADACHE

Chen, John K. *Chinese Medical Herbology and Pharmacology.* Los Angeles: Art of Medicine Press, 2003.

De Benedittis, G. and R. Massei. 1985. Serotonin precursors in chronic primary headache. A double-blind cross-over study with L-5-hydroxytryptophan vs. placebo. *J. Neurosurg. Sci.* 29:239–48.

Johnson, E.S., et al. 1985. Efficacy of feverfew as a prophylactic treatment of migraine. *British Medical Journal.* 291:569–73.

Longo, G., et al. 1984. Treatment of essential headache in developmental age with L-5-HTP (cross over double-blind study versus placebo). *Pediatr. Med. Chir.* 6:241–45.

Ni, M. *Self Healing Qi Gong Video.* Los Angeles: Seven Star, 1992.

Ni, M., and C. McNease. *The Tao of Nutrition.* Los Angeles: Seven Star, 1987.

HEARING LOSS

Dobie, R. A. 2007. Folate supplementation and age-related hearing loss. *Ann. Int. Med.* 146:63–64.

Durga, J. 2007. Effects of folic acids supplementation on hearing in older adults. *Ann. Int. Med.* 146:1–9.

Jones, N.S., and A. Davis. 2000. A retrospective case-controlled study of 1490 consecutive patients presenting to a neuro-otology clinic to examine the relationship between blood lipid levels and sensorineural hearing loss. *Clin. Otolaryngol.* 25 (6):511-17.

Ni, H. *Attune Your Body with Dao In.* Los Angeles: Seven Star, 1989.

Ni, M., and C. McNease. *The Tao of Nutrition*. Los Angeles: Seven Star, 1987.

Pillsbury, H.C. 1986. Hypertension, hyperlipoproteinemia, chronic noise exposure: Is there synergism in cochlear pathology? *Laryngoscope* 96:1112–37.

Suzuki, K., M. Kaneko, and K. Murai. 2000. Influence of serum lipids on auditory function. *Laryngoscope* 110 (10 pt 1):1736–38.

HEMORRHOIDS

Boisseau, M.R., et al. 1995. Fibrinolysis and hemorrheology in chronic venous insufficiency: a double-blind study of troxerutin efficiency. *J. Cardiovasc. Surg.* 36:369–74.

Ghiringhelli, C., et al. 1978. Capillarotropic activity of anthocyanosides in high doses in phlebopathic stasis. *Minerva Cardioangiol.* 26:255–76.

Ni, H. *Attune Your Body with Dao In*. Los Angeles: Seven Star, 1989.

Ni, M. *Self Healing Qi Gong Video*. Los Angeles: Seven Star, 1992.

Ni, M., and C. McNease. *The Tao of Nutrition*. Los Angeles: Seven Star, 1987.

Wijayanegara, H., et al. 1992. A clinical trial of hydroxyethylrutosides in the treatment of hemorrhoids of pregnancy. *J. Int. Med. Res.* 20:54–60.

HIGH BLOOD PRESSURE

Benskey, D., and R. Barolet. *Chinese Herbal Medicine*. Seattle: Eastland, 1990.

Chen, J. K. *Chinese Medical Herbology and Pharmacology*. Los Angeles: Art of Medicine Press, 2003.

Murray, M., and J. Pizzorno. *Encyclopedia of Natural Medicine*. Roseville, CA: Prima, 2001.

Ni, M. *Self Healing Qi Gong Video*. Los Angeles: Seven Star, 1992.

Ni, M., and C. McNease. *The Tao of Nutrition*. Los Angeles: Seven Star, 1987.

Pate, R. R., et al. 1995. Physical activity and public health. *JAMA*. 273:404.

HIGH CHOLESTEROL

Benskey, D., and R. Barolet. *Chinese Herbal Medicine*. Seattle: Eastland, 1990.

Chen, J. K. *Chinese Medical Herbology and Pharmacology*. Los Angeles: Art of Medicine Press, 2003.

Murray, M., and J. Pizzorno. *Encyclopedia of Natural Medicine*. Roseville, CA: Prima, 2001.

Ni, M. *Self Healing Qi Gong Video*. Los Angeles: Seven Star, 1992.

Ni, M., and C. McNease. *The Tao of Nutrition.* Los Angeles: Seven Star, 1987.

Pate, R. R., et al. 1995. Physical activity and public health. *JAMA.* 273:404.

HIVES

Balch, P. A. *Prescription for Nutritional Healing.* 4th ed. New York: Avery, 2006.

Beers, M.H., and R. Berkow, eds. *The Merck Manual of Diagnosis and Therapy.* 17th ed. Whitehouse Station, NJ: Merck Research, 1999.

Blumenthal, M., A. Goldberg, and J. Brinckmann, eds. *Herbal Medicine: Expanded Commission E Monographs.* Newton, MA: Integrative Medicine, 2000, 230–39, 253–63, 419–23.

Cummings, S., and D. Ullman. *Everybody's Guide to Homeopathic Medicines.* 3rd ed. New York: Putnam, 1997, 227, 319–20, 345–46.

Dambro, M.R. *Griffith's 5 Minute Clinical Consult.* Baltimore: Lippincott Williams & Wilkins, 1999.

Ni, H. *Attune Your Body with Dao In.* Los Angeles: Seven Star, 1989.

Ni, M., and C. McNease. *The Tao of Nutrition.* Los Angeles: Seven Star, 1987.

INCONTINENCE

Bartram, T. *Encyclopedia of Herbal Medicine.* Dorset, England: Grace, 1995, 247.

Blumenthal, M., ed. *The Complete German Commission E Monographs: Therapeutic Guide to Herbal Medicines.* Boston: Integrative Medicine, 1998, 432.

Dambro, M.R., ed. *Griffith's 5 Minute Clinical Consult.* Baltimore: Williams & Wilkins, 1998.

Ni, M. *The Eight Treasures: Energy Enhancement Exercises.* Los Angeles: Seven Star, 1996.

Thom, D.H., S. K. Van den Eeden, and J. S. Brown. 1997. Evaluation of parturition and other reproductive variables as risk factors for urinary incontinence. *Obstet. Gynecol.* 90:983–89.

INDIGESTION AND HEARTBURN

DeVault, K.R., and D. O. Castell. 1999. Updated guidelines for the diagnosis and treatment of gastroesophageal reflux disease. The Practice Parameters Committee of the American College of Gastroenterology. *Am. J. Gastroenterol.* 94:1434–42.

Kaltenbach, T., S. Crockett, and L. B. Gerson. 2006. Are lifestyle measures effective in patients with gastroesophageal reflux disease? An evidence-based approach. *Arch. Intern. Med.* 166:965–71.

Ni, H. *Attune Your Body with Dao In.* Los Angeles: Seven Star, 1989.

Ni, M. *Self Healing Qi Gong Video.* Los Angeles: Seven Star, 1992.

Ni, M., and C. McNease. *The Tao of Nutrition.* Los Angeles: Seven Star, 1987.

Zuschlag, J.M. 1988. Double blind clinical study using certain proteolytic enzyme mixtures in karate fighters. Working paper. Mucos Pharma (Germany): 1–5.

INSECT BITES

Blumenthal, M., A. Goldberg, and J. Brinckmann, eds. *Herbal Medicine: Expanded Commission E Monographs.* Newton, MA: Integrative Medicine, 2000, 230–32, 379–84.

Cavanagh, H.M., and J. M. Wilkinson. 2002. Biological activities of lavender essential oil. *Phytother. Res.* 16(4):301–08.

Conforti, A., S. Bertani, H. Metelmann, S. Chirumbolo, S. Lussignoli, and P. Bellavite. 1997. Experimental studies of the anti-inflammatory activity of a homeopathic preparation. *BiolTher.* 15(1):28–31.

Coverman, M.H. 1989. Alternative therapies for acne, aphthae, insect bites, and callous diseases. *Dermatol Clin.* 7(1):71–72.

Ni, M. *Self Healing Qi Gong Video.* Los Angeles: Seven Star, 1992.

1998. Bromelain. *Alt Med Rev.* 3:302–05.

INSOMNIA

Benson, H., D. Goleman, and J. Gurin, eds. *The Relaxation Response.* New York: Consumer Reports Books, 1993, 233–57.

Chen, J. K. *Chinese Medical Herbology and Pharmacology.* Los Angeles: Art of Medicine Press, 2004.

Chen, J. *Clinical Manual of Oriental Medicine.* Los Angeles: Lotus Institute of Integrative Medicine, 2002.

Hazelhoff, B. et al. 1982. Antispasmodic effects of valerian compounds. *Arch. Int. Pharmacodyn.* 257:274.

Maciocia, G. *The Practice of Chinese Medicine.* London: Churchill Livingstone, 2000.

Ni, M. *Meditation for Stress Release.* Audio CD. Los Angeles: Seven Star, 2003.

Ni, M., and C. McNease. *The Tao of Nutrition.* Los Angeles: Seven Star, 1987.

Palatnik, A., K. Frolov, M. Fux, and J. Benjamin. 2001. Double-blind, controlled, crossover trial of inositol versus fluvoxamine for the treatment of panic disorder. *Clin. Psychopharma Col.* 21(3):335–39.

IRRITABLE BOWEL SYNDROME

Atkinson, W., T. A. Sheldon, N. Shaath, and P. J. Whorwell. 2004. Food elimination based on IgG antibodies in irritable bowel syndrome: a randomized controlled trial. *Gut* 53(10):1459–64.

Drossman, D., J. Leserman, G. Nachman, Z. Li, H. Gluck, T. Toomey, and C. Mitchell. 1990. Sexual and physical abuse in women with functional or organic gastrointestinal disorders. *Ann. Intern. Med.* 113(11):828–33.

Lim, B., E. Manheimer, L. Lao, E. Ziea, J. Wisniewski, J. Liu, and B. Berman. Acupuncture for treatment of irritable bowel syndrome. *Cochrane Database Syst. Rev:* CD005111.

Ni, M. *Self Healing Qi Gong Video.* Los Angeles: Seven Star, 1992.

Ni, M., and C. McNease. *The Tao of Nutrition.* Los Angeles: Seven Star, 1987.

JET LAG

Baker, S. M., and K. Baar. *The Circadian Prescription: Get in Step with Your Body's Natural Rhythms to Maximize Energy, Vitality and Longevity.* New York: Berkley, 2000.

Ehret, C. F. *Overcoming Jetlag.* New York: Berkley, 1987.

Ni, H. *Attune Your Body with Dao In.* Los Angeles: Seven Star, 1989.

Smolensky, M., and L. Lamberg. *The Body Clock Guide to Better Health.* New York: Holt, 2000.

LOW ENERGY

Balch, P. A. *Prescription for Nutritional Healing.* 4th ed. New York: Avery, 2006.

Ni, H. *Attune Your Body with Dao In.* Los Angeles: Seven Star, 1989.

Ni, M., and C. McNease. *The Tao of Nutrition.* Los Angeles: Seven Star, 1987.

Penninx, B.W. 2003. Anemia and decline in physical performance among older persons. *Am. J. Med.* 115(2):104–10.

Ressel, G.W. 2003. National Institutes of Health. NIH releases statement on managing pain, depression, and fatigue in cancer. *Am. Fam. Physician* 67(2):423–24.

Williams, R.H., and P. R. Larsen, eds. *Williams Textbook of Endocrinology.* Amsterdam: Elsevier, 2003.

LOW IMMUNE FUNCTION

Allard, J.P., et al. 1998. Effects of vitamin E and C supplementation on oxidative stress and viral load in HIV-infected subjects. *AIDS.* 13:1653–59.

Balch, P. A. *Prescription for Nutritional Healing.* 4th ed. New York: Avery, 2006.

Blumenthal, M., ed. *The Complete German Commission E Monographs: Therapeutic Guide to Herbal Medicines.* Boston: Integrative Medicine, 1998, 119–20, 134, 169–170.

Elion, R.A., and C. Cohen. Complementary medicine and HIV infection. *Primary Care* 4:905–19.

Fauci, A.S., E. Braunwald, and K. J. Isselbacher, et al., eds. *Harrison's Principles of Internal Medicine.* 14th ed. New York: McGraw-Hill, 1998, 1110–11, 1818–40.

Ni, M. *Self Healing Qi Gong Video.* Los Angeles: Seven Star, 1992.

Ni, M., and C. McNease. *The Tao of Nutrition.* Los Angeles: Seven Star, 1987.

Wynia, M.K., D. M. Eisenberg, and I. B. Wilson. 1999. Physician-patient communication about complementary and alternative medical therapies: a survey of physicians caring for patients with human immunodeficiency virus. *J. Altern. Comp. Med.* 5:447–56.

LOW LIBIDO

Chapple, C.R. 2003. Clinical study of benign prostatic disease, current concepts and future prospects randomized controlled trials versus real life practice. *Curr. Opin. Urol.* 13(1):1–5.

Denis, L., M. S. Morton, and K. Griffiths. 1999. Diet and its preventive role in prostatic disease. *Eur. Urol.* 35(5–6):377–87.

Di Silverio, F., G. D'Eramo, C. Lubrano, et al. 1992. Evidence that Serenoa repens extract displays an antiestrogenic activity in prostatic tissue of benign prostatic hypertrophy patients. *Eur. Urol.* 21:309–14.

Ernst, E. 1999. Herbal medications for common ailments in the elderly. *Drugs Aging.* 15(6):423–28.

Feinblatt, H.M., and J. C. Gant. 1958. Palliative treatment of benign prostatic hypertrophy: value of glycine, alanine, glutamic acid combination. *J. Maine Med. Assoc.* 46:99–102.

Koch, E. 2001. Extracts from fruits of saw palmetto (Sabal serrulata) and roots of stinging nettle (Urtica dioica): viable alternatives in the medical treatment of benign prostatic hyperplasia and associated lower urinary tract symptoms. *Planta Med.* 67(6):489–500.

Ni, H. *Workbook for Spiritual Development for All People.* Los Angeles: Seven Star, 1995.

Ni, M., and C. McNease. *The Tao of Nutrition.* Los Angeles: Seven Star, 1987.

Schiebel-Schlosser, G., and M. Friederich. 1998. Phytotherapy of BPH with pumpkin seeds—a multicenter clinical trial. *Zeits Phytother.* 19:71–76.

LOWER BACK PAIN

Balch, P. A. *Prescription for Nutritional Healing.* 4th ed. New York: Avery, 2006.

Cherkin, D.C., D. Eisenberg, and K. J. Sherman, et al. 2001. Randomized trial comparing traditional Chinese medical acupuncture, therapeutic massage, and self-care education for chronic low back pain. *Arch. Intern. Med.* 161:1081–88.

Levine, M., S.C. Rumsey, R. Daruwala, J.B. Park, and Y. Wang. 1999. Criteria and recommendations for vitamin C intake. *JAMA* 281(15):1415–53.

Morrison, R. *Desktop Guide to Keynotes and Confirmatory Symptoms.* Albany, CA: Hahnemann Clinic, 1993, 36–39, 59–61.

Mowrey, D. *The Scientific Validation of Herbal Medicine.* New Canaan, CT: Keats, 1986, 223–27.

Murray, M.T., and J. E. Pizzorno. *Encyclopedia of Natural Medicine.* 2nd ed. Rocklin, CA: Prima, 1998, 338.

Ni, H. *Attune Your Body with Dao In.* Los Angeles: Seven Star, 1989.

Smith, L., A. D. Oldman, H. J. McQuay, and R. A. Moore. 2000. Teasing apart quality and validity in systematic reviews: an example from acupuncture trials in chronic neck and back pain. *Pain.* 86:119–32.

Snider, R.K., ed. *Essentials of Musculoskeletal Care.* Rosemont, IL: American Academy of Orthopaedic Surgeon, 1997.

MEMORY LOSS

Bludau, J., M.D., et al. 2007. Cognitive impairment over the age of 85: hospitalization and mortality. *Arch. Gerontol. Geriatr.* (May 9).

Kanowski, S., et al. 1996. Proof of efficacy of the Ginkgo biloba special extract EGb 761 in outpatients suffering from mild to moderate primary degenerative dementia of the Alzheimer type or multi-infarct dementia. *Pharmacopsychiatry* 29:47–56.

Ni, M. *Self Healing Qi Gong Video.* Los Angeles: Seven Star, 1992.

Ni, M., and C. McNease. *The Tao of Nutrition.* Los Angeles: Seven Star, 1987.

Schulz, V., et al. *Rational Phytotherapy.* New York: Springer, 1998.

MENOPAUSE

Albertazzi, P., F. Pansini, and G. Bonaccorsi, et al. 1998. The effect of dietary soy supplementation on hot flushes. *Obstet Gynecol.* 91:6–11.

Haggans, C.J., A. M. Hutchins, and B. M. Olson, et al. 1999. Effect of flaxseed consumption on urinary estrogen metabolites in postmenopausal women. *Nutr Cancer.* 33(2):188–95.

Hammar, M., G. Berg, and R. Lindgren. 1990. Does physical exercise influence the frequency of postmenopausal hot flushes? *Acta. Obstet. Gynecol. Scand.* 69(5):409–12.

Heller, H.J., A. Stewart, and S. Haynes, et al. 1999. Pharmacokinetics of calcium absorption from two commercial calcium supplements. *J. Clin. Pharmacol.* 39:1151–54.

Kass-Annese, B. 2000. Alternative therapies for menopause. *Clin. Obstet. Gynecol.* 43(1):162–83.

Kelley, G.A. 1998. Exercise and regional bone mineral density in postmenopausal women. *Am. J. Phys. Med. Rehabil.* 77:76–87.

Lianzhong, W., and Z. Xiu. 1998. 300 cases of menopausal syndrome treated by acupuncture. *J. Trad. Chin. Med.* 18(4):259–62.

Lieberman, S. 1998. A review of the effectiveness of Cimicifuga racemosa (black cohosh) for the symptoms of menopause. *J. Womens Health.* 7(5):525–29.

Ni, M. *The Eight Treasures: Energy Enhancement Exercises.* Los Angeles: Seven Star, 1996.

Ni, M., and C. McNease. *The Tao of Nutrition.* Los Angeles: Seven Star, 1987.

MENSTRUAL DISORDERS

Berkow, R. ed. *The Merck Manual of Diagnosis and Therapy.* 16th ed. Rahway, NJ: Merck Research, 1992.

Helms, J.M. 1987. Acupuncture for the management of primary dysmenorrhea. *Obstet. Gynecol.* 69(1):51–56.

Jonas, W.B., and J. Jacobs. *Healing with Homeopathy: The Doctors' Guide.* New York: Warner, 1996, 185–86.

Ni, M. *The Eight Treasures: Energy Enhancement Exercises.* Los Angeles: Seven Star, 1996.

Ni, M., and C. McNease. *The Tao of Nutrition.* Los Angeles: Seven Star, 1987.

NIH Consensus Statement: Acupuncture. 1997. National Institutes of Health, Office of the Director. 15(5):1–34. Accessed at PubMed.

Penland, J.G., and P. E. Johnson. 1993. Dietary calcium and manganese effects on menstrual cycle symptoms. *Am. J. Obstet. Gynecol.* 168:1417–23.

Werbach, M.R. *Nutritional Influences on Illness.* New Canaan, CT: Keats, 1987.

MIGRAINES

Chen, J. K. *Chinese Medical Herbology and Pharmacology.* Los Angeles: Art of Medicine Press, 2004.

Gao, X., and X. Liu. 1979. Kudzu, Radix puerariae in migraine. *Chinese Med. Journal,* 92(1):260–62.

Lipton, R. 2004. News release, Albert Einstein "CoQ10 reduces migraine occurrence"—American Academy of Neurology's annual meeting report. *Neurology.* 63:2240–44.

Ni, M. *Self Healing Qi Gong Video.* Los Angeles: Seven Star, 1992.

Ni, M., and C. McNease. *The Tao of Nutrition.* Los Angeles: Seven Star, 1987.

Tuchin, P. J., H. Pollard, and R. Bonello. 2000. A randomized controlled trial of chiropractic spinal manipulative therapy. *J. Manipulative Physiol. Ther.* 23(2):91–95.

MORNING SICKNESS

Balch, P. A. *Prescription for Nutritional Healing.* 4th ed. New York: Avery, 2006.

Ni, M. *Meditation for Stress Release* (audio CD). Los Angeles: Seven Star, 2003.

Ni, M., and C. McNease. *The Tao of Nutrition.* Los Angeles: Seven Star, 1987.

MUSCLE PAIN AND SPASM

Balch, P. A. *Prescription for Nutritional Healing.* 4th ed. New York: Avery, 2006.

Ni, M. *Meditation for Pain Management* (audio CD). Los Angeles: Seven Star, 1995.

Ni, M., and C. McNease. *The Tao of Nutrition.* Los Angeles: Seven Star, 1987.

NAUSEA

Habek, D., et al. 2004. Success of acupuncture and acupressure of the Pc 6 acupoint in the treatment of hyperemesis gravid arum. *Forscho Komplement. Klass. Naturheilkd.* (1):20–23.

Johnson, J. A., PhD. *Chinese Medical Qigong Therapy.* Palm Desert, CA: International Institute of Medical Qi Gong, 2000.

Ni, M. *Self Healing Qi Gong Video.* Los Angeles: Seven Star, 1992.

Ni, M., and C. McNease. *The Tao of Nutrition.* Los Angeles: Seven Star, 1987.

Pitchford, P. *Healing with Whole Foods.* 3rd ed. Berkeley, CA: North Atlantic, 2002.

NOSEBLEED

Bunney, S., ed. *The Illustrated Encyclopedia of Herbs: Their Medicinal and Culinary Uses.* New York: Dorset, 1984.

Maclean, W., and J. Littleton. *Clinical Handbook of Internal Medicine.* Sydney: Sydney University Press, 2003.

Newall, C., et al. *Herbal Medicines: A Guide for Health-Care Professionals.* London: Pharmaceutical Press, 1996, 272.

Ni, M., and C. McNease. *The Tao of Nutrition.* Los Angeles: Seven Star, 1987.

OBESITY

Gibney, M. J., H. H. Vorster, and J. K. Frans, *Introduction to Human Nutrition.* Oxford: Blackwell, 2002.

McArdle, W. D., F. I. Katch, and V. L. Katch, *Exercise Physiology: Energy, Nutrition, and Human Performance.* Philadelphia: Lea and Febiger, 1986.

Morrill, A., and C. Chinn. 2004. The obesity epidemic in the United States. *J. Public Health Policy* 25:353–66.

Ni, H. *Attune Your Body with Dao In.* Los Angeles: Seven Star, 1989.

Ni, M., and C. McNease. *The Tao of Nutrition.* Los Angeles: Seven Star, 1987.

U.S. Department of Health and Human Services, National Institutes of Health. *The Practical Guide: Identification, Evaluation and Treatment of Overweight and Obesity in Adults 5,* 2000.

PAINFUL BLADDER SYNDROME

Cummings, S., and D. Ullman. *Everybody's Guide to Homeopathic Medicines.* 3rd ed. New York: Putnam, 1997, 193–195.

Engel, J.D., and A. J. Schaeffer. 1998. Evaluation of and antimicrobial therapy for recurrent urinary tract infections in women. *Urol. Clin. North. Am.* 25:685–701.

Goodman-Gilman, A., T. Rall, A. Nies, and T. Palmer. *The Pharmacological Basis of Therapeutics.* 8th ed. New York: Pergamon, 1990.

Howell, A., N. Vorsa, A. Der Marderosian, and Yeap Foo Lai. 1998. Inhibition of the adherence of P-fimbriated Escherichia coli to uroepithelial-cell surfaces by proanthocyanidin extracts from cranberries. *N. Engl. J. Med.* 339:1085–86.

JAMA Patient Page. 1999. How much vitamin C do you need? *JAMA* 281(15):1460.

Ni, M. *The Eight Treasures: Energy Enhancement Exercises.* Los Angeles: Seven Star, 1996.

Ni, M., and C. McNease. *The Tao of Nutrition.* Los Angeles: Seven Star, 1987.

POISON IVY AND POISON OAK

Bartram, T. *Encyclopedia of Herbal Medicine.* Dorset, England: Grace, 1995, 144.

Habif, T.P. *Clinical Dermatology.* 3rd ed. St. Louis, MO: Mosby–Year Book, 1996.

Middleton E., ed. *Allergy: Principles and Practice.* 5th ed. St. Louis, MO: Mosby–Year Book, 1998.

Ni, M. *Self Healing Qi Gong Video.* Los Angeles: Seven Star, 1992.

PSORIASIS

Behrendt, M. 1998. Reduction of psoriasis in a patient under network spinal analysis care: a case report. *J. Vertebr. Sublux. Res.* 2(4):196–200.

Blumenthal, M., ed. *The Complete German Commission E Monographs: Therapeutic Guide to Herbal Medicines.* Boston: Integrative Medicine, 1998, 169–70.

Cummings, S., and D. Ullman. *Everybody's Guide to Homeopathic Medicines.* 3rd ed. New York: Putnam, 1997, 227, 319–20, 345–46.

Ergil, K.V. *Medicines from the Earth: Protocols for Botanical Healing.* Harvard, MA: Gaia Herbal Research Institute, 1996, 207–11.

Gruenwald, J., T. Brendler, and C. Jaenicke, et al., eds. *PDR for Herbal Medicines.* Montvale, NJ: Medical Economics, 1998, 903–04, 1114, 1157.

Jonas, W.B., and J. Jacobs. *Healing with Homeopathy: The Doctors' Guide.* New York: Warner, 1996, 263–65.

Ni, M. *Self Healing Qi Gong Video.* Los Angeles: Seven Star, 1992.

Ni, M., and C. McNease. *The Tao of Nutrition.* Los Angeles: Seven Star, 1987.

Syed, T.A., et al. 1996. Management of psoriasis with aloe vera extract in a hydrophilic cream: a placebo-controlled, double-blind study. *Trop. Med. Int. Health* 1:505–09.

Time-Life Books, eds. *The Medical Advisor.* Alexandria, VA: Time-Life, 1996.

RINGING IN THE EAR

Axelsson, A., S. Andersson, and L. D. Gu. 1994. Acupuncture in the management of tinnitus: a placebo-controlled study. *Audiology* 33:351–60.

Ni, M. *Self Healing Qi Gong Video.* Los Angeles: Seven Star, 1992.

Nielsen, O.J., K. Moller, and K. E. Jorgensen. 1999. The effect of traditional Chinese acupuncture on severe tinnitus. A double-blind, placebo-controlled clinical study with an open therapeutic surveillance [in Danish]. *Ugeskr. Laeger.* 161:424–29.

Rosenberg, S.I., H. Silverstein, P. T. Rowan, and M. J. Olds. 1998. Effect of melatonin on tinnitus. *Laryngoscope* 108:305–10.

Vilholm, O.J., K. Moller, and K. Jorgensen. 1998. Effect of traditional Chinese acupuncture on severe tinnitus: a double-blind, placebo-controlled, clinical investigation with open therapeutic control. *Br. J. Audiol.* 32:197–204.

ROSACEA

Behrendt, M. 1998. Reduction of psoriasis in a patient under network spinal analysis care: a case report. *J. Vertebr. Sublux. Res.* 2(4):196–200.

Blumenthal, M., ed. *The Complete German Commission E Monographs: Therapeutic Guide to Herbal Medicines.* Boston: Integrative Medicine, 1998, 169–70.

Cummings, S., and D. Ullman. *Everybody's Guide to Homeopathic Medicines.* 3rd ed. New York: Putnam, 1997, 227, 319–20, 345–46.

Ergil, K. V. *Medicines from the Earth: Protocols for Botanical Healing.* Harvard, MA: Gaia Herbal Research Institute, 1996, 207–11.

Gruenwald, J., T. Brendler, and C. Jaenicke, et al., eds. *PDR for Herbal Medicines.* Montvale, NJ: Medical Economics, 1998, 903–04, 1114, 1157.

Jonas, W.B., and J. Jacobs. *Healing with Homeopathy: The Doctors' Guide.* New York: Warner, 1996, 263–65.

Ni, M. *Self Healing Qi Gong Video.* Los Angeles: Seven Star, 1992.

Syed, T.A., et al. 1996. Management of psoriasis with aloe vera extract in a hydrophilic cream: a placebo-controlled, double-blind study. *Trop. Med. Int. Health.* 1:505–09.

Time-Life Books, eds. *The Medical Advisor.* Alexandria, VA: Time-Life, 1996.

SCIATICA

Balch, P. A. *Prescription for Nutritional Healing,* 4th ed., New York: Avery, 2006.

Duvall, R. Sciatica, what causes and how to treat it effectively. http://holisticonline.com/remedies/sciatica/sciaticaduvall.htm

Ni, H. *Attune Your Body with Dao In.* Los Angeles: Seven Star, 1989.

Prevention magazine, eds. *Doctors' Book of Home Remedies II.* Emmaus, PA: Rodale, 1993.

SINUS PROBLEMS

Eby, G.A. 1997. Zinc ion availability—the determinant of efficacy in zinc lozenge treatment of common colds. *J. Antimicrob. Chemother.* 40(4):483–93.

Ni, H. *Attune Your Body with Dao In.* Los Angeles: Seven Star, 1989.

Ogasawara, H., and E. Middleton, Jr. 1985. Effect of selected flavonoids on histamine release (HR) and hydrogen peroxide (H_2O_2) generation by human leukocytes. *J. Allergy Clin. Immunol.* 75:184.

Yoshimoto, T., et al. 1983. Flavonoids: Potent inhibitors of arachidonate 5-lipoxygenase. *Biochem. Biophys. Res. Commun.* 116:612–18.

SNORING

Caldwell J.P. *Sleep: Everything You Need to Know.* Buffalo, NY: Firefly, 1997.

Cummings, S., and D. Ullman. *Everybody's Guide to Homeopathic Medicines.* 3rd ed. New York: Putnam, 1997, 237–39, 306, 320–21, 331–32.

Dunkell, S. *Goodbye Insomnia, Hello Sleep.* New York: Carol, 1994.

Ni, H. *Attune Your Body with Dao In.* Los Angeles: Seven Star, 1989.

SORE THROAT

Braunig, B., et al. 1992. Echinacea purpurea root for strengthening the immune response in flu-like infections. *Z. Phytother.* 13:7–13.

Brinkeborn, R. M., et al. 1999. Echinacea preparations in the treatment of common colds. *Phytomedicine.* 6(1):1–6.

Ni, H. *Power of Natural Healing.* Los Angeles: Seven Star, 1995.

Zakay-Rones, Z., et al. 1995. Inhibition of several strains of influenza virus and reduction of symptoms by an elderberry extract (*Sambucus nigra L.*) during an outbreak of influenza B Panama. *J. Altern. Complement. Med.* 1(4):361–69.

SUNBURN

Abramowitz, A.I., K. S. Resnik, and K. R. Cohen. 1993. Margarita photodermatitis [letter]. *N. Engl. J. Med.* 328(12):891.

Adamski, H., L. Benkalfate, and Y. Delaval, et al. 1998. Photodermatitis from nonsteroidal anti-inflammatory drugs. *Contact Dermatitis.* 38(3):171–74.

American Academy of Pediatrics. 1999. Ultraviolet light: a hazard to children. *Pediatrics.* 104(2):328–33.

Ni, M. *Meditation for Stress Release* (audio CD). Los Angeles: Seven Star, 2003.

Rhodes, L.E., and S.I. White. 1998. Dietary fish oil as a photoprotective agent in hydroa vacciniforme. *Br. J. Dermatol.* 138(1):173–78.

Ross, J.B., and M. A. Moss. 1990. Relief of the photosensitivity of erythropoietic protoporphyria by pyridoxine. *J. Am. Acad. Dermatol.* 22(2 pt 2):340–42.

Scholzen, T.E., T. Brzoska, and D. H. Kalden, et al. 1999. Effect of ultraviolet light on the release of neuropeptides and neuroendocrine hormones in the skin: mediators of photodermatitis and cutaneous inflammation. *J. Invest. Dermatol. Symp. Proc.* 4(1):55–60.

TENDINITIS

Gimblett, P.A., J. Saville, and P. Ebrall. 1999. A conservative management protocol for calcific tendonitis of the shoulder. *J. Manipulative Physiol. Ther.* 22(9):622–27.

Jensen, R., O. Gothesen, K. Liseth, and A. Baerheim. 1999. Acupuncture treatment of patellofemoral pain syndrome. *J. Altern. Complement. Med.* 5(6):521–27.

Johnston, C.S. 1999. Recommendations for vitamin C intake. *JAMA* 282(22): 2118–19.

Kelly, W. N., E. D. Harris, Jr., S. Ruddy, and C. B. Sledge. *Textbook of Rheumatology.* 5th ed. Philadelphia: Saunders, 1997, 372–73, 386, 422–29, 462–63, 486, 558–59, 598–99, 603–06, 642.

Kleinhenz, J., K. Streitberger, J. Windeler, A. Gubbacher, G. Mavridis, and E. Martin. 1999. Randomised clinical trial comparing the effects of acupuncture and a newly designed placebo needle in rotator cuff tendinitis. *Pain.* 83:235–41.

Koopman, W. J. *Arthritis and Allied Conditions: A Textbook of Rheumatology.* 13th ed. Baltimore: Williams & Wilkins, 1997, 44, 1769–71, 1795, 1894–96.

Levine, M., S. C. Rumsey, R. Daruwala, J. B. Park, and Y. Wang. 1999. Criteria and recommendations for vitamin C intake. *JAMA* 281(15):1415–53.

Millar, A. P. *Sports Injuries and Their Management.* Sydney: Maclennan & Petty, 1994, 10–14, 84–85, 101–03, 111–12, 118–19, 130–31.

Ni, M. *The Eight Treasures: Energy Enhancement Exercises.* Los Angeles: Seven Star, 1996.

ULCERS

Beil, W., et al. 1995. Effects of flavonoids on parietal cell acid secretion, gastric mucosal prostaglandin production and *Helicobacter pylori* growth. *Arzneimittelforschung Drug. Res.* 45(6):697–700.

Levenstein, S. 1999. Stress and peptic ulcer. *JAMA* 281:10–11.

Ni, H. *Attune Your Body with Dao In.* Los Angeles: Seven Star, 1989.

Ni, M. *Self Healing Qi Gong Video.* Los Angeles: Seven Star, 1992.

Ni, M., and C. McNease. *The Tao of Nutrition.* Los Angeles: Seven Star, 1987.

Rees, W. D. W., J. Rhodes, and J. E. Wright, et al. 1979. Effect of deglycyrrhizinated liquorice on gastric mucosal damage by aspirin. *Scand. J. Gastroenterol.* 14(5):605–7.

Thaly, H. 1965. A new therapy of peptic ulcer: the anti-ulcer factor of cabbage. *Gaz. Med. Fr.* 72:1992–93.

Yeoh, K. G., J. Y. Kang, and I. Yap, et al. 1995. Chili protects against aspirin-induced gastroduodenal mucosal injury in humans. *Dig. Dis. Sci.* 40(3):580–83.

VARICOSE VEINS AND SPIDER VEINS

Johnson, J. A., PhD. *Chinese Medical Qigong Therapy.* International Institute of Medical Qi Gong. Palm Desert, CA: 2000.

Neiss, A., and C. Bohm. 1976. Proof of the efficacy of horse chestnut seed extract in the treatment of varicose syndrome [translated from German]. *Münch. Med. Wochenschr.* 118(7):213–16.

Ng, M., T. Andrew, T. Spector, and S. Jeffery. 2005. Linkage to the FOXC2 region of chromosome 16 for varicose veins in otherwise healthy, unselected sibling pairs. *J. Med. Genet.* 42(3):235–39.

Ni, H. *Attune Your Body with Dao In.* Los Angeles: Seven Star, 1989.

Ni, M. *Self Healing Qi Gong Video.* Los Angeles: Seven Star, 1992.

Ni, M., and C. McNease. *The Tao of Nutrition.* Los Angeles: Seven Star, 1987.

WARTS

Bairati, I., K. J. Sherman, and B. McKnight, et al. 1994. Diet and genital warts: a case-control study. *Sex. Transm. Dis.* 21:149–54.

Barker, L. R., et al., eds. *Principles of Ambulatory Medicine.* 4th ed. Baltimore: Williams & Wilkins, 1995, 1467–69.

Jonas, W.B., and J. Jacobs. *Healing with Homeopathy: The Doctors' Guide.* New York: Warner, 1996, 236.

Ni, M. *Self-Healing Qi Gong* (video). Los Angeles: Seven Star, 1992.

Schneider, A., A. Morabia, U. Papendick, and R. Kirchmayr. 1990. Pork intake and human papillomavirus-related disease. *Nutr. Cancer.* 13:209–11.

Walker, L.P., and E. H. Brown. *The Alternative Pharmacy.* Paramus, NJ: Prentice Hall, 1998, 353–54.

YEAST INFECTIONS

Balch, P. A. *Prescription for Nutritional Healing.* 4th ed. New York: Avery, 2006.

Berkow, R., and A. J. Fletcher, eds. *The Merck Manual of Diagnosis and Therapy.* Rahway, NJ: Merck, 1992.

Blumenthal, M., ed. *The Complete German Commission E Monographs: Therapeutic Guide to Herbal Medicines.* Boston: Integrative Medicine, 1998, 463.

Ni, M. *Self-Healing Qi Gong* (video). Los Angeles: Seven Star, 1992.

Ni, M., and C. McNease. *The Tao of Nutrition.* Los Angeles: Seven Star, 1987.

. . . .

for obesity, 434–435
for painful bladder syndrome, 440–441
for poison ivy/poison oak, 445
for psoriasis, 450–451
for ringing in the ear, 456
for rosacea, 460–461
for sciatica, 466
for sinus problems, 471
for snoring, 476–477
for sore throat, 481
for sunburn, 485
for tendinitis, 490
for ulcers, 496
USDA Food Guide Pyramid, 70–71
for varicose/spider veins, 501
for warts, 505
for yeast infections, 510
yin-yang zones, 74–75
digestive system, 79–80, 280, 471
dioxin, 136
disease, 43–45, 137
disharmony, 43–45
Divine Farmer's Materia Medica, The, 84–85
dizziness, 275–279
doctor, 45–46
dong quai, 93
drugs, 94–95

ears, 60–61
earth archetype, 31–32
earth element, 27
east (wood), 140–141
eating mindfully, 78
ecology, 26
eczema, 279–285
eight extraordinary channels, 127–129
electroencephalogram (EEG), 22
electrolyte imbalance, 418
emotions, 29, 155
  balancing, 158–160
  damage from, 44–45
  and five-element network, 155–158
  negative, 154, 172
  suppressing, 358
endorphins, 120
energy, 20
  five transformation phases, 26–29
  flow, 122
  in human body, 22, 159
  individual, 154
  meridians, 15, 138–139
  rotation, 145

subtle, 16, 21–23
universal, 154
entrainment, 150
estrogen, 396–397
euphorbia, 98
exercise, 106–107
  for acne, 183–184
  and acupressure, 12–14
  for allergies, 189
  for arterial plaque, 194
  for arthritis, 200–201
  for asthma, 205–206
  for bad breath, 210–211
  for bone loss, 215–216
  for bronchitis, 221–222
  for candida, 227
  for carpal tunnel syndrome, 232–233
  for chronic fatigue syndrome, 238–239
  circularity of movement, 111–112
  for cold and flu, 243–244
  for cold hands and feet, 248
  for constipation, 253
  for cough, 257–259
  for dandruff, 263
  for diabetes, 268–269
  for diarrhea, 273–274
  for dizziness, 278
  for eczema, 283–284
  for flatulence, 288–289
  for floaters, 292–293
  for gout, 297–298
  for gum disease, 302–303
  for hair loss, 307
  for headache, 311–312
  health benefits of, 107–108
  for hearing loss, 316–317
  for hemorrhoids, 321–322
  for high blood pressure, 327–328
  for high cholesterol, 333
  for hives, 337–338
  for incontinence, 341–342
  for indigestion/heartburn, 346
  for insect bites, 350–351
  for insomnia, 355–356
  for irritable bowel syndrome, 361
  for jet lag, 365–367
  for low energy, 372
  for low immune function, 377–378
  for low libido, 382–384
  for lower back pain, 388–390
  for memory loss, 394–395
  for menopause, 400–401

intestinal flora, 224, 509
intestinal gas, 285–290
intravenous immunoglobulin therapy, 375
irritable bowel syndrome (IBS), 270, 357–362
isolates, 94
isothiocyanates, 77

jet lag, 362–368
Journal of the American Medical Association, 98
joy, 29, 156

KID-6 (Illuminate the Sea point), 132
kidney-bladder network, 41–43, 157, 314, 339,
    385, 391, 397, 455
Kidney Channel (KID), 124, 126
Knowles, John H., 135
kukoamines, 3

lactic acidosis, 109
Large Intestine Channel (LI), 123, 125
late summer, 144
L-carnitine, 102
left cheek, 56
licensed acupuncturist, 97
life, 21
life force, 20–22, 118, 122, 134
life processes, 26
life span, 146
lifestyle and environment, 14–15
ligaments, 489
Liver Channel (L), 124, 126
liver-gallbladder network, 37–38, 156, 286,
    374, 418, 489
local foods, 79
love, 17
low-density lipoprotein (LDL), 329
low energy, 368–373
low immune function, 373–379
low libido, 379–385
lower back pain, 385–391
LU-7 (Branching Crevice point), 129–130
Lung Channel (LU), 123, 125
lung–large intestine network, 40–41, 156–157,
    186, 280, 470
lutein, 77
lycopene, 78

ma huang, 98
macrocosm, 136
macronutrients, 100
malaria, 12
matter, 21

medicinal herbs, 94–97
    potent, 97–98
meditation
    Awareness Exercise, 50–51
    General Cleansing, 263, 283–284, 350–351,
        447–448, 453, 507–508, 512–513
    light sitting, 416
    nausea treatment, 426–427
    Six Healing Sounds, 483
    stress-release, 355–356, 487–488
    White Light, 312, 411–412
melatonin, 103
memory loss, 391–396
Menière's disease, 314
menopause, 396–402
    instant, 176–177
menstrual disorders, 402–408
Merry-Go-Round Circle Walk, 268–269, 333
metabolic waste, 294
metal archetype, 32
metal element, 27, 140
microcosm, 136
micronutrients, 99
middle finger, 63
migraines, 408–413
milk thistle, 89
mind, 16–17, 29, 161
    yin and yang of, 162–163
mind-body exercises, 13, 110–111
mindfulness in movement, 114–115
minerals, 73
mint, 92
morning sickness, 413–417
Mother Nature, 103
movement, 106–107
    circularity of, 111–112
    gentle rhythmic, 116
    mindfulness in, 114–115
    tai chi and qi gong, 112–117
    yin and yang in, 115
movement arts, 13
mucus, 255
mulberry leaf, 89
muscle pain/spasm, 417–423

National Institutes of Health (NIH), 120, 323,
    413, 424
natural killer (NK) cells, 16
natural law, 26, 139, 143
natural remedies, 3. *See also* home remedies
nausea, 424–428
negative emotions, 154, 172, 455